Anne E. Dixon · Emmanuelle M. Clerisme-Beaty
Editors

Obesity and Lung Disease

A Guide to Management

Humana Press

Editors
Anne E. Dixon
Department of Medicine
University of Vermont College of Medicine
Burlington, VT, USA

Emmanuelle M. Clerisme-Beaty
Clinical Development Medical Affairs, Respiratory
Boehringer Ingelheim Pharmaceuticals, Inc.
Ridgefield, CT, USA

ISBN 978-1-62703-938-3 ISBN 978-1-62703-053-3 (eBook)
DOI 10.1007/978-1-62703-053-3
Springer New York Heidelberg Dordrecht London

Printed on acid-free paper

Humana Press is a brand of Springer
Springer is part of Springer Science+Business Media (www.springer.com)

Respiratory Medicine

Series editor:
Sharon I.S. Rounds

For further volumes:
http://www.springer.com/series/7665

Preface

The prevalence of obesity is increasing at an alarming rate, with more than 300 million obese people worldwide. The increase in the prevalence of obesity has been most pronounced in developed countries. For example, in the United States, the prevalence of obesity has doubled over the past 30 years, with more than a third of adults meeting criteria for obesity based on a body mass index (BMI) >30 kg/m^2. This number is likely to continue to increase in the coming decade, as more than two-thirds of US adults have been shown to be overweight and at risk for becoming obese.

Unfortunately, the obesity epidemic has not been limited to adults and developed countries. There has also been parallel increase in the prevalence of obesity among children over the past few decades. Despite controversies regarding the definition of obesity in children, childhood obesity has become a major public health concern worldwide, with nearly 43 million children under the age of 5 being overweight or obese as of 2010. In the United States, the prevalence of childhood obesity has almost tripled over the past two decades with approximately 17% of children (12.5 million) aged 2–19 being obese. The obesity epidemic has also affected developing countries, with as much as a 40% increase in obesity prevalence noted in some countries over the past 20 years. Although the obesity epidemic has affected men, women, and children, several demographic factors have been linked with an increased prevalence of obesity worldwide, including increasing age, female gender, urban lifestyle, and socioeconomic status. However, the association between socioeconomic status and obesity risk has been shown to vary between developed and developing countries, with a higher prevalence of obesity being noted among higher socioeconomic class in developing countries, as opposed to developed countries where lower socioeconomic status is linked to higher obesity risk.

Obesity is a risk factor for several chronic diseases, including cardiovascular disease, diabetes, arthritis, cancer, and as such is associated with significant morbidity and mortality. In addition, the obesity epidemic has placed a significant burden on national health-care systems, as a result of direct and indirect costs associated with the diagnosis and treatment of obesity-related chronic conditions, with an estimated 41.5% higher medical expenditure cost. Obesity also contributes to a significant increase in indirect cost due to loss of productivity, absenteeism, disability, and premature death, with a projected cumulative indirect cost due to premature death of $208 billion over the next 30–40 years. Accordingly, there has been increasing scientific and public health interest aimed at understanding the effect of obesity on the prevalence, management, and clinical outcomes of chronic illnesses, including pulmonary diseases.

The obesity epidemic has had a major impact on the epidemiology of pulmonary diseases. Obesity has impacted not only the type of diseases commonly encountered by the pulmonary clinician, but has also had a profound impact on the pathophysiology of common pulmonary diseases. Increased body mass index is associated with changes in resting lung volumes that can lead to respiratory complaints, such as dyspnea. However, aside from its mechanical effects on the lung, increased adiposity is associated with neural, metabolic, and inflammatory dysregulation that can contribute to modifications in risk profile, clinical presentation, response to therapy, and clinical outcomes. We have known for many years that obesity is a risk factor for sleep disordered breathing. More recently it has also become increasingly evident that obesity is also a major risk factor for asthma, with 250,000 cases of asthma per year in the United States thought to be related to obesity. Obesity is thought to contribute to worse asthma, severity of asthma, decreased response to treatment, and is likely a major modifier of the phenotype of asthma. It also appears to affect response to pathogens, and as such has a major influence on response to pneumonia as well as having a significant impact on outcomes pertaining to acute lung injury in the intensive care unit. As a result, this has led scientists and clinicians to struggle in trying to understand how to deal with the obese patient and their pulmonary health.

Given the increasing prevalence of obesity and overweight people worldwide and the negative effects of obesity on health, this book is intended to serve as a resource for clinicians and scientists involved in the care and evaluation of pulmonary, critical care, and sleep disorders in the twenty-first century.

Burlington, VT, USA — Anne E. Dixon
Ridgefield, CT, USA — Emmanuelle M. Clerisme-Beaty

Contents

Contributors

Norbert Berend, MBBS, M.D. Woolcock Institute of Medical Research, Glebe, NSW, Australia

Sydney Medical School, University of Sydney, Sydney, NSW, Australia

Anne E. Dixon, M.A., BM, BCh. Department of Medicine, University of Vermont College of Medicine, Burlington, VT, USA

Frits M.E. Franssen, M.D., Ph.D. Program Development Center, Ciro+, Center of Expertise for Chronic Organ Failure, Limburg, NM, The Netherlands

Anna Ryan Hemnes, M.D. Department of Medicine, Vanderbilt University Medical Center, Nashville, TN, USA

Gregory G. King, MB ChB, Ph.D. Woolcock Institute of Medical Research, Glebe, NSW, Australia

Sydney Medical School, University of Sydney, Sydney, NSW, Australia

Department of Respiratory Medicine, Royal North Shore Hospital, St. Leonards, NSW, Australia

Jason Paul Kirkness, Ph.D. Division of Pulmonary and Critical Care Medicine, Johns Hopkins School of Medicine, Baltimore, MD, USA

Jason E. Lang, M.D. Department of Pulmonology, Allergy & Immunology, Center for Pharmacogenomics & Translational Research, Mayo Clinic College of Medicine, Nemours Children's Clinic, Jacksonville, FL, USA

Mikhail Litinski, M.D. Department of Surgery, Saint Barnabas Medical Center, Livingston, NJ, USA

Stephen W. Littleton, M.D. Pulmonary, Critical Care, and Sleep Medicine, Cook County Hospital and Rush University Medical Center, Chicago, IL, USA

Atul Malhotra, M.D. Department of Medicine, Brigham and Women's Hospital and Harvard Medical School, Boston, MA, USA

Peter Mancuso, M.S., Ph.D. Environmental Health Sciences and Graduate Program in Immunology, Ann Arbor, MI, USA

Babak Mokhlesi, M.D., M.Sc. Department of Medicine/Section of Pulmonary and Critical Care, University of Chicago Pritzker School of Medicine, Chicago, IL, USA

Robert L. Owens, M.D. Divisions of Sleep and Pulmonary and Critical Care Medicine, Brigham and Women's Hospital, Boston, MA, USA

Susheel P. Patil, M.D., Ph.D. Division of Pulmonary and Critical Care Medicine, Johns Hopkins School of Medicine, Baltimore, MD, USA

Ivan M. Robbins, M.D. Department of Medicine, Vanderbilt University Medical Center, Nashville, TN, USA

Cheryl M. Salome, B.Sc., Ph.D. Woolcock Institute of Medical Research, Glebe, NSW, Australia

Sydney Medical School, University of Sydney, Sydney, NSW, Australia

Stephanie A. Shore, Ph.D. Environmental Health, Harvard School of Public Health, Boston, MA, USA

Akshay Sood, M.D., M.PH. Department of Medicine, University of New Mexico Health Sciences Center School of Medicine, Albuquerque, NM, USA

Renee D. Stapleton, M.D., Ph.D. Department of Medicine, Division of Pulmonary and Critical Care Medicine, University of Vermont College of Medicine, Burlington, VT, USA

Benjamin T. Suratt, M.D. Department of Medicine, Division of Pulmonary and Critical Care Medicine, University of Vermont College of Medicine, Burlington, VT, USA

E. Rand Sutherland, M.D., M.P.H. Department of Medicine, National Jewish Health, Denver, CO, USA

Emiel F.M. Wouters, M.D., Ph.D. Department of Respiratory Medicine, Maastricht University Medical Center, Limburg, HX, The Netherlands

Chapter 1
Effects of Obesity on Lung Function

Cheryl M. Salome, Gregory G. King, and Norbert Berend

Abstract Obesity causes significant changes in lung function, many of which are secondary to the reduction in operating lung volume caused by a stiffening of the respiratory system. In addition, reductions in the volume of the intrathoracic cavity, due to the presence of adipose tissue and changes in other structures, may also contribute to an overall reduction in lung volume. Thus, the primary effects of obesity on lung function arise from the mechanical effects of adipose tissue on the respiratory system. However, some studies have reported changes in airway function associated with obesity that appear to be independent of lung volumes, though the causes of these abnormalities are unknown. It is unclear whether the mechanical effects of obesity on lung function can increase the risk of respiratory symptoms in otherwise healthy individuals. However, in respiratory disease, a reduction in operating lung volume may increase symptoms during bronchoconstriction in asthma and protect against symptoms during exercise in COPD.

Keywords Adiposity • Respiratory compliance • Lung volumes • Expiratory flow limitation • Ventilation distribution • Gas exchange • Breathlessness

---

C.M. Salome, B.Sc., Ph.D. (✉) • N. Berend, MBBS, M.D.
Woolcock Institute of Medical Research, 431 Glebe Point Road, Glebe, NSW 2037, Australia

Sydney Medical School, University of Sydney, Sydney, NSW 2006, Australia
e-mail: cms@woolcock.org.au; nberend@woolcock.org.au

G.G. King, MB ChB, Ph.D.
Woolcock Institute of Medical Research, 431 Glebe Point Road, Glebe, NSW 2037, Australia

Sydney Medical School, University of Sydney, Sydney, NSW 2006, Australia

Department of Respiratory Medicine, Royal North Shore Hospital, St Leonards, NSW 2065, Australia
e-mail: ggk@woolcock.org.au

A.E. Dixon and E.M. Clerisme-Beaty (eds.), *Obesity and Lung Disease: A Guide to Management*, Respiratory Medicine, DOI 10.1007/978-1-62703-053-3_1,

Objectives

- Evaluate the effects adiposity on respiratory mechanics
- Assess the mechanism by which obesity leads to impairment in lung function
- Evaluate how obesity may impact clinical presentation and physiology of obstructive and restrictive lung diseases
- Examine the impact of obesity on pulmonary function testing interpretation

Introduction

The accumulation of adipose tissue, leading to the development of obesity, has a profound effect on human physiology, including significant effects on respiratory function due to the mechanical effects of excess adipose tissue on the balance of forces that normally act on the lung. In addition, adipose tissue produces hormones and other mediators, collectively termed adipokines, which are associated with low-grade systemic inflammation that can act indirectly on the respiratory system. However, at present it is unclear whether this causes any measurable impairment in respiratory function. The changes in lung function associated with obesity can lead to respiratory symptoms in otherwise healthy people, which are accentuated in those with respiratory disease, as a result of interaction between disease pathophysiology and the direct and indirect effects of obesity. The outcomes of this interaction are complex and differ according to the disease and the outcome of interest. The major effects of obesity on lung function are summarized in Fig. 1.1 and suggest that many of the changes in lung function result from changes in respiratory system mechanics and subsequent reduction in operating lung volume, whereas others may be associated with reduced thoracic volume, or may be due to other non-volume-related factors. In this chapter, the effects of obesity on lung function and the relationships summarized in Fig. 1.1 will be reviewed along with the effects of these impairments on respiratory symptoms.

Adipose Tissue and Respiratory Mechanics

Obesity is defined as a body mass index >30 kg/m^2. However, body mass index is a non-specific measure of body mass that includes both fat and lean mass, without any account of differences in fat distribution. Central obesity is associated with increased adipose tissue in the anterior chest and abdominal walls and visceral organs, whereas peripheral obesity reflects adiposity located peripherally on limbs, or in subcutaneous tissue. The effect of obesity on respiratory function is likely to be determined by the distribution of fat mass. Abdominal and thoracic fat are likely to have direct effects on the downwards movement of the diaphragm and on chest wall properties, while

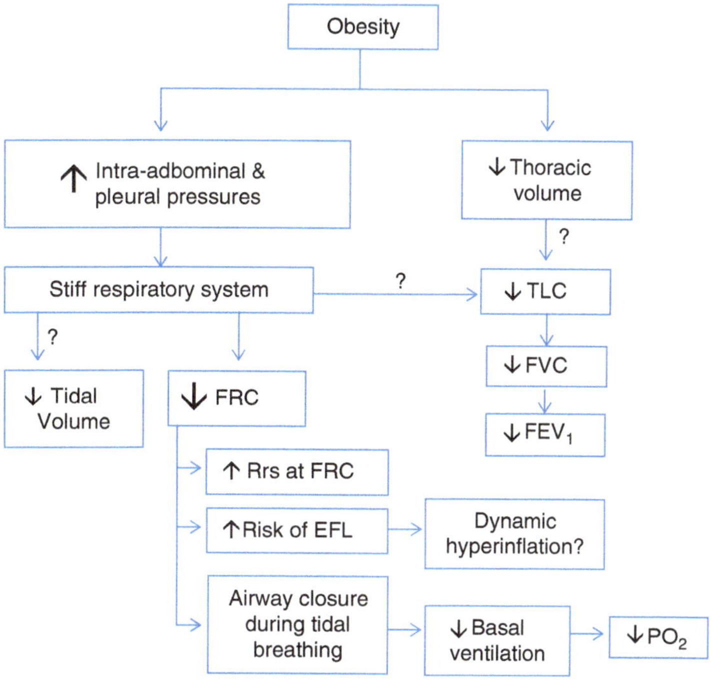

Fig. 1.1 The effects of obesity on lung function, illustrating likely mechanisms. *Question marks* indicate mechanisms for which further research evidence is needed. See text for more detailed discussion. *TLC* total lung capacity, *FRC* functional residual capacity, *Rrs* respiratory system resistance, *EFL* expiratory flow limitation

subcutaneous fat on the hips and limbs is unlikely to have any direct mechanical effect on the lungs. In addition, visceral fat is more metabolically active than subcutaneous fat and may therefore make a greater contribution to low-grade systemic inflammation in obesity. Because central obesity is more common in men than in women, the effect of obesity on respiratory function is also influenced by gender. Adipose tissue is also found inside the thoracic cavity, predominantly as pericardial fat, which, when combined with obesity-associated increase in the volume of the heart and major blood vessels, can reduce the volume of the thoracic cavity [1].

Intra-abdominal and Intrathoracic Pressures

Obesity is associated with chronic increases in intra-abdominal pressure that may affect the pleural space by altering pressure across the diaphragm. Intra-abdominal pressure is increased in obese subjects compared to non-obese [2, 3] and is greater in men than women [3], likely due to the greater prevalence of central obesity in men. Indeed, intra-abdominal pressure correlates with markers of central obesity, such as the sagittal abdominal diameter [2, 3]. Although pleural pressures are also increased in obese subjects compared to non-obese and may exceed atmospheric pressure at FRC in some patients [2], there were no gender related differences observed. In addition, in contrast to intra-abdominal pressure, studies in supine anaesthetized subjects [2] have shown that abdominal obesity, measured by waist circumferences and by sagittal abdominal diameter, was not correlated with pleural pressures. Since the relationship between abdominal pressure and pleural pressure is mediated by the diaphragm, the lack of correlation between the two may be due to compensatory increase in passive tension in the diaphragm in response to increased intra-abdominal pressure in the obese. Alternatively, factors other than increased abdominal pressures, such as changes in the properties of the chest wall, may also contribute to the altered respiratory system mechanics associated with obesity. Imaging studies of abdominal and thoracic fat have shown that both regions make a significant contribution to impairments of lung function in the obese [4].

Respiratory System Compliance

Obesity has consistently been associated with a reduction in the compliance of the total respiratory system [2, 5], likely due to reduction in the compliance of the chest wall and lungs. However, despite numerous studies of the compliance of the chest wall and lungs in obese subjects, the mechanisms that lead to a stiffening of the respiratory system in the obese remain poorly understood.

Measurement of chest wall compliance is challenging since the respiratory muscles must be relaxed and inactive to allow for accurate measurement. Studies of conscious, spontaneously breathing subjects, in which changes in lung volumes were induced using externally applied changes in pressures in a plethysmograph, suggest that there is a reduction in chest wall compliance in obesity [5, 6]. However, since respiratory muscle relaxation was assessed using EMG measurements, this may not adequately reflect muscle relaxation across the whole of the chest wall. In contrast, normal chest wall compliance has been reported in studies of supine anaesthetized, paralysed subjects with mild [7] or severe [2, 8] obesity, as well as in studies of upright conscious subjects [9]. Alteration in chest wall mechanics from being in the supine position [10] may account for some of the differences in findings between studies. However, a definitive understanding of the effect of obesity on chest wall mechanics remains elusive.

Although some studies have reported that lung compliance, measured by full P-V curves to TLC, is normal in some obese subjects [11], there is more consistent evidence that lung compliance is decreased in obese individuals [6–8, 12], and lung compliance appears to be exponentially related to BMI [7]. The mechanism for decreased lung compliance in obesity remains unclear; however, increased pulmonary blood volume [13], closure of dependent airways resulting in small areas of atelectasis [8], and increased alveolar surface tension due to a reduction in functional residual capacity (FRC) have been implicated as potential contributors to increased stiffness of the lung tissue.

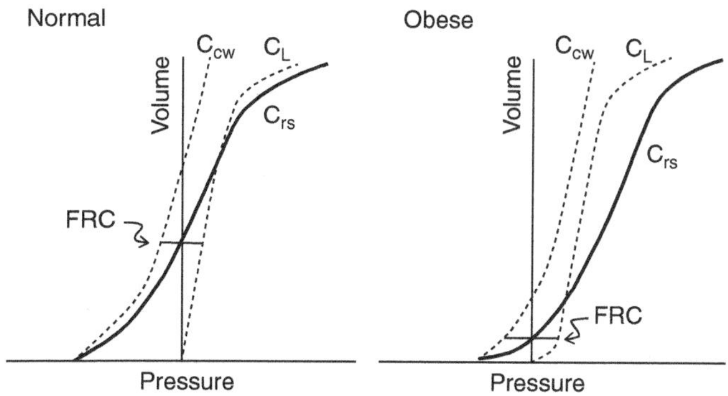

Fig. 1.2 Compliance curves for the chest wall (C_{CW}), lung (C_L) and respiratory system (C_{RS}) in normal weight and obese individuals. Functional residual capacity (FRC) is reduced in the obese individual

An alternative hypothesis for altered respiratory mechanics in the obese has been proposed by Behazin et al. [2], who suggest that the apparent stiffening of the chest wall may simply reflect the mass loading of the chest wall due to an increased volume of intra-abdominal and mediastinal fat [1]. This hypothesis is consistent with findings from an experimental study by Sharp et al. [14], which showed that mass loading of the thorax in normal weight conscious or anaesthetized/paralysed subjects produced a parallel rightward shift of the chest wall pressure-volume curve without any effect on compliance. Furthermore, Behazin et al. [2] suggest that high pleural pressures, which are often above atmospheric pressure at FRC, would lead to closure of small airways. As a result, there would be an apparent reduction in lung compliance at FRC since the pressure-volume relationship would reflect both lung stiffness and the opening pressures of small airways. Thus, obesity could be associated with apparent changes in chest wall and lung compliance without actually causing any changes in the stiffness of either the chest wall or lung tissue. Figure 1.2 shows compliance curves for the chest wall (C_{CW}), lung (C_L) and respiratory system (C_{RS}) in normal weight and obese individuals. In the obese, although the shape of the C_{CW} curve is normal, it is shifted to the right, consistent with the effect of an inspiratory threshold load. The C_L curve has an inflection point reflecting the increased pressure required to open airways that are closed just below FRC. As a result, the C_{RS} curve, which is the summation of the C_{CW} and C_L curves, is flattened, indicating reduced compliance of the respiratory system in the obese. The volume at which the C_{RS} curve crosses zero on the pressure axis (i.e. where there is a balance between inflationary and deflationary pressures) is FRC and occurs at a lower volume in the obese.

Consequences of Altered Respiratory Mechanics in Obesity

Alterations in respiratory mechanics in the obese, leading to an overall stiffening of the respiratory system, lead directly to changes in breathing pattern and resting lung volumes (Fig. 1.1).

Breathing Pattern

Increased stiffness of the respiratory system is likely to induce a rapid shallow pattern of tidal breathing, which is a typical response to an elastic load [15]. Indeed, previous studies have shown that tidal volumes are often reduced in severe obesity, and breathing follows a rapid, shallow pattern [16]. This alteration to breathing pattern is most apparent during exercise, when obese subjects preferentially increase their breathing frequency more, and tidal volumes less, than non-obese subjects [17, 18]. During bronchoconstriction, there is a greater decrease in tidal volumes in overweight or obese subjects than in normal weight subjects [19]. However, in mild-moderate obesity, tidal volumes at rest are often in the normal range [18, 20–22], and the frequency and magnitude of regular sighs and deep inspirations appear similar to that in normal weight subjects [20, 22]. Thus, increased respiratory system stiffness has a minor effect on breathing pattern and is only seen in severe obesity or when the system is under stress, such as during exercise or bronchoconstriction.

Resting Lung Volume

Aside from its effect on breathing pattern, increased respiratory system stiffness also has a major effect on resting lung volume, causing a reduction lung volume at relaxation, when the recoil pressures of the lung and chest wall are equal and opposite (Fig. 1.2). The relaxation volume of the lung usually equates to the functional residual capacity (FRC), which is very commonly reduced in obesity [7, 23]. FRC is exponentially related to BMI [7, 23], with reduction in FRC being detected even in overweight individuals [23]. This is illustrated in Fig. 1.3, which shows the relationship between BMI and FRC in a study of young adults, aged 28–30 years [24]. The reduction in FRC is also manifested by an increase in inspiratory capacity (IC). With increasing severity of obesity, the reduction in FRC may become so marked that the FRC approaches residual volume (RV), leaving the individual with a negligible expiratory reserve volume (ERV) [23]. In fact, in many studies, the reduction in ERV is one of the earliest and most marked changes in lung function that occurs with increasing weight [25]. In contrast, the effects of obesity on the upper and lower limits of lung volumes, total lung capacity (TLC) and RV are modest. Increasing body weight is associated with only small decrease in TLC [23, 26, 27], and RV is usually well preserved [16, 26, 28–30]. As a result, the RV/TLC ratio remains normal or slightly increased in obese individuals [23, 29].

The relationship between BMI and FRC, shown in Fig. 1.3, is steeper in men than in women. This difference in slope is likely to result from differences in the prevalence of central obesity between men and women. Central obesity, associated with greater fat deposition on the trunk and abdomen, is likely to have a greater effect on respiratory system compliance than peripheral fat distribution. Reductions in lung volumes are associated with both abdominal fat, measured by waist circumference [31], waist to hip ratio [32] or abdominal height [33], and thoracic or upper

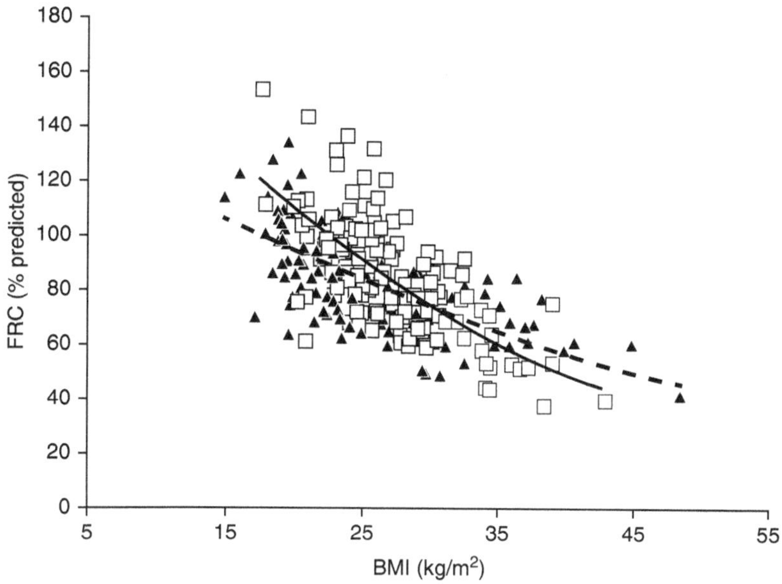

Fig. 1.3 Relationship between BMI and FRC in young men (*open squares, solid line*) and women (*solid triangles, dashed line*)

body fat, measured by sub-scapular skinfold thickness [34] or biceps skinfold thickness [26]. Several studies have used dual-energy X-ray absorptiometry (DXA) to quantify fat and lean mass in different regions of the body and relate these findings to lung function [4, 35]. Sutherland et al. [4] used a wide range of body fat variables to determine the effect of fat distribution on lung volumes in healthy adults. Lung volumes were only loosely associated with BMI; however, both DXA and non-DXA-derived measures of upper body fat showed highly significant negative correlations with FRC and ERV in both men and women. Both abdominal obesity and thoracic fat mass were similarly correlated with lung volumes, making it difficult to differentiate between the effects of abdominal and thoracic fat. Similarly, improvements in lung volumes such as FVC, FRC and ERV, following moderate weight loss, were related to the cumulative loss of fat from areas impinging on the chest wall, such as chest, subcutaneous abdominal or visceral fat, rather than from any specific region [36].

Consequences of Reduced FRC

In the causal pathway shown in Fig. 1.1, low operating lung volume due to reduced respiratory system compliance leads to effects on airway resistance, expiratory flow limitation, ventilation distribution and gas exchange.

Airway Resistance and Reactance

Since airway calibre is related to lung volume, reduction in FRC in the obese has significant effects on the mechanical properties of the airway and on expiratory flows during tidal breathing. Respiratory system resistance and airway resistance are increased in the obese [37], indicating that airway calibre is reduced throughout the breathing cycle. However, measurement of specific airway resistance in obese subjects, which is adjusted for lung volume, is in the normal range [30, 37–39], suggesting that the reduction in airway calibre at FRC in the obese is attributable to the reduction in lung volumes rather than to airway obstruction. Respiratory system reactance is also abnormal in the obese [21], but the mechanism for this is not clear.

Similarly, expiratory flows also decrease with increasing weight [29, 38] in proportion to changes in lung volumes [30]. As such, decrease in expiratory flows in an obese individual is unlikely to indicate bronchial obstruction unless the flow measurements have been normalized for the reduction in vital capacity. In a large sample of obese and normal weight non-smokers, reductions in expiratory flows at 50% (V'_{50}) and 25% (V'_{25}) of vital capacity were found in obese men, but not in obese women [38]. Although the difference between obese and normal weight men in V'_{50} disappeared after normalization for vital capacity, the difference in V'_{25} persisted after normalization, suggesting the presence of peripheral airway obstruction in obese men. It is not clear why this was only detected in men in this study, but increased peripheral airway obstruction in obesity is consistent with findings from other studies, in both men and women, showing that obesity is associated with increased frequency dependence of resistance [30] and increased frequency dependence of compliance [11].

Expiratory Flow Limitation During Tidal Breathing

Expiratory flow rates are closely related to lung volumes, so that maximal flow decreases rapidly as expired volume approaches RV. As shown in Fig. 1.4, the predicted maximal flow, shown in the dashed line, is maintained well above the flows generated during tidal expiration at normal FRC, but the obese subject, breathing tidally at very low FRC, has very little expiratory flow reserve available during tidal breathing. For the obese individual, breathing at low lung volume places the tidal flow volume loop in a region where it may encroach on the maximal flow, thus increasing the risk of tidal expiratory flow limitation. It is not clear whether tidal expiratory flow limitation is a common occurrence in the obese. Two studies [40, 41], using the negative expiratory pressure technique, have found evidence of expiratory flow limitation in only 20% of severely obese subjects when upright. However, both expiratory flow limitation and breathlessness substantially increased when the subjects were placed supine. Quantification of expiratory flow limitation from the flow volume loop, as the percentage of the tidal volume that encroached on

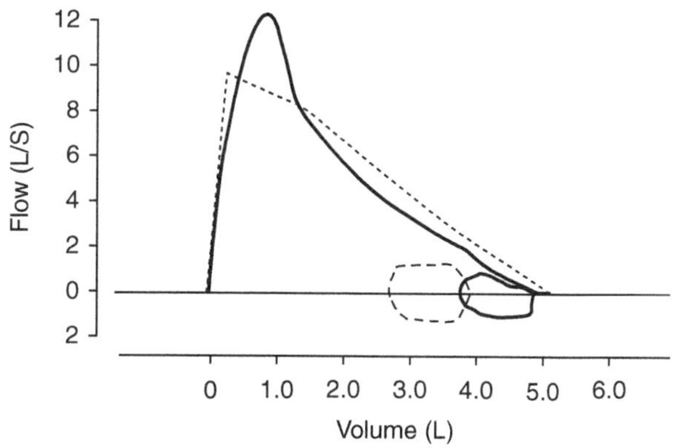

Fig. 1.4 Flow volume loop from a healthy, obese individual (BMI=43). The *dashed lines* show the predicted normal flow volume and tidal loops. There is minimal airway obstruction, but because FRC is low, the tidal loop encroaches onto the maximal loop, putting this individual at risk of expiratory flow limitation during tidal breathing

the maximal flow envelope, shows highly significant differences between obese and normal weight women when seated at rest [18]. However, the accuracy of comparisons of tidal and maximal flow volume curves may be limited by effects of dynamic compression of the airways during maximal forced expiratory manoeuvres. New techniques are available for measuring expiratory flow limitation during tidal breathing, based on the forced oscillation technique [42], that would allow larger studies to determine the extent of expiratory flow limitation in obese populations.

Intrinsic PEEP and Dynamic Hyperinflation

The presence of expiratory flow limitation during tidal breathing promotes the development of intrinsic positive end-expiratory pressure (PEEPi) and dynamic hyperinflation in obstructive airway disease, where it is an important determinant of respiratory symptoms. Pankow et al. [40] were able to detect PEEPi in all six severely obese subjects in whom they were able to make the measurement, even in the absence of expiratory flow limitation. The mechanism for PEEPi in the absence of EFL is unknown, but could be due to persistent post-inspiratory activity of the diaphragm, which has previously been observed in severely obese subjects [16]. PEEPi is a potential cause of respiratory symptoms in the obese since it is an additional elastic load that must be overcome at the beginning of each inspiration.

Although dynamic hyperinflation is usually closely associated with expiratory flow limitation and PEEPi, it might be expected that the decrease in respiratory system compliance associated with obesity would reduce the risk of dynamic hyperinflation in the obese. Indeed, the relationship between BMI and FRC is curvilinear and tends to flatten at high BMI (Fig. 1.3). We can speculate that the development of expiratory flow limitation and PEEPi in severely obese individuals might counteract, at least to a small degree, the effects of the stiffened respiratory system on lung volumes.

Airway Closure and Ventilation Distribution

It has been postulated that breathing at low lung volume, particularly in the setting of marked reduction in ERV seen in obesity, could lead to closure of peripheral airways in dependent lung zones [2, 11]. However, indicators of gas trapping and airway closure, such as RV [16, 28] and closing capacity [43], are not usually noted to be increased in obesity at rest. On the other hand, there is consistent evidence that if the FRC is very low, closing capacity exceeds the FRC and airway closure can occur within the tidal breaths [43–46]. Closing capacity, and particularly the extent to which closure occurs within the range of tidal breathing, has been correlated with arterial PO_2 [43, 46] raising the possibility that airway closure during tidal breathing may be associated with under-ventilation of some regions of the lung.

Abnormalities of regional ventilation have been observed in obese individuals using lung imaging to determine the distribution of ventilation [47–49]. Holley et al. [47] found that in obese subjects with marked reductions in ERV to around 20% predicted, ventilation was preferentially distributed to the upper zones of the lung, leaving the lower, dependent zones relatively under-ventilated. Similarly, Demedts [49] found that ventilation was significantly lower in the lung bases and tended to be higher in the apical regions in obese subjects compared to normal weight controls. The findings were consistent with a reduced expansion of the basal zone, possibly due to limitations in chest wall and diaphragm movements. However, global measures of ventilation heterogeneity, measured by the slope of phase III from single-breath washouts or by lung clearance index, are normal even in severely obese individuals [43].

Gas Exchange

Mild hypoxemia and increased alveolar-arterial oxygen difference are frequently reported, even in eucapnic obese individuals [7, 8, 43, 50, 51], and have been associated with abdominal obesity in the morbidly obese [52]. Reduction in oxygenation is unlikely to be due to abnormalities of gas transfer since most studies suggest that DLCO is normal [6, 17, 27, 53], even in morbid obesity [29]. Indeed, some studies suggest that DLCO is increased in extremely obese subjects [27, 38], probably as a result of the increase in blood volume [27]. Regional ventilation-perfusion mismatch in the dependent zones of the lung is a potential determinant of hypoxemia in obese individuals. Although an increase in blood volume in the obese could improve the homogeneity of perfusion and increase perfusion in the apices of the lung, the distribution of perfusion is predominantly to the lower zones, and individuals with reduced ventilation in the lung bases are likely to be at risk of ventilation-perfusion mismatch [47]. The extent to which gas exchange abnormalities in the obese are reversible is unclear, since some weight loss studies show improvements in arterial oxygen tensions [51, 54] while others report no change [44, 55]. Hakala et al. [44] found no increase in oxygenation with weight loss, even though there were significant improvements in FRC and most subjects no longer had closing capacities above FRC.

Consequences of Reduced Intrathoracic Volume

The effect of obesity on lung function is often described in terms of a restrictive rather than obstructive pattern, characterized by reduction in total lung capacity and vital capacity. The mechanisms for the reduction in total lung capacity in the obese are not well understood, but, as proposed in Fig. 1.1, may be due to reduced intrathoracic volume, as outlined below, or decreased respiratory system compliance.

Total Lung Capacity

The magnitude of the reduction in TLC with increasing weight is proportionally smaller than the effect on FRC, at least until BMI exceeds 35 kg/m^2 [23], with TLC usually maintained above the lower limit of normal even in severe obesity [23, 26, 28]. Lung restriction of the magnitude associated with restrictive lung disease, defined as TLC below the lower limit of normal, is not commonly associated with obesity in the absence of other disease. Nonetheless, evidence from prospective studies showing increases in TLC with weight loss in both mild [55] and morbidly obese [51] subjects, and decreases in vital capacity with weight gain [56], is consistent with the development of mild restrictive patterns of lung function in obesity.

The reasons for the reduction in TLC in the obese are unknown. It may be due to a reduction in the downwards movement of the diaphragm, due to increased abdominal mass, which could decrease TLC by limiting the room for lung expansion on inflation. Alternatively, deposition of fat in sub-pleural spaces [57] or elsewhere in the intrathoracic cavity might directly reduce lung volume by reducing the volume of the chest cavity. An exploratory study to investigate the mechanism for reduced TLC in obesity used MRI to measure intrathoracic volumes in obese and non-obese men and found increased mediastinal volume in the obese due to an increase in the volume of intrathoracic fat, the heart and major blood vessels [1]. At full inflation, the proportion of the intrathoracic volume occupied by inflated lungs was only 78% of the total in the obese compared with 88% in the controls, suggesting that the increased mediastinal volume may prevent full lung expansion in the obese, and may therefore explain the slight loss of TLC with increasing BMI. However, the marked loss of TLC in obese subjects with lung restriction (TLC < 80% predicted) was not explained by increased mediastinal volume, suggesting that other factors, such as reduced expansion of the thoracic cage, may also be important in this subgroup [1]. Since respiratory muscle strength and maximum inspiratory and expiratory pressures have been shown to be intact in obesity [16, 37, 58], it is unlikely that these would be an important determinant of obesity-related reduction in TLC.

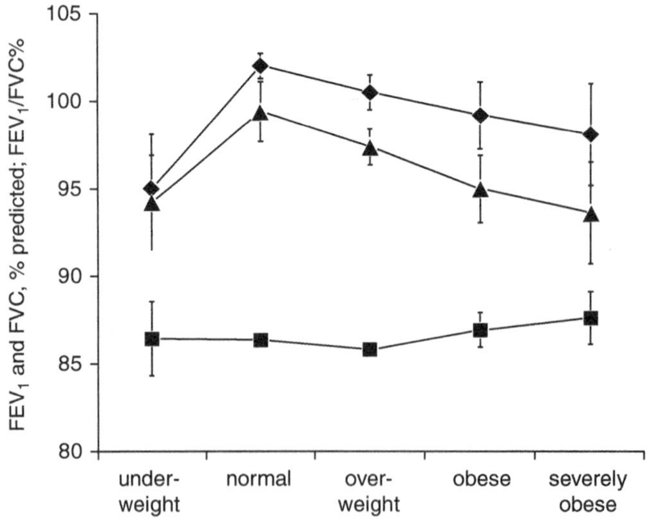

Fig. 1.5 Mean spirometric values, according to weight category, in adults (Adapted from data in Schachter et al. [60]). FEV_1 (*diamonds*) and FVC (*triangles*), as percent predicted, and FEV_1/FVC (*squares*) as a percentage

Spirometry

A reduction in total lung capacity, in the absence of any change in residual volume, indicates a reduction in vital capacity (VC). Consistent with a mild restrictive pattern of lung function in the obese, there is a progressive linear decrease in VC with increasing BMI that parallels the decrease in TLC [23]. Similarly, increasing BMI is also associated with a decrease in both FEV_1 and FVC [30, 59, 60]. However, this effect is small and both FEV_1 and FVC are usually within the normal range in healthy obese adults [59, 60] and children [61]. As a result, the FEV_1/FVC ratio, which is a marker of airway obstruction, is usually well preserved or increased [30, 34, 38, 59, 60], even in morbid obesity [29]. Figure 1.5 shows data from a population of 1,971 adults aged between 17 and 73 years [60] based on per cent of predicted values. Although FVC is affected to a greater extent than FEV_1 as BMI increases, FEV_1/FVC ratio remains normal across the weight groups, even in the severely obese group. Studies looking at the effect of body fat distribution on spirometry have shown that abdominal obesity is a stronger predictor than either weight or BMI of reductions in FEV_1 and FVC [33, 62], with one very large study of over 130,000 people suggesting that abdominal obesity may also be a risk for reduced FEV_1/FVC ratio [62]. Moreover, weight gain following smoking cessation [63] or with increasing age [56] is associated with reductions in both FEV_1 and FVC; the effect is greater on FVC than on FEV_1 and greater in men than women, presumably because men gain more abdominal fat than women.

Volume-Independent Effects on Airway Function

Although many of the effects of obesity on airway function can be attributed to the mechanical effects of breathing at low lung volume, as illustrated in Fig. 1.1, some studies have reported effects that appear to be independent of lung volume. In a population study of young adults, King et al. [24] found that obesity was associated with a persistent decrease in airway calibre, measured by respiratory system conductance, even after adjustment for lung volumes. This effect was present in men, but not in women. Another study by Watson et al. [28] comparing obese and control subjects sitting and supine found that differences in lung volume could only partly explain the differences in airflow resistance between obese and controls [28] or the increase in resistance associated with recumbency [28, 37]. Also, as discussed above, in the studies by Rubinstein et al. [38], although adjustment for vital capacity normalized V'_{50}, there were significant differences in V'_{25} which persisted after normalization. Lastly, the effect of obesity on spirometry increases with increasing duration of obesity, independent of the severity of obesity [64].

The cause of these volume-independent abnormalities of airway function is unknown. In addition, it is unclear whether there are any structural changes in the airways of the obese. It is possible that airway structures could be remodelled by chronic exposure to pro-inflammatory adipokines or systemic inflammation, or damaged by the continual opening and closing of small airways throughout the breathing cycle [45]. However, it is unlikely that fat is present in the airways of obese people or has any direct effect on airway structure, but studies of diet-induced obesity in rats have reported changes in lipid deposition in the lungs [65] which may affect surfactant function [66]. There are no reports of biopsy, pathological or imaging studies of the airway walls of obese subjects to indicate whether there are any cellular or structural abnormalities of the airways that might explain abnormal airway function.

Effects of Altered Ventilatory Mechanics on Symptoms, Performance and Clinical Presentation

Breathlessness at Rest and During Exercise

Breathlessness at rest is usually regarded as uncommon in healthy obese subjects, particularly in those with mild to moderate obesity. One study found that 15 of 23 mildly obese men reported breathing difficulties at rest associated with lower maximum voluntary ventilation and maximal expiratory flows at low lung volumes. However, the dyspnoeic group included a greater proportion of smokers, which may account for some of the symptoms and differences in lung function [67]. In morbidly obese subjects ($BMI > 40\ kg/m^2$) [68], dyspnoea scores at rest correlate with both inspiratory muscle endurance and lung function.

In contrast, breathlessness during exercise is a common complaint among obese individuals. In population studies, subjects with the highest BMI quintile have the greatest risk of dyspnoea with exertion, despite being at least risk of airway obstruction [59]. Standardized weight-bearing exercise tests, such as the 6-minute walk test, show that exercise capacity is reduced in obese adults [69, 70] and children [71] compared to normal weight controls. However, increased exertional symptoms in the obese are most likely due to the increased metabolic cost of the energy needed to move heavy limbs and drive the respiratory muscles [18, 72, 73], rather than to deconditioning or to abnormalities of airway or lung mechanics. Studies using weight-supported exercise, such as with a cycle ergometer, show that peak exercise capacity, in terms of both peak work rate and oxygen consumption, is normal in healthy obese subjects suggesting that they are not deconditioned [18, 72, 74]. The ventilatory response to inhaled CO_2 [17] and the relationships between oxygen consumption and minute ventilation, and between breathlessness and both oxygen consumption and minute ventilation are all normal in the obese [18]. Breathing at low lung volume could increase exertional breathlessness by preventing obese subjects from decreasing their end-expiratory volume during exercise [75, 76], but, in fact, because they breathe at low lung volumes, obese subjects have enough inspiratory reserve to increase their end-expiratory lung volume, to minimize expiratory flow limitation, but still increase tidal volumes to meet ventilatory demands [18]. Taken together, these observations suggest that the ability of the obese to increase ventilation in response to increasing metabolic demand is not impaired and that changes in lung volumes or airway mechanics due to obesity make little contribution to respiratory discomfort during exercise.

Effects of Obesity on Respiratory Function in Disease

The detrimental effects of obesity on lung function may have an impact on the outcomes of respiratory disease, although the effects are complex. In asthma, obesity is associated with greater prevalence and incidence of the disease [60, 61, 77] and may also be associated with worse clinical outcomes [78, 79], particularly in mild [80] or well-controlled [81] disease. In COPD, increasing BMI is associated with a reduced risk of death in patients with more severe disease, but not in those with mild COPD [82]. Although these relationships appear paradoxical, the mechanical effects of obesity on lung function are likely to be important contributing factors to many of the effects of obesity in respiratory disease.

How could the mechanical effects of obesity on lung function modify asthma pathophysiology? Asthma is characterized by airway obstruction, airway inflammation and airway hyperresponsiveness. One hypothesis suggests that breathing at reduced tidal volumes could affect the modulation of airway smooth muscle contractility by regular tidal stretching and deep inspirations [83], and increase the responsiveness of the muscle. Tidal volumes are not usually abnormal in mild to moderate obesity [18, 20–22]. However, breathing at low lung volumes means that airway calibre, and thus the length of airway smooth muscle, is reduced throughout the breathing cycle. It is not clear whether this leads to clinically meaningful increases in airway hyperresponsiveness in the obese. In studies of asthmatic subjects, there is little evidence that the severity of AHR is systematically increased in the obese [39, 80, 84, 85]. Moreover, there is inconsistent evidence of an association between BMI and airway responsiveness in studies of random populations [60, 61, 86]. An alternative hypothesis is that the reduction in operating lung volume in the obese has the potential to amplify the symptoms associated with bronchoconstriction. Bronchoconstriction in the obese is associated with increased airway closure compared to non-obese controls [87] and thus could increase gas trapping and alter ventilation distribution. Bronchoconstriction at low lung volume increases the risk of expiratory flow limitation and causes greater dynamic hyperinflation in obese asthmatic [84] and non-asthmatic [21] subjects, which may increase the severity of dyspnoea [88]. Nicolacakis et al. [39] suggest that obesity and asthma have additive, rather than synergistic effects, on outcomes such as spirometry and lung volumes. We can speculate that, in more severe or uncontrolled asthma, symptoms are likely to be dominated by the effects of uncontrolled airway inflammation and airway hyperresponsiveness. However, as these effects diminish with treatment and better asthma control, the effects of obesity on the development of airway closure, expiratory flow limitation and dynamic hyperinflation during episodes of mild bronchoconstriction may become more apparent. The occurrence of these additional elastic loads during bronchoconstriction, reflected by greater changes in respiratory system reactance in obese than non-obese subjects [21, 22], are often not well reflected by spirometry and may explain why some obese asthmatics have more severe symptoms than their lean counterparts, despite similar spirometry [89].

In COPD, it has been proposed that reduced operating lung volumes in obese patients may provide a mitigating influence on the intensity of exertional dyspnoea, by counterbalancing the negative mechanical consequences of severe lung hyperinflation [90, 91]. Because the obese COPD patients start from a much reduced FRC, dynamic hyperinflation during exercise does not result in such severe loss of inspiratory reserve as in non-obese COPD patients. The interactions between obesity and respiratory disease are discussed in detail in later chapters.

In restrictive lung disease, there are few available data about the effects of obesity on lung function. However, one study suggests increased BMI is associated with better survival in patients with idiopathic pulmonary fibrosis [92].

Impact of Obesity on the Interpretation of Pulmonary Function Tests

Obesity modifies many aspects of pulmonary function, even in people without respiratory disease, so the interpretation of pulmonary function tests in obese individuals can present problems. As outlined in this chapter, obesity in people without respiratory disease is typically associated with marked reductions in expiratory reserve volume and FRC, and modest reductions in TLC, VC, FEV_1 and FVC. However, reductions in FEV_1/FVC ratio, indicating airway obstruction, are not typical and would require further investigation. Measurements of expiratory flows and airway resistance may be abnormal and must be adjusted for lung volume before interpretation. The effect of obesity on pulmonary function tests in people at the extremes of age and height, where predicted values are less reliable, may be difficult to interpret.

In restrictive lung disease, TLC is, by definition, below the lower limit of normal. Although obesity is associated with a mild restrictive pattern of lung function, reductions of TLC of this magnitude are uncommon, even in severe obesity, and causes other than obesity should be sought for this restrictive pattern. Furthermore, in diseases such as idiopathic pulmonary fibrosis, diffusing capacity is reduced and both hypoxia and hypercapnia may be present. Some obese subjects have mild hypoxia on blood gas analysis, despite normal diffusing capacity. However, the presence of hypercapnia is uncommon and would suggest obesity hypoventilation syndrome (discussed in Chap. 5).

References

1. Watson RA, Pride NB, Thomas EL, et al. Reduction of total lung capacity in obese men: comparison of total intrathoracic and gas volumes. J Appl Physiol. 2010;108:1605–12.
2. Behazin N, Jones SB, Cohen RI, Loring SH. Respiratory restriction and elevated pleural and esophageal pressures in morbid obesity. J Appl Physiol. 2010;108:212–8.
3. Sugerman H, Windsor A, Bessos M, Wolfe L. Intra-abdominal pressure, sagittal abdominal diameter and obesity comorbidity. J Intern Med. 1997;241:71–9.
4. Sutherland TJT, Goulding A, Grant AM, et al. The effect of adiposity measured by dual-energy x-ray absorptiometry on lung function. Eur Respir J. 2008;32:85–91.
5. Naimark A, Cherniack RM. Compliance of the respiratory system and its components in health and obesity. J Appl Physiol. 1960;15:377–82.
6. Sharp JT, Henry JP, Swaeny SK, Meadows WR, Pietras RJ. The total work of breathing in normal and obese men. J Clin Invest. 1964;43:728–39.
7. Pelosi P, Croci M, Ravagnan I, et al. The effects of body mass on lung volumes, respiratory mechanics, and gas exchange during general anesthesia. Anesth Analg. 1998;87:654–60.
8. Hedenstierna G, Santesson J. Breathing mechanics, dead space and gas exchange in the extremely obese, breathing spontaneously and during anaesthesia with intermittent positive pressure ventilation. Acta Anaesthesiol Scand. 1976;20:248–54.
9. Suratt PM, Wilhoit SC, Hsiao HS, Atkinson RL, Rochester DF. Compliance of chest wall in obese subjects. J Appl Physiol. 1984;57:403–7.
10. Steier J, Jolley CJ, Seymour J, et al. Neural respiratory drive in obesity. Thorax. 2009;64:719–25.
11. Douglas FG, Chong PY. Influence of obesity on peripheral airways patency. J Appl Physiol. 1972;33:559–63.
12. Pelosi P, Croci M, Ravagnan I, Vicardi P, Gattinoni L. Total respiratory system, lung, and chest wall mechanics in sedated-paralyzed postoperative morbidly obese patients. Chest. 1996;109:144–51.
13. Rochester DF, Enson Y. Current concepts in the pathogenesis of the obesity hypoventilation syndrome. Mechanical and circulatory factors. Am J Med. 1974;57:402–20.

14. Sharp JT, Henry JP, Swaeny SK, Meadows WR, Pietras RJ. Effects of mass loading the respiratory system in man. J Appl Physiol. 1964;19:959–66.
15. Axen K, Haas SS, Haas F, Gaudino D, Haas A. Ventilatory adjustments during sustained mechanical loading in conscious humans. J Appl Physiol. 1983;55:1211–8.
16. Sampson MG, Grassino AE. Load compensation in obese patients during quiet tidal breathing. J Appl Physiol. 1983;55:1269–76.
17. Dempsey JA, Reddan W, Rankin J, Balke B. Alveolar-arterial gas exchange during muscular work in obesity. J Appl Physiol. 1966;21:1807–14.
18. Ofir D, Laveneziana P, Webb KA, O'Donnell DE. Ventilatory and perceptual responses to cycle exercise in obese women. J Appl Physiol. 2007;102:2217–26.
19. Mansell AL, Walders N, Wamboldt MZ, et al. Effect of body mass index on response to methacholine bronchial provocation in healthy and asthmatic adolescents. Pediatr Pulmonol. 2006; 41:434–40.
20. Boulet L-P, Turcotte H, Boulet G, Simard B, Robichaud P. Deep inspiration avoidance and airway response to methacholine: influence of body mass index. Can Respir J. 2005;12: 371–6.
21. Salome CM, Munoz PA, Berend N, et al. Effect of obesity on breathlessness and airway responsiveness to methacholine in non-asthmatic subjects. Int J Obes. 2008;32:502–9.
22. Torchio R, Gobbi A, Gulotta C, et al. Mechanical effects of obesity on airway responsiveness in otherwise healthy humans. J Appl Physiol. 2009;107:408–16.
23. Jones RL, Nzekwu M-MU. The effects of body mass index on lung volumes. Chest. 2006;130:827–33.
24. King GG, Brown NJ, Diba C, et al. The effects of body weight on airway calibre. Eur Respir J. 2005;25:896–901.
25. Sin DD, Sutherland ER. Obesity and the lung: 4. Obesity and asthma. Thorax. 2008;63: 1018–23.
26. Collins LC, Hoberty PD, Walker JF, Fletcher EC, Peiris AN. The effect of body fat distribution on pulmonary function tests. Chest. 1995;107:1298–302.
27. Ray CS, Sue DY, Bray G, Hansen JE, Wasserman K. Effects of obesity on respiratory function. Am Rev Respir Dis. 1983;128:501–6.
28. Watson RA, Pride NB. Postural changes in lung volumes and respiratory resistance in subjects with obesity. J Appl Physiol. 2005;98:512–7.
29. Biring M, Lewis M, Liu JT, Mohsenifar Z. Pulmonary physiologic changes of morbid obesity. Am J Med Sci. 1999;318:293–7.
30. Zerah F, Harf A, Perlemuter L, et al. Effects of obesity on respiratory resistance. Chest. 1993;103:1470–6.
31. Chen Y, Rennie D, Cormier YF, Dosman JA. Waist circumference is associated with pulmonary function in normal-weight, overweight, and obese subjects. Am J Clin Nutr. 2007; 85:35–9.
32. Canoy D, Luben R, Welch A, et al. Abdominal obesity and respiratory function in men and women in the EPIC-Norfolk Study, United Kingdom. Am J Epidemiol. 2004;159:1140–9.
33. Ochs-Balcom HM, Grant BJ, Muti P, et al. Pulmonary function and abdominal obesity in the general population. Chest. 2006;129:853–62.
34. Lazarus R, Sparrow D, Weiss ST. Effects of obesity and fat distribution on ventilatory function. Chest. 1997;111:891–8.
35. De Lorenzo A, Maiolo C, Mohamed EI, et al. Body composition analysis and changes in airways function in obese adults after hypocaloric diet. Chest. 2001;119:1409–15.
36. Babb TG, Wyrick BL, Chase PJ, et al. Weight loss via diet and exercise improves exercise breathing mechanics in obese men. Chest. 2011;140:454–60.
37. Yap JC, Watson RA, Gilbey S, Pride NB. Effects of posture on respiratory mechanics in obesity. J Appl Physiol. 1995;79:1199–205.
38. Rubinstein I, Zamel N, DuBarry L, Hoffstein V. Airflow limitation in morbidly obese, nonsmoking men. Ann Int Med. 1990;112:828–32.
39. Nicolacakis K, Skowronski ME, Coreno AJ, et al. Observations on the physiological interactions between obesity and asthma. J Appl Physiol. 2008;105:1533–41.

40. Pankow W, Podszus T, Gutheil T, et al. Expiratory flow limitation and intrinsic positive end-expiratory pressure in obesity. J Appl Physiol. 1998;85:1236–43.
41. Ferretti A, Giampiccolo P, Cavalli A, Milic-Emili J, Tantucci C. Expiratory flow limitation and orthopnea in massively obese subjects. Chest. 2001;119:1401–8.
42. Dellaca RL, Santus P, Aliverti A, et al. Detection of expiratory flow limitation in COPD using the forced oscillation technique. Eur Respir J. 2004;23:232–40.
43. Hedenstierna G, Santesson J, Norlander O. Airway closure and distribution of inspired gas in the extremely obese, breathing spontaneously and during anaesthesia with intermittent positive pressure ventilation. Acta Anaesthesiol Scand. 1976;20:334–42.
44. Hakala K, Mustajoki P, Aittomaki J, Sovijarvi AR. Effect of weight loss and body position on pulmonary function and gas exchange abnormalities in morbid obesity. Int J Obes. 1995;19:343–6.
45. Milic-Emili J, Torchio R, D'Angelo E. Closing-volume: a reappraisal (1967–2007). Eur J Appl Physiol. 2007;99:567–83.
46. Farebrother MJB, McHardy GJR, Munro JF. Relation between pulmonary gas exchange and closing volume before and after substantial weight loss in obese subjects. Br Med J. 1974;3: 391–3.
47. Holley HS, Milic-Emili J, Becklake MR, Bates DV. Regional distribution of pulmonary ventilation and perfusion in obesity. J Clin Invest. 1967;46:475–81.
48. Hurewitz A, Susskind H, Harold W. Obesity alters regional ventilation in lateral decubitus position. J Appl Physiol. 1985;59:774–83.
49. Demedts M. Regional distribution of lung volumes and of gas inspired at residual volume: influence of age, body weight and posture. Bull Eur Physiopathol Respir. 1980;16:271–85.
50. Jenkins SC, Moxham J. The effects of mild obesity on lung function. Respir Med. 1991;85: 309–11.
51. Thomas PS, Milledge JS. Respiratory function in the morbidly obese before and after weight loss. Thorax. 1989;44:382–6.
52. Zavorsky GS, Murias JM, Kim DJ, et al. Waist-to-hip ratio is associated with pulmonary gas exchange in the morbidly obese. Chest. 2007;131:362–7.
53. Sutherland TJT, Cowan JO, Young S, et al. The association between obesity and asthma: interactions between systemic and airway inflammation. Am J Respir Crit Care Med. 2008;178:469–75.
54. Refsum HE, Holter PH, Lovig T, Stadaas JO. Pulmonary function and energy expenditure after marked weight loss in obese women: observations before and one year after gastric banding. Int J Obes. 1990;14:175–83.
55. Womack CJ, Harris DL, Katzel LI, et al. Weight loss, not aerobic exercise, improves pulmonary function in older obese men. J Gerontol A Biol Sci Med Sci. 2000;55:M453–7.
56. Chen Y, Horne SL, Dosman JA. Body weight and weight gain related to pulmonary function decline in adults: a six year follow up study. Thorax. 1993;48:375–80.
57. Sargent EN, Boswell Jr WD, Ralls PW, Markovitz A. Subpleural fat pads in patients exposed to asbestos: distinction from non-calcified pleural plaques. Radiology. 1984;152:273–7.
58. Kelly TM, Jensen RL, Elliott CG, Crapo RO. Maximum respiratory pressures in morbidly obese subjects. Respiration. 1988;54:73–7.
59. Sin DD, Jones RL, Man SF. Obesity is a risk factor for dyspnea but not for airflow obstruction. Arch Intern Med. 2002;162:1477–81.
60. Schachter LM, Salome CM, Peat JK, Woolcock AJ. Obesity is a risk for asthma and wheeze but not airway hyperresponsiveness. Thorax. 2001;56:4–8.
61. Schachter LM, Peat JK, Salome CM. Asthma and atopy in overweight children. Thorax. 2003;58:1031–5.
62. Leone N, Courbon D, Thomas F, et al. Lung function and metabolic syndrome: the critical role of abdominal obesity. Am J Respir Crit Care Med. 2008;179:509–16.
63. Wise RA, Enright PL, Connett JE, et al. Effect of weight gain on pulmonary function after smoking cessation in the Lung Health Study. Am J Resp Crit Care Med. 1998;157:866–72.

64. Santamaria F, Montella S, Greco L, et al. Obesity duration is associated to pulmonary function impairment in obese subjects. Obesity (Silver Spring). 2011;19:1623–8.
65. Inselman LS, Spencer H. Obesity-induced hyperplastic lung growth. Am Rev Respir Dis. 1987;135:613–6.
66. Inselman LS, Chander A, Spitzer AR. Diminished lung compliance and elevated surfactant lipids and proteins in nutritionally obese young rats. Lung. 2004;182:101–17.
67. Sahebjami H. Dyspnea in obese healthy men. Chest. 1998;114:1373–7.
68. Collett F, Mallart A, Bervar JF, et al. Physiologic correlates of dyspnea in patients with morbid obesity. Int J Obes. 2007;31:700–6.
69. Larsson UE, Reynisdottir S. The six-minute walk test in outpatients with obesity: reproducibility and known group validity. Physiother Res Int. 2008;13:84–93.
70. Beriault K, Carpentier AC, Gagnon C, et al. Reproducibility of the 6-minute walk test in obese adults. Int J Sports Med. 2009;30:725–7.
71. Morinder G, Mattsson E, Sollander C, Marcus C, Larsson UE. Six-minute walk test in obese children and adolescents: reproducibility and validity. Physiother Res Int. 2009;14:91–104.
72. Babb TG, Ranasinghe KG, Comeau LA, Semon TL, Schwartz B. Dyspnea on exertion in obese women. Association with increased oxygen cost of breathing. Am J Respir Crit Care Med. 2008;178:116–23.
73. Kress JP, Pohlman AS, Alverdy J, Hall JB. The impact of morbid obesity on oxygen cost of breathing (VO2RESP) at rest. Am J Respir Crit Care Med. 1999;160:883–6.
74. Babb TG, DeLorey DS, Wyrick BL, Gardner PP. Mild obesity does not limit change in end-expiratory lung volume during cycling in young women. J Appl Physiol. 2002;92: 2483–90.
75. Babb TG, Buskirk ER, Hodgson JL. Exercise end-expiratory lung volumes in lean and moderately obese women. Int J Obes. 1989;13:11–9.
76. DeLorey DS, Wyrick BL, Babb TG. Mild-to-moderate obesity: implications for respiratory mechanics at rest and during exercise in young men. Int J Obes. 2005;29:1039–47.
77. Beuther DA, Sutherland ER. Overweight, obesity, and incident asthma: a meta-analysis of prospective epidemiologic studies. Am J Respir Crit Care Med. 2007;175:661–6.
78. Mosen DM, Schatz M, Magid DJ, Camargo Jr CA. The relationship between obesity and asthma severity and control in adults. J Allergy Clin Immunol. 2008;122:507–11. e6.
79. Vortmann M, Eisner MD. BMI and health status among adults with asthma. Obesity (Silver Spring). 2008;16:146–52.
80. Raviv S, Dixon AE, Kalhan R, Shade D, Smith LJ. Effect of obesity on asthma phenotype is dependent upon asthma severity. J Asthma. 2011;48:98–104.
81. Farah CS, Kermode JA, Downie SR, et al. Obesity is a determinant of asthma control, independent of inflammation and lung mechanics. Chest. 2011;140:659–66.
82. Landbo C, Prescott E, Lange P, Vestbo J, Almdal TP. Prognostic value of nutritional status in chronic obstructive pulmonary disease. Am J Respir Crit Care Med. 1999;160:1856–61.
83. Fredberg J, Inouye D, Mijailovich M, Butler J. Perturbed equilibrium of myosin binding in airway smooth muscle and its implications in bronchospasm. Am J Resp Crit Care Med. 1999;159:959–67.
84. Sutherland TJT, Cowan JO, Taylor DR. Dynamic hyperinflation with bronchoconstriction: differences between obese and nonobese women with asthma. Am J Respir Crit Care Med. 2008;177:970–5.
85. van Veen IH, ten Brinke A, Sterk PJ, Rabe KF, Bel EH. Airway inflammation in obese and non-obese patients with difficult-to-treat asthma. Allergy. 2008;63:570–4.
86. Chinn S, Jarvis D, Burney P. Relation of bronchial responsiveness to body mass index in the ECRHS. Thorax. 2002;57:1028–33.
87. Chapman DG, Berend N, King GG, Salome CM. Increased airway closure is a determinant of airway hyperresponsiveness. Eur Respir J. 2008;32:1563–9.
88. Lougheed MD, Lam M, Forkert L, Webb KA, O'Donnell DE. Breathlessness during acute bronchoconstriction in asthma. Am Rev Respir Dis. 1993;148:1452–9.

89. Thomson CC, Clark S, Camargo Jr CA. Body mass index and asthma severity among adults presenting to the emergency department. Chest. 2003;124:795–802.
90. Guenette JA, Jensen D, O'Donnell DE. Respiratory function and the obesity paradox. Curr Opin Clin Nutr Metab Care. 2010;13:618–24.
91. Ora J, Laveneziana P, Wadell K, et al. Effect of obesity on respiratory mechanics during rest and exercise in COPD. J Appl Physiol. 2011;111:10–9.
92. Alakhras M, Decker PA, Nadrous HF, Collazo-Clavell M, Ryu JH. Body mass index and mortality in patients with idiopathic pulmonary fibrosis. Chest. 2007;131:1448–53.

Chapter 2
Effects of Obesity on Airway Responsiveness

Stephanie A. Shore

Abstract Although obesity is a risk factor for asthma, the mechanistic basis for this relationship is not established. In this chapter, we review data from human subjects and animal models examining how obesity impacts a characteristic feature of asthma airway hyperresponsiveness. We focus on two aspects of obesity that may affect airway responsiveness: the impact of obesity on the mechanical properties of the lungs and chest wall, and the low-grade systemic inflammation that results from interactions between adipocytes and leukocytes that are recruited to obese adipose tissue. We also discuss the possibility that diet may contribute to airway hyperresponsiveness, either through direct effects of dietary constituents or by altering the gut microbiome. Determining how obesity promotes asthma may uncover novel therapeutic strategies that are effective in the obese asthmatic.

Keywords Mice • Adipokines • Inflammation • Chest wall • Functional residual capacity

Objectives

- Review the epidemiological and cohort studies that have examined airway responsiveness in obese human subjects.
- Describe the outcome of studies that have examined airway responsiveness in obese mice.

S.A. Shore, Ph.D. (✉)
Environmental Health, Harvard School of Public Health, 665 Huntington Ave,
Boston, MA 02115, USA
e-mail: sshore@hsph.harvard.edu

A.E. Dixon and E.M. Clerisme-Beaty (eds.), *Obesity and Lung Disease: A Guide to Management*, Respiratory Medicine, DOI 10.1007/978-1-62703-053-3_2,

- Understand the mechanisms by which obesity may contribute to airway responsiveness.
- Describe the adipose tissue, systemic, and pulmonary inflammation extant in obesity.

Introduction

As described elsewhere in this book, obesity is an important risk factor for asthma. Numerous epidemiological studies performed in adults and children throughout the world have consistently established a role for obesity in asthma prevalence and incidence [1–4] and in worsening asthma control [5–7]. In contrast, evidence for an effect of obesity on airway responsiveness, a characteristic feature of asthma, is less consistent. In this chapter, we describe the complexities in the relationship between obesity and airway hyperresponsiveness (AHR). We also discuss possible mechanisms by which obesity might promote AHR, including effects of obesity on the mechanical properties of the lungs and chest wall and the potential role of obesity-related inflammation. In addition, we consider the possibility that alterations in dietary factors may be contributing to this relationship.

Obesity and Airway Responsiveness in Human Subjects

Studies reporting the impact of obesity on airway responsiveness in adults are summarized in Table 2.1. It is notable that the first study of this type was published only 10 years ago, as the tide of the obesity epidemic began to swell. The results of these studies are mixed, with some showing that obesity is a risk factor for AHR, and others showing no impact of obesity on AHR. Essentially similar results have been reported in children (see [8]).

Epidemiological and Cohort Studies

Among the epidemiological studies addressing the relationship between obesity and AHR, that of Litonjua et al. [9] deserves special mention here, because it is the only prospective longitudinal cohort study in adults to address this issue. The authors used the Normative Aging Study population, which consisted of mostly older Caucasian males from the greater Boston area. Airway responsiveness was assessed twice in each subject with an interval of approximately 4 years. Subjects were chosen who had negative methacholine challenges on the first visit. Cases were subjects who had positive challenges on the second visit (i.e., they developed AHR) and were matched with controls whose methacholine responsiveness remained negative

Table 2.1 Studies describing the impact of obesity on airway responsiveness in adults

Authors (year)	No. of subjects	Nationality of subjects	Gender of subjects	Nature of study	Outcome(s)
Celedon et al. (2001) [11]	7,109	Chinese	Men and women	Cross-sectional analysis of families with at least one asthmatic	U-shaped relationship between BMI and symptomatic AHR in both men and women
Schachter et al. (2001) [13]	1,971	Australian	Men and women	Cross-sectional analysis of randomly selected population	No effect of BMI on AHR
Litonjua et al. (2002) [9]	300	American	Men	Prospective study of older men who developed AHR over a 3–4-year period	U-shaped relationship between initial BMI and risk of developing AHR; positive linear relationship between weight gain and development of AHR
Chinn et al. (2002) [10]	11,277	European	Men and women	Cross-sectional analysis of randomly selected population	AHR increased with BMI in men; similar trend in women but did not reach statistical significance
Aaron et al. (2004) [28]	58	American	Women	Study of the effects of weight loss on airway responsiveness in obese asthmatics and nonasthmatics	Diet-induced weight loss did not affect airway responsiveness but did improve lung function
Sood et al. (2006) [12]	1,725	American	Men and women	Cross-sectional analysis of subjects referred to a pulmonary function lab for diagnosis	BMI increases AHR in nonasthmatics but not in asthmatics
Bustos et al. (2006) [14]	1,232	Chilean	Men and women	Cross-sectional analysis of randomly selected population	BMI was negatively associated with AHR
Nicolacakis et al. (2008) [15]	210	American	Men and women	Comparison of obese and nonobese asthmatic and nonasthmatic subjects	No effect of obesity on AHR in either asthmatics or nonasthmatics
Salome et al. (2008) [19]	49	Australian	Men and women	Comparison of obese and nonobese nonasthmatics with normal airway responsiveness	No effect of obesity on AHR as measured by FEV1 or respiratory system resistance, whereas methacholine-induced changes in respiratory system reactance were greater in obese subjects

(continued)

Table 2.1 (continued)

Authors (year)	No. of subjects	Nationality of subjects	Gender of subjects	Nature of study	Outcome(s)
Sharma et al. (2008) [16]	861	Canadian	Men and women	Cross-sectional analysis of subjects referred to a pulmonary function lab for asthma diagnosis	Obesity was a significant risk factor for AHR in subjects suspected of having asthma. The relative risk increased with the magnitude of obesity
Torchio et al. (2009) [17]	41	Italian	Men and women	Comparison of obese and nonobese nonasthmatics	Airway responsiveness increased with increasing BMI. Breathing at low lung volume explained this relationship in men but not in women
Skloot et al. (2011) [18]	36	American	Men and women	Comparison of obese and nonobese nonasthmatics	Obese subjects had greater airway responsiveness especially when measures of changes in small airways were used as the outcome indicator but not with FEV1. The obesity-related difference was attenuated when deep breaths were withheld
Farah et al. (2011) [55]	49	Australian	Men and women	Study compared the effects of steroid treatment in obese and nonobese asthmatics	Obese asthmatics had greater airway responsiveness than nonobese asthmatics. Treatment with high-dose inhaled steroids reduced airway responsiveness in both normal weight and obese asthmatics. Only 1 nonatopic asthmatic was included in the obese group
Dixon et al. (2011) [27]	40	American	Men and women	Study of the effect of bariatric surgery on airway responsiveness in obese asthmatics	Weight loss caused reduced airway responsiveness in nonatopic but not in atopic asthmatics

The table is ordered by year of publication. Modified from Shore [8] on the second visit. The authors reported that after controlling for age, smoking, serum IgE, and initial FEV_1, there was an increased risk for AHR with increasing initial body mass index (BMI). Similarly, weight gain was related to the risk of developing AHR.

In addition to the study of Litonjua et al. [9], three other large cross-sectional epidemiological studies also noted a greater prevalence of AHR or symptomatic AHR in obese versus normal weight adults [10–12], although in the study of Chinn et al. [10], a relationship was observed in males but not in females. In the study of Celedon et al. [11], the odds ratio for symptomatic AHR in obese versus normal weight individuals was approximately the same in men (2.3) and in women (2.5). In contrast, others have reported no increase in airway responsiveness with increasing BMI [13, 14]. It is perhaps notable that in the study by Schachter et al. [13], airway responsiveness was not assessed in any subjects with severe obesity (BMI ≥ 35) who were also nonatopic. As described below, it is this group in which obesity-related AHR may be particularly prevalent. In the study of Chinn et al., the relationship between BMI and AHR became stronger after adjusting for atopy [10].

There are some methodological issues that need consideration in interpreting these data. Some studies have reported a U-shaped relationship between BMI and AHR [9, 11]: both underweight and obesity were associated with increased airway responsiveness, although the effect of underweight has received little attention. Schachter et al. [13] also noted an increase in airway responsiveness in underweight (BMI < 18.5) individuals even though they did not find an increase in responsiveness in overweight or obese individuals. Failure to account for the effects of low BMI could confound the interpretation of the data relating AHR to BMI. For example, in the study of Bustos et al. [14], much of the apparent trend toward a *reduction* in responsiveness with increasing BMI is driven by these underweight individuals.

The method by which subjects are enrolled may also affect the outcome of these studies. For example, the nonasthmatic obese subjects in the study of Nicolacakis et al. [15] described above were chosen because they were free of lung disease. Such a choice would lessen the likelihood of detecting an effect of obesity on AHR, since the presence of AHR might manifest in symptoms suggestive of lung disease. In contrast, in the two studies which evaluated populations sent to the pulmonary function clinic for measurement of AHR for diagnostic purposes (i.e., populations that likely had symptoms suggestive of AHR), there was a positive relationship between obesity and airway responsiveness [12, 16].

The outcome indicator used to assess airway narrowing is also important to consider. Torchio et al. [17] were able to observe increased airway responsiveness in obese versus lean nonasthmatic subjects. To assess bronchoconstriction, they did not use FEV_1 but rather maximum expiratory flow at 60% of total lung capacity (TLC) corrected for thoracic gas compression volume. They argued that the correction for gas compression was important, especially since the TLC tends to decline with obesity. Skloot et al. [18] reported no difference between obese and lean subjects when FEV_1 was used as the outcome indicator, but did observe greater airway responsiveness in the obese when measures of small airways were used instead. Similarly, in a study of obese versus nonobese nonasthmatics, Salome et al. [19]

reported no obesity-related differences in methacholine-induced changes in FEV_1 or total respiratory system resistance. They did, however, observe greater increases in respiratory system reactance in the obese subjects, an observation that has been reproduced by others [17, 18]. Increased respiratory system reactance is consistent with greater hyperinflation, and the Salome group subsequently confirmed greater airway closure and consequent hyperinflation in the obese versus lean subjects after methacholine challenge [20]. Sutherland et al. [21] also noted greater hyperinflation following methacholine challenge in obese versus lean asthmatics. Notably, in obese subjects, small airway closure occurs in the dependent regions of the lung even without administration of any bronchoconstricting agonist [22–25]. The situation may be even more complicated in obese asthmatics, who may have additional areas of airway closure consequent to airway disease. It is significant that airway closure in some parts of the lung results in dilation of the airways in the rest of the lung, which now receive a greater portion of the tidal volume. Greater volume causes more stretch of airway smooth muscle and subsequent bronchodilation in those regions [26]. The FEV_1 is unlikely to capture the complexity of such heterogeneous airway changes. Nevertheless, Sood et al. [12] were able to observe an increase in the prevalence of AHR in obese versus nonobese nonasthmatics using FEV_1 as the outcome indicator. However, the effect was small and may have been observable only because their sample size was much greater than in the studies described immediately above where an effect of obesity on AHR could not be detected using FEV_1. Environmental, genetic, and epigenetic factors can all affect AHR, and such factors may obscure any additional effect of obesity without the use of such large sample sizes when a blunt tool such as the FEV_1 is used for assessment. Interestingly, Sood et al. [12] did not detect any impact of obesity on airway responsiveness in subjects with asthma. These subjects already had hyperresponsive airways, and it is possible that the additional effect of obesity was too small to be observed under these conditions.

Weight Loss Studies

There are only two reports of the impact of weight loss on AHR [27, 28]. In the study of Dixon et al. [27], obese asthmatic subjects underwent bariatric surgery and lost an average 27% of their initial body weight. This weight loss was associated with a significant reduction in airway responsiveness. Importantly, the atopic status of the subjects predicted the impact of weight loss on airway responsiveness. In the 9 atopic subjects (atopy was ascertained on the basis of serum IgE), weight loss had no significant effect on AHR. These subjects had asthma of long duration and likely had AHR of allergic origin. Since serum IgE did not change with weight loss, it is perhaps not surprising that in these subjects, AHR was not affected either. In contrast, in the 14 nonatopic subjects, there was a significant loss of responsiveness with weight loss. These subjects had asthma with an onset later in life and had more obesity-related comorbidities, suggesting a different asthma phenotype, with the asthma (and AHR) more directly related to obesity.

In the weight loss study of Aaron et al. [28], there was a trend toward an improvement in AHR after 6 months on a diet-induced weight reduction program, but the effect was not significant, even though subjects lost an average 17.4% of their initial body weight and did have improved flow rates and symptoms. The reason for the discrepant effects of weight loss in the two studies is not clear, but there were some noteworthy differences in the two study populations. In the study of Aaron et al. [28], the subjects were not as obese initially, and while they had approximately the same percentage of atopic subjects as did Dixon et al. [27], their population included only 41% of asthmatics. Importantly, despite the overall lack of improvement in AHR, there were several individuals in their study who did have reduced airway responsiveness after weight loss, but it is not possible to determine from the report whether these were nonatopic subjects.

Obese Mice Exhibit Innate AHR

AHR is a common feature of murine obesity. Regardless of how mice become obese, they exhibit increased responses to intravenous methacholine [29–34] (Fig. 2.1). In mice, obesity-related AHR is also observed with another bronchoconstricting agonist, serotonin [31], consistent with the nonspecific AHR of asthma. Obese mice also develop greater increases in airway responsiveness following ozone exposure [29, 31, 32, 35] or allergen sensitization and challenge [36, 37] than lean mice. As previously discussed [8], the more consistent effect of obesity in mice than in humans may be the consequence of the more consistent environmental, genetic, and epigenetic influences on AHR in the mice, since the studies were performed on animals often born to the same mothers and housed together.

In contrast to the situation in obese humans described by Salome et al. (see above), we observed AHR in obese mice when changes in airway resistance (Raw) were used as the outcome indicator, but not with outcomes that reflect changes in the lung tissues [30, 32–34]. Two factors may contribute to this human/mouse difference. First, we made measurements in mice with the chest wall open, and we applied 3-cm H_2O positive end-expiratory pressure (PEEP). Second, measurements were made using intravenous rather than inhaled methacholine. Both factors may limit the airway closure that appears to explain the obesity-related augmentation of methacholine-induced changes in lung tissue properties observed in obese humans [19]. Using a histological system, Saraiva et al. [36] observed an increase in the proportion of the lung with collapsed alveoli even in the absence of any bronchoconstricting agonist in lungs of mice with diet-induced obesity versus lean controls, suggesting an increased tendency toward airway closure. In their system, PEEP was not applied.

In mice, AHR is affected by the extent of the obesity (Fig. 2.1). For example, *ob/ob* and *db/db* mice that lack leptin or the leptin receptor, respectively, are massively obese by 8 weeks of age. They exhibit AHR even at this early age, and the magnitude of this hyperresponsiveness is substantial [29, 31]. The increase in body weight

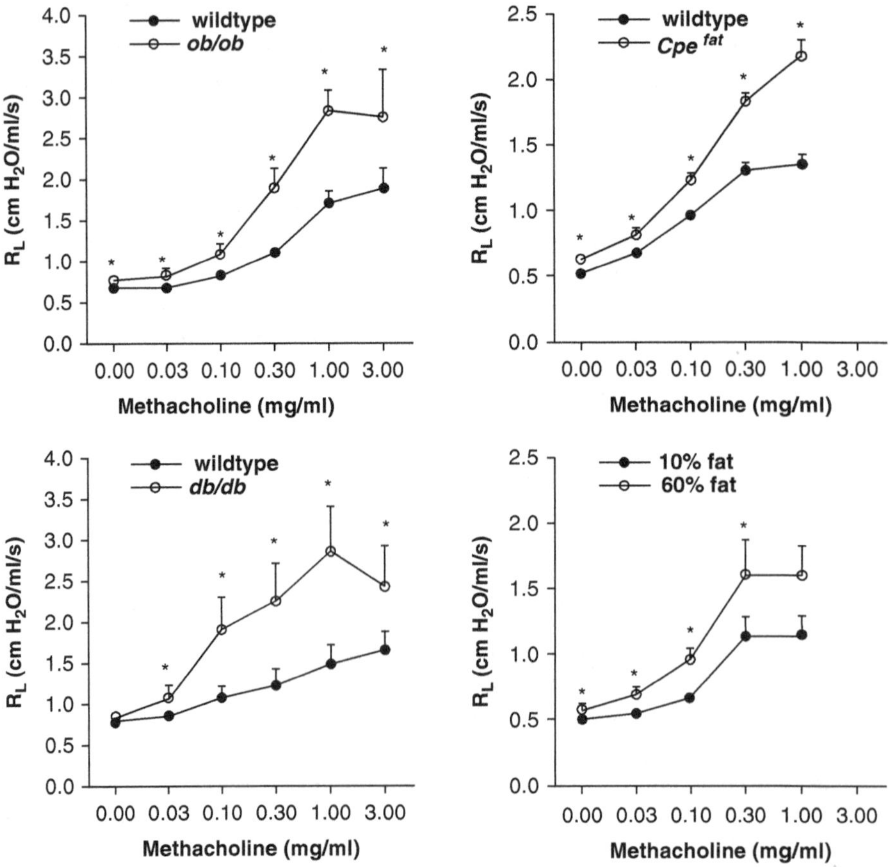

Fig. 2.1 Changes in pulmonary resistance (R_L) induced by i.v. methacholine in four types of obese mice and their lean controls. Data are mean ± SE. $^*p<0.05$ versus wild-type or low-fat-diet-fed control mice (Data are from previous publications from the author's lab and are reproduced from the American Physiological Society [8])

in Cpe^{fat} mice, which are obese because of a genetic defect in an enzyme that regulates satiety neuropeptides, is slower in onset. At 7 weeks of age, Cpe^{fat} mice weigh approximately 25% more than wild-type controls and are not hyperresponsive. By 10 weeks of age, body weight averages 61% more than wild-type controls, and hyperresponsiveness is apparent [35]. The magnitude of obesity continues to increase, and AHR is sustained with increasing age [32]. The duration of obesity may also play a role in the induction of hyperresponsiveness. Mice become obese when high-fat diets are initiated at the time of weaning, although the magnitude of this obesity is not as great as with the genetic obesities [38]. Interestingly, even though the magnitude of obesity is approximately the same in 23- and 35-week-old mice with dietary obesity, only the older obese mice develop AHR. Perhaps with milder obesity, longer durations are required to elicit effects.

Mechanistic Basis for Airway Hyperresponsiveness in Obesity

Several factors may contribute to AHR in the obese. Among these, two factors have received considerable attention and are the focus of the discussion below: (1) mechanical changes in the lungs and chest wall and (2) aspects of the low-grade systemic inflammation that occurs in obesity. We also discuss the potential for diet to contribute to obesity-related AHR.

Mechanical Factors

In the absence of asthma, obesity reduces the functional residual capacity (FRC). For example, Jones et al. [39] reported declines in FRC of 10%, 22%, and 33% predicted in overweight, mild, and morbidly obese individuals. The pressure volume relationship of the respiratory system changes in obesity, and the relaxation volume of the respiratory system, the volume at which the outward recoil of the relaxed chest wall balances the inward recoil of the lung (V_{rel}), declines (Fig. 2.2). FRC usually occurs at V_{rel}, though in obesity, other factors may also contribute (see below).

There is ample evidence that a decline in FRC can promote AHR. Ding et al. [40] instructed normal human subjects to breath (1) at their regular FRC, (2) at a volume 0.5 L below FRC, or (3) at a volume 0.5 L above FRC. They observed that the extent of bronchoconstriction induced by methacholine declined significantly as the lung

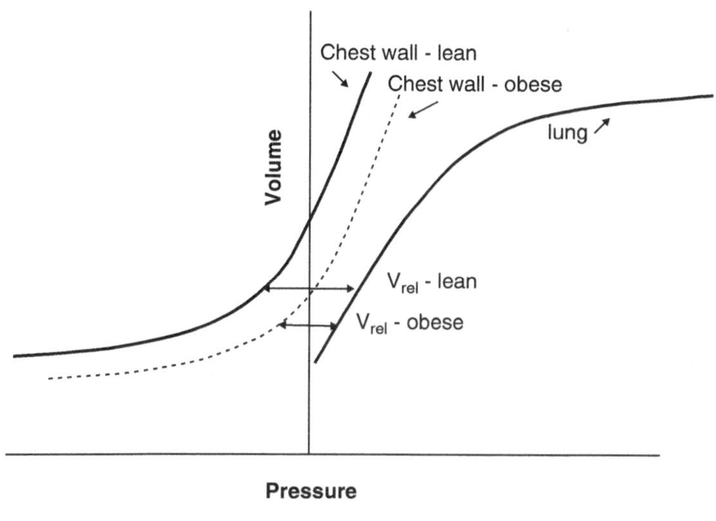

Fig. 2.2 Obesity-related alterations in the pressure volume curve of the chest wall lead to changes in static lung volumes, including a reduction in the relaxation volume of the respiratory system (V_{rel}), the volume at which the inward recoil of the lung balances the outward recoil of the chest wall (Reproduced from the American Physiological Society [147])

volume increased. Airway responsiveness also increases when declines in FRC are caused by adopting the supine posture [41] or by chest strapping [42]. Ding et al. argued that the increased responsiveness observed at low lung volumes was the result of loss of the retractive forces that the lung parenchyma exerted on the airways. In other words, breathing at low lung volume reduced the load on the airway smooth muscle (ASM). Consequently, it shortened more. Loss of this load also reduces the resting length of the ASM, which should place it at a less favorable position on its length tension relationship. However, Torchio et al. [42] argued that the ability of ASM to rapidly adapt its cytoskeletal structure to changes in length allowed it to generate increased force despite its shorter length at low lung volume. Indeed, McClean et al. [43] observed that ASM from sheep that had had their FRC restricted for 4 weeks by means of a leather corset had a velocity of shortening that was almost double that of sheep maintained at normal FRC.

As previously discussed [8], there are other ways in which a reduction in FRC might promote AHR. The propensity for small airways to close increases as FRC declines. Indeed, airway closure is observed in many obese subjects at FRC [22, 23, 44]. The repeated opening and closing of these airways during normal tidal breathing could cause rupture of alveolar attachments to bronchioles [45], further reducing the load on ASM.

In addition to reductions in absolute lung volume, reductions in tidal volume (V_T) or in the frequency of sighing might also promote AHR in the obese. During tidal breathing, and especially during sighs, ASM is stretched, causing actin-myosin crossbridges to detach, relaxing the muscle, and dilating the airways [46]. Crossbridge detachment also reduces the stiffness of ASM, making it easier to stretch, further promoting bronchodilation. Obesity does not alter the frequency of sighing [17]. However, in both obese humans [47] and obese mice [3], V_T is reduced. Such reductions could lead to sustained ASM contraction and airway narrowing (see [3] for more details).

Skloot et al. [18] recently reported that in obese subjects, airway responsiveness was not altered when deep breaths were withheld during methacholine challenge. In contrast, in lean subjects withholding deep breaths increased airway responsiveness to levels comparable to the obese subjects. Others have also reported reduced responses to the bronchodilating effects of a deep breath in obese subjects [17, 48, 49]. Factors that uncouple the airways from the parenchyma, such as reductions in lung volume, fluid cuffing around airways, or stiffening of the airways consequent to reduced V_T (see above), would be expected to attenuate the salutary effects of a deep breath on the airways. Importantly, a similar reduced bronchodilatory effect of a deep breath is also observed in asthma [50].

Only one study has directly addressed the importance of reductions in FRC for AHR in obesity. Torchio et al. [17] measured airway responsiveness and FRC in men and women with varying degrees of obesity. In men, airway responsiveness increased progressively as FRC declined with obesity. Indeed, the decline in FRC alone accounted for a substantial proportion of the AHR observed in the obese. However, in women, even though obesity did lead to AHR and did reduce FRC, there was no relationship between the magnitude of AHR and the decline in lung volume, suggesting that other factors, perhaps differences in inflammation, must account for obesity-related AHR in women.

There are additional factors that require consideration in any discussion of obesity and its impact on FRC. In a substantial proportion of obese individuals, FRC is not statically determined. Instead, up to 50% of obese subjects exhibit expiratory flow limitation during tidal breathing (tidal flows overlap the maximal expiratory flow volume loop) [51–53]. With flow limitation, expiration may be incomplete when the next inspiration is initiated, so that lung volume gradually ratchets up until expiratory flow rates are sufficient to permit full expiration. In obesity, such dynamic hyperinflation may prevent even greater reductions in FRC than would otherwise occur. Inspiratory muscle braking during early expiration also occurs in most obese subjects breathing quietly in the upright posture [47], and may also serve to attenuate declines in FRC. Dynamic hyperinflation also occurs in asthmatics [54] and may explain why FRC is elevated rather than reduced in individuals who are both obese and asthmatic [21, 55]. If obesity-related reductions in FRC do indeed contribute to promoting AHR in obesity, this may also explain why some investigators have had difficulty discerning differences in AHR between obese and nonobese asthmatics [12, 15] since measurements of FRC do not differ between obese and nonobese asthmatics [21, 55].

While it is possible that the mechanical effects of obesity on the lung may contribute to obesity-related AHR in humans, such effects do not appear to explain the AHR observed in obese mice. In obese mice, measurements of airway responsiveness were performed with the chest open and with a fixed PEEP, in order that absolute lung volume not be influenced by obesity. In addition, the mice were mechanically ventilated with tidal volumes that were the same in the obese and lean mice. The lungs of obese *db/db* and *ob/ob* mice are smaller than those of age- and gender-matched lean wild-type mice, and this could impact airway responsiveness [38]. However, lung size is similar in mice with diet-induced obesity and their lean controls, but obese mice still exhibit AHR [33].

Inflammation

The adipose tissue of obese humans and obese rodents is infiltrated with macrophages and other immune/inflammatory cells (Fig. 2.3). Importantly, products of these cells appear to spill over into the blood, leading to a state that has been termed low-grade systemic inflammation. This inflammatory state appears to contribute to many obesity-related conditions, and it is conceivable that circulating inflammatory moieties also affect the lungs in such a way as to augment airway responsiveness. Below we review current concepts regarding the systemic inflammation of obesity and its importance. We also review evidence regarding inflammation in the lungs of obese individuals.

Fig. 2.3 Summary of the effects of obesity on immune and inflammatory cells within adipose tissue. See text for details

Cell type	Impact of Obesity
Macrophages	↑
Cytotoxic T cells	↑
CD4+ cells	
•Th1 cells	↑
•Th2 cells	↓
•T regs	↓
NKT cells	↔
Mast cells	↑
Eosinophils	↓

Adipose Tissue Inflammation: There are numerous effects of obesity on the types and activation state of immune and inflammatory cells that infiltrate the adipose tissue (Fig. 2.3). Adipose tissue macrophages (ATM) infiltrate the adipose tissue of obese humans and obese mice. Some ATM exist even in lean individuals [56, 57], but in obesity, ATM account for up to 50% of the cells isolated from adipose tissue [58]. These ATM cluster in crown-like structures around necrotic adipocytes [59], consistent with one of the classic roles of macrophages in phagocytosing dead cells. Areas of macrophage infiltration are also hypoxic [60]. One hypothesis consistent with these observations is that enlargement of adipocytes increases the distance between adipocytes and capillaries, leading to adipose tissue hypoxia and consequent adipocyte death [60–62].

The ATM of lean individuals are of the alternatively activated M2 phenotype [56, 57], which are largely anti-inflammatory. However, in obesity, adipose M2 gene expression declines, and proinflammatory macrophages are recruited from precursors in the blood [57, 59, 63]. Mgl1, MCP-1, and C3a have each been shown to be important in this recruitment [64]. The expression of a variety of other inflammatory genes, including many cytokines, chemokines, complement proteins, and acute phase proteins, is also increased in the adipose tissue of obese versus lean individuals [58, 65]. The term "adipokine" was coined to describe substances derived from adipose tissue. ATM are the source of much of this inflammatory gene expression, perhaps as a result of TLR4 stimulation via fatty acids [63].

In addition to macrophages, there are also changes in the numbers and types of adipose tissue lymphocytes with obesity. CD8+ T cells increase, particularly in the inflammatory infiltrates that form around necrotic adipocytes [60]. Interestingly, during the development of obesity, the recruitment of CD8+ cells to adipose tissue actually precedes macrophage recruitment [66]. Importantly, genetic depletion and adoptive transfer experiments in mice indicate that these cells are required for subsequent macrophage recruitment to adipose tissue [67]. CD4+ cells also increase in adipose tissue of mice with dietary obesity [68]. These cells appear to be of the Th1 lineage, whereas Th2 cells and Foxp3-expressing regulatory T cells (Tregs) decline with obesity, contributing to the loss of M2 macrophage phenotype [68, 69]. NKT cells that recognize lipid antigens are also present in obese adipose tissue [70] but do not appear to change in numbers in obesity [71]. Nevertheless, NKT cells are important for the obese phenotype. Obese mice lacking NKT cells have reduced ATMs, whereas administration of α-galactosylceramide, an activator of NKT cells, increases ATMs and adipose expression of inflammatory genes, indicating that NKT cells also play a role in adipose tissue inflammation. IL-17 is also expressed in T cells infiltrating adipose tissue, but the great majority of these IL-17-expressing T cells are $\gamma\delta$ TCR positive cells that are both CD4 and CD8 negative, rather than Th17 cells [72].

There are also changes in adipose tissue mast cells and eosinophils in obesity [73, 74]. The mast cells accumulate around microvessels in obese adipose tissue and appear to play a role in the angiogenesis required for sustaining expansion of adipose tissue [73]. In contrast, eosinophils are typically present in normal lean adipose tissue where they constitute a major source of the IL-4 required for biasing ATM toward a Th2 phenotype [74], though adipocytes themselves are important sources of IL-13 that can also serve this function [75]. Adipose tissue eosinophils decline in mice with diet-induced obesity [74]. Understanding what factors contribute to this reduction in eosinophils may be important for the obese lung, since airway eosinophils are also reduced in obese versus lean asthmatics (see below).

Systemic Inflammation: Many of the inflammatory moieties expressed in obese adipose tissue are produced in sufficient quantities that they leak into the systemic circulation. Levels of IL-8, MCP-1, TNFα, and IL-6 are elevated in the serum of obese versus lean humans or mice and decline with weight loss [76–79]. The number of circulating leukocytes is also higher in blood from obese versus lean individuals [80], and the neutrophils are in an activated state [81]. In addition, serum concentrations of many adipose-derived, energy-regulating hormones are also affected by obesity in such a manner as to promote inflammation. For example, concentrations of leptin, which has proinflammatory activities, increase in obesity, whereas concentrations of adiponectin, which is largely anti-inflammatory, decline. Finally, in both obese rodents and obese humans, there is systemic oxidative stress, as indicated by increases in reactive oxygen species (ROS) and declines in antioxidants [82–87].

The systemic inflammation and oxidative stress that accompany obesity affect many organs and tissues. For example, circulating leukocytes become activated [88]. Endothelial cell expression of endothelin is increased, while nitric oxide production is reduced, events that promote increased vascular reactivity [89]. There is also substantial evidence that the systemic inflammation and increased oxidative stress of obesity contribute to many obesity-related conditions. In obese humans, elevations in serum leptin, TNFα, IL-6, and MCP-1 have each been shown to correlate with the

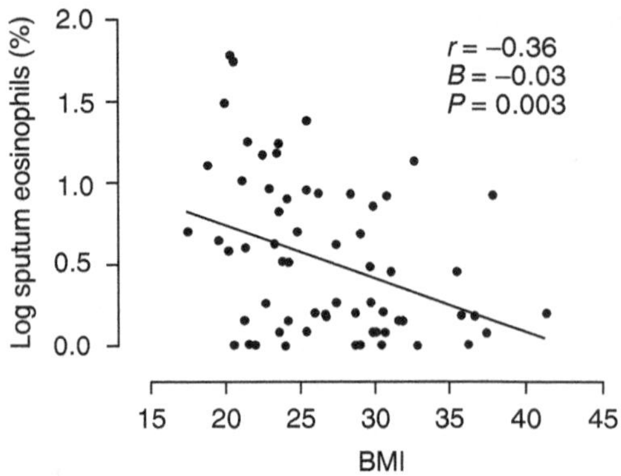

Fig. 2.4 Sputum eosinophils as a function of body mass index (BMI) in asthmatics. *r* correlation coefficient; *B* slope of regression line (From van Veen et al. [100])

presence of obesity-related diseases such as type 2 diabetes and atherosclerosis (see [90, 91] for reviews), while there is an inverse correlation with serum adiponectin. Markers of systemic oxidative stress also predict diabetes and cardiovascular disease [84]. In animal models, aspects of the systemic inflammation and oxidative stress of obesity are required for several obesity-related conditions. For example, the reduction in insulin resistance observed in obese mice with myeloid specific knockout of IkappaB kinase beta, a central regulator of inflammatory responses, establishes the functional importance of inflammation derived from ATM in obesity [92]. In obese rats and mice, attenuating TNF signaling either by genetic manipulation or by antibody administration attenuates insulin resistance and hepatic steatosis [93–95]. Diabetic renal injury is reduced in obese mice deficient in MCP-1 [96]. Similarly, mice with dietary obesity treated with an inhibitor of CCR2, the receptor that binds MCP-1, have improved glucose tolerance and insulin sensitivity and reduced hepatic triglycerides [97]. In obese mice, treatment with an NADPH oxidase inhibitor reduces ROS production, attenuates hyperlipidemia and hepatic steatosis, and improves insulin sensitivity [85]. Administration of cobalt protoporphyrin, which induces the antioxidant, heme oxygenase 1, attenuates hypertension and glucose intolerance in obese mice [98].

Pulmonary Inflammation: While airway inflammation, particularly eosinophilic inflammation, is a common feature of allergic asthma, it is increasingly apparent that the asthma associated with obesity is noneosinophilic in nature [99]. Indeed, in asthmatics, the percentage of sputum eosinophils is inversely related to BMI [100] (Fig. 2.4), which may explain why exhaled nitric oxide, a common marker of airway eosinophilia, is also lower in obese versus lean asthmatics [100–102]. In contrast, Scott et al. reported that the percentage of neutrophils in sputum increases with increasing BMI in asthmatics, especially in women [103]. Other investigators have reported similar trends that did not reach statistical significance [104–106].

Consistent with the declines in sputum eosinophils observed in obese asthmatics, examination of BAL fluid of mice that have been sensitized and challenged with allergen also indicates a decline in airway eosinophils in obese versus lean mice

[37, 107, 108]. Nevertheless, the obese mice exhibit greater allergen-induced AHR [37]. Histological sections of allergen-challenged genetically obese mice also indicate a decline in eosinophils around airways [37], whereas airway eosinophils are augmented in mice that have been rendered obese by high-fat feeding, despite reductions in BAL eosinophils [108]. There are also greater increases in airway smooth muscle mass and in airway fibrosis in mice with dietary obesity [36]. The results suggest that airway biopsies may ultimately provide more definitive information about airway inflammation in obese asthmatics than sputum and BAL, which sample only those cells that have migrated to the airspaces.

In the absence of allergen challenge, there is no overt cellular inflammation either around the airways in other parts of the lung of obese mice [31, 32]. However, even these unchallenged obese mice are hyperresponsive compared to their lean controls (Fig. 2.1). The results suggest that cellular inflammation is not required for the AHR of obesity, though we cannot rule out the possibility that the obesity causes changes in the activation status of resident immune cells such as macrophages, $\gamma\delta$ T cells, and iNKT cells.

There are also obesity-related changes in lung lymphocytes in obese asthmatics. Dixon et al. reported an increase in BAL lymphocytes in obese asthmatics 12 months after bariatric surgery induced weight loss [27]. Reductions in BAL lymphocytes have also been observed in obese versus lean allergen-challenged mice [37, 107]. Dixon et al. also observed a profound increase in cytokine production from peripheral blood CD4+ lymphocytes after weight loss in obese asthmatics, suggesting that obesity attenuates rather than augments CD4+ lymphocyte activation. A similar reduced cytokine release upon activation has been observed in cells of lymph nodes draining the lungs of obese versus lean mice [107]. In the mice, the reduction in lymphocyte activation was not the result of changes in Tregs, which were similar in number in the lymph nodes of the obese and lean mice. Taken together, the data suggest suppressed adaptive immunity in the obese asthmatic lung.

Other aspects of airway inflammation have also been assessed in the obese. For example, 8-isoprostane in the exhaled breath condensate increases with BMI in asthmatics but not in nonasthmatics [102]. We have also noted increased 8-isoprostane in BAL fluid of obese versus nonobese mice (unpublished observations). 8-Isoprostane is a non-cyclooxygenase-dependent product of arachidonic acid and is a marker of oxidative stress. Urinary LTE_4 also correlates with BMI in asthmatics [109]. It is possible that obesity-related elevations in leukotrienes are the result of increases in the proinflammatory adipokine, leptin, which has been shown to augment leukotriene production in alveolar macrophages [110]. Concentrations of leptin are higher in BAL fluid and sputum of obese versus nonobese individuals [111, 112], consistent with elevations in serum leptin. Indeed, BAL leptin correlates with serum leptin in both asthmatics and nonasthmatics [111]. It is likely that the elevated lung concentrations in obesity are consequent to passive diffusion into the lung of higher blood leptin in the obese. Both BAL and serum concentrations of the anti-inflammatory adipokine, adiponectin, increase with weight loss [27]. BAL and serum concentrations of adiponectin are also correlated in asthmatics but not in nonasthmatics [111]. In contrast, in nonasthmatics, there is no significant correlation between BAL and serum adiponectin. Adiponectins, especially the high molecular weight isoforms of adiponectin, which are the dominant forms in serum, are extremely large molecules and likely require a transport molecule for transit from the blood into the lung. The adiponectin-binding protein, T-cadherin, may serve this function [113]. Thus, increases in serum adiponectin may not necessarily lead to increases in adiponectin in lung fluids unless there is a marked increase in the permeability of the alveolar/capillary barrier, an event which may occur secondary to airway inflammation in asthma.

Inflammation and AHR: While the systemic inflammation of obesity may not necessarily translate into airway inflammation, especially cellular inflammation, it may, nevertheless, have the capacity to augment airway responsiveness. For example, many of the inflammatory moieties that are elevated in serum of obese individuals, including IL-6, TNFα, PAI-1, eotaxin, VEGF, and MCP-1, have been associated with altered airway responsiveness in various models (see recent reviews [3, 38, 114, 115]). Obesity-related increases in leptin and declines in adiponectin also have the capacity to contribute, since exogenous administration of leptin augments [116], while adiponectin inhibits [117] allergen-induced AHR in mice.

An additional aspect of the systemic inflammation of obesity is an increase in the serum concentration of endothelin [118, 119]. Endothelin contributes to the hypertension of obesity [89, 120, 121] and may also play a role in obesity-related AHR. Endothelin is among the most potent known constrictors of airway smooth muscle [122, 123] and also causes AHR when administered intranasally in mice [124]. Endothelin is also required for allergen-induced AHR in some animal models [125].

Recent evidence also points to IL-17 as a component of the systemic inflammation of obesity. IL-17A is increased in the serum of obese versus lean individuals [126]. Similar elevations in serum IL-17A are observed in severe versus moderate or mild asthmatics [127]. IL-17A and Th17 cells are increased in spleens of mice with diet-induced obesity versus lean controls, whereas other CD4+ lymphocyte populations are not affected [128, 129]. Consistent with these observations, in obesity, susceptibility is increased for several autoimmune diseases in which Th17 is known to play a significant role. Th17 cells are not the only source of IL-17, and there is also increased IL-17A expression in neutrophils in the peritoneal cavity of obese versus lean mice undergoing zymosan-induced peritonitis [130]. As noted above, increases in serum IL-6 are common in obesity. IL-6 is important for induction of Th17 cells, and obesity-related increases in Th17 cells are not observed in IL-6-deficient mice [128]. However, neutrophil expression of IL-17 in experimental peritonitis is not affected by IL-6 neutralization.

It is conceivable that elevations in IL-17 could play a role in obesity-related AHR. The role of IL-17 in allergic models of asthma is somewhat controversial [131], but IL-17 is expressed in the lungs following ozone exposure and contributes to ozone-induced neutrophil recruitment and AHR in mice [132]. Obesity-related elevations in IL-17 might therefore contribute to the augmented ozone-induced AHR that is observed in obese mice [29, 31, 32, 35].

Diet

It is conceivable that the apparent alterations in airway responsiveness associated with obesity are actually secondary to dietary factors. Indeed, the observed heterogeneity in the effects of obesity on AHR (Table 2.1) may reflect regional differences in dietary constituents. Obese individuals tend to consume not just more calories but also a less healthy diet [133]. There is evidence that dietary antioxidants and omega-3 fatty acids, which are plentiful in fruits, vegetables, nuts, and marine fish, can positively impact lung function [134]. In contrast, high dietary fat intake is associated with AHR [135]. In a variety of cell types, certain fatty acids cause TLR4 activation, leading to increased NF-κB activation and proinflammatory cytokine release [136]. Indeed, in obese individuals, plasma levels of IL-6 rise after a high-fat meal [137]. In contrast, consumption of orange juice or a supplement containing resveratrol and muscadine, components of red grapes, reduces TLR4 activation and oxidative stress within circulating mononuclear cells [138, 139]. Indeed, even a single high-fat meal can have an impact on the lung [140]. Compared to consumption of a low-fat meal, consumption of a high-fat meal increased the percentage of neutrophils in sputum in asthmatics and attenuated bronchodilator responsiveness.

Interestingly, Ghanim et al. [141] reported that consumption of a high-fat, high-carbohydrate meal increased plasma endotoxin concentrations, whereas consumption of a meal rich in fruits and fiber did not [141], even though both meals contained the same amount of endotoxin. Plasma endotoxin also increased in obese mice fed a high-fat diet [142]. The rise in plasma endotoxin was secondary to an increase in intestinal permeability and increased absorption into the blood of endotoxin derived from intestinal bacteria. Importantly, plasma endotoxin correlated with indices of adipose tissue inflammation and macrophage infiltration in these mice, whereas treatment with antibiotics suppressed this adipose tissue inflammation along with metabolic complications including insulin resistance. High-fat feeding also reduced the number of intestinal bifidobacteria, a population whose presence improves mucosal barrier function [143]. Genetically obese *ob/ob* mice also exhibit endotoxemia [142], alterations in gut microbiota [144], and improved adipose tissue inflammation upon treatment with antibiotics [142]. In fact, alterations in the gut microbiome in obesity result in bacterial species with an increased capacity to harvest energy from the diet, thus perpetuating the obese state [144]. The lungs are not sterile, and there are differences in the populations of bacteria in lungs of asthmatics versus controls [145]. It is conceivable that obesity may also lead to alterations in lung bacterial populations that promote AHR.

Colonic bacteria also ferment dietary fiber leading to the generation of short-chain fatty acids (SCFA) with anti-inflammatory activities. Many of these SCFA signal via the G-protein-coupled receptor Gpr43, and gpr43-deficient mice have augmented allergic airways responses [146]. Thus, diets low in fiber may promote asthma via loss of the anti-inflammatory effects of SCFA generation in the colon. Interestingly, *Bacteroidetes* bacteria, which are major producers of SCFA, are reduced both in the GI tract in obesity [144] and in the lungs of subjects with asthma [145].

Conclusions

A growing body of evidence indicates that obesity does promote AHR, especially when sensitive measures of airway function are employed in assessing responsiveness. Obesity results in reductions in the FRC, which may contribute to AHR in males. However, in females, who make up the majority of obese asthmatics, other factors appear to dominate. Even in lean subjects, adipose tissue is infiltrated with numerous immune and inflammatory cells. With obesity, the relative numbers and activation state of these cells change, leading to increased circulating levels of several inflammatory moieties. Many of these moieties have the capacity to promote AHR. Diet is often different in obese versus lean individuals, and some dietary components, including dietary fat and fiber, have been shown to influence lung function and airway responsiveness. Moreover, there are changes in the gut microbiome with obesity that may interact with the diet to exacerbate systemic inflammation. Understanding how obesity promotes AHR may lead to better treatment modalities for asthma in this difficult-to-treat population.

Acknowledgments This work was supported by National Institute of Environmental Health Sciences Grants ES-013307 and ES-000002, and National Heart, Lung, and Blood Institute Grant HL-084044.

References

1. Beuther DA, Sutherland ER. Overweight, obesity, and incident asthma: a meta-analysis of prospective epidemiologic studies. Am J Respir Crit Care Med. 2007;175(7):661–6.
2. Ford ES. The epidemiology of obesity and asthma. J Allergy Clin Immunol. 2005;115(5): 897–909.
3. Shore SA, Johnston RA. Obesity and asthma. Pharmacol Ther. 2006;110(1):83–102.
4. Litonjua AA, Gold DR. Asthma and obesity: common early-life influences in the inception of disease. J Allergy Clin Immunol. 2008;121(5):1075–84.
5. Mosen DM, Schatz M, Magid DJ, Camargo Jr CA. The relationship between obesity and asthma severity and control in adults. J Allergy Clin Immunol. 2008;122(3):507–11.
6. Peters-Golden M, Swern A, Bird SS, Hustad CM, Grant E, Edelman JM. Influence of body mass index on the response to asthma controller agents. Eur Respir J. 2006;27(3):495–503.
7. Saint-Pierre P, Bourdin A, Chanez P, Daures JP, Godard P. Are overweight asthmatics more difficult to control? Allergy. 2006;61(1):79–84.
8. Shore SA. Obesity, airway hyperresponsiveness, and inflammation. J Appl Physiol. 2010; 108(3):735–43.
9. Litonjua AA, Sparrow D, Celedon JC, DeMolles D, Weiss ST. Association of body mass index with the development of methacholine airway hyperresponsiveness in men: the Normative Aging Study. Thorax. 2002;57(7):581–5.
10. Chinn S, Jarvis D, Burney P. Relation of bronchial responsiveness to body mass index in the ECRHS. European Community Respiratory Health Survey. Thorax. 2002;57(12):1028–33.
11. Celedon JC, Palmer LJ, Litonjua AA, Weiss ST, Wang B, Fang Z, et al. Body mass index and asthma in adults in families of subjects with asthma in Anqing, China. Am J Respir Crit Care Med. 2001;164(10 Pt 1):1835–40.

12. Sood A, Verhulst SJ, Varma A, Eagleton LE, Henkle JQ, Hopkins-Price P. Association of excess weight and degree of airway responsiveness in asthmatics and non-asthmatics. J Asthma. 2006;43(6):447–52.
13. Schachter LM, Salome CM, Peat JK, Woolcock AJ. Obesity is a risk for asthma and wheeze but not airway hyperresponsiveness. Thorax. 2001;56(1):4–8.
14. Bustos P, Amigo H, Oyarzun M, Rona RJ. Is there a causal relation between obesity and asthma? Evidence from Chile. Int J Obes Relat Metab Disord. 2005;29(7):804–9.
15. Nicolacakis K, Skowronski ME, Coreno AJ, West E, Nader NZ, Smith RL, et al. Observations on the physiological interactions between obesity and asthma. J Appl Physiol. 2008;105(5): 1533–41.
16. Sharma S, Tailor A, Warrington R, Cheang M. Is obesity associated with an increased risk for airway hyperresponsiveness and development of asthma? Allergy Asthma Clin Immunol. 2008;4(2):51–8.
17. Torchio R, Gobbi A, Gulotta C, Dellaca R, Tinivella M, Hyatt RE, et al. Mechanical effects of obesity on airway responsiveness in otherwise healthy humans. J Appl Physiol. 2009;107(2):408–16.
18. Skloot G, Schechter C, Desai A, Togias A. Impaired response to deep inspiration in obesity. J Appl Physiol. 2011;111(3):726–34.
19. Salome CM, Munoz PA, Berend N, Thorpe CW, Schachter LM, King GG. Effect of obesity on breathlessness and airway responsiveness to methacholine in non-asthmatic subjects. Int J Obes (Lond). 2008;32(3):502–9.
20. Chapman DG, Berend N, King GG, Salome CM. Increased airway closure is a determinant of airway hyperresponsiveness. Eur Respir J. 2008;32(6):1563–9.
21. Sutherland TJ, Cowan JO, Taylor DR. Dynamic hyperinflation with bronchoconstriction: differences between obese and nonobese women with asthma. Am J Respir Crit Care Med. 2008;177(9):970–5.
22. Hakala K, Mustajoki P, Aittomaki J, Sovijarvi AR. Effect of weight loss and body position on pulmonary function and gas exchange abnormalities in morbid obesity. Int J Obes Relat Metab Disord. 1995;19(5):343–6.
23. Hedenstierna G, Santesson J, Norlander O. Airway closure and distribution of inspired gas in the extremely obese, breathing spontaneously and during anaesthesia with intermittent positive pressure ventilation. Acta Anaesthesiol Scand. 1976;20(4):334–42.
24. Behazin N, Jones SB, Cohen RI, Loring SH. Respiratory restriction and elevated pleural and esophageal pressures in morbid obesity. J Appl Physiol. 2010;108(1):212–8.
25. Benedik PS, Baun MM, Keus L, Jimenez C, Morice R, Bidani A, et al. Effects of body position on resting lung volume in overweight and mildly to moderately obese subjects. Respir Care. 2009;54(3):334–9.
26. Winkler T, Venegas JG. Complex airway behavior and paradoxical responses to bronchoprovocation. J Appl Physiol. 2007;103(2):655–63.
27. Dixon AE, Pratley RE, Forgione PM, Kaminsky DA, Whittaker-Leclair LA, Griffes LA, et al. Effects of obesity and bariatric surgery on airway hyperresponsiveness, asthma control and inflammation. J Allergy Clin Immunol. 2011;128(3):508–15.
28. Aaron SD, Fergusson D, Dent R, Chen Y, Vandemheen KL, Dales RE. Effect of weight reduction on respiratory function and airway reactivity in obese women. Chest. 2004;125(6): 2046–52.
29. Shore SA, Rivera-Sanchez YM, Schwartzman IN, Johnston RA. Responses to ozone are increased in obese mice. J Appl Physiol. 2003;95(3):938–45.
30. Rivera-Sanchez YM, Johnston RA, Schwartzman IN, Valone J, Silverman ES, Fredberg JJ, et al. Differential effects of ozone on airway and tissue mechanics in obese mice. J Appl Physiol. 2004;96(6):2200–6.
31. Lu FL, Johnston RA, Flynt L, Theman TA, Terry RD, Schwartzman IN, et al. Increased pulmonary responses to acute ozone exposure in obese db/db mice. Am J Physiol Lung Cell Mol Physiol. 2006;290(5):L856–65.

32. Johnston RA, Theman TA, Shore SA. Augmented responses to ozone in obese carboxypeptidase E-deficient mice. Am J Physiol Regul Integr Comp Physiol. 2006;290:R126–33.
33. Johnston RA, Theman TA, Lu FL, Terry RD, Williams ES, Shore SA. Diet-induced obesity causes innate airway hyperresponsiveness to methacholine and enhances ozone-induced pulmonary inflammation. J Appl Physiol. 2008;104(6):1727–35.
34. Shore SA, Williams ES, Zhu M. No effect of metformin on the innate airway hyperresponsiveness and increased responses to ozone observed in obese mice. J Appl Physiol. 2008;105(4):1127–33.
35. Johnston RA, Zhu M, Hernandez CB, Williams ES, Shore SA. Onset of obesity in carboxypeptidase E-deficient mice and effect on airway responsiveness and pulmonary responses to ozone. J Appl Physiol. 2010;108(6):1812–9.
36. Saraiva SA, Silva AL, Xisto DG, Abreu SC, Silva JD, Silva PL, et al. Impact of obesity on airway and lung parenchyma remodeling in experimental chronic allergic asthma. Respir Physiol Neurobiol. 2011;177(2):141–8.
37. Johnston RA, Zhu M, Rivera-Sanchez YM, Lu FL, Theman TA, Flynt L, et al. Allergic airway responses in obese mice. Am J Respir Crit Care Med. 2007;176(7):650–8.
38. Shore SA. Obesity and asthma: lessons from animal models. J Appl Physiol. 2007;102(2):516–28.
39. Jones RL, Nzekwu MM. The effects of body mass index on lung volumes. Chest. 2006;130(3):827–33.
40. Ding DJ, Martin JG, Macklem PT. Effects of lung volume on maximal methacholine-induced bronchoconstriction in normal humans. J Appl Physiol. 1987;62(3):1324–30.
41. Meinero M, Coletta G, Dutto L, Milanese M, Nova G, Sciolla A, et al. Mechanical response to methacholine and deep inspiration in supine men. J Appl Physiol. 2007;102(1):269–75.
42. Torchio R, Gulotta C, Ciacco C, Perboni A, Guglielmo M, Crosa F, et al. Effects of chest wall strapping on mechanical response to methacholine in humans. J Appl Physiol. 2006;101(2):430–8.
43. McClean MA, Matheson MJ, McKay K, Johnson PR, Rynell AC, Ammit AJ, et al. Low lung volume alters contractile properties of airway smooth muscle in sheep. Eur Respir J. 2003;22(1):50–6.
44. Rorvik S, Bo G. Lung volumes and arterial blood gases in obesity. Scand J Respir Dis Suppl. 1976;95:60–4.
45. Milic-Emili J, Torchio R, D'Angelo E. Closing volume: a reappraisal (1967–2007). Eur J Appl Physiol. 2007;99(6):567–83.
46. Gump A, Haughney L, Fredberg J. Relaxation of activated airway smooth muscle: relative potency of isoproterenol vs. tidal stretch. J Appl Physiol. 2001;90(6):2306–10.
47. Sampson MG, Grassino AE. Load compensation in obese patients during quiet tidal breathing. J Appl Physiol. 1983;55(4):1269–76.
48. Holguin F, Cribbs S, Fitzpatrick AM, Ingram Jr RH, Jackson AC. A deep breath bronchoconstricts obese asthmatics. J Asthma. 2010;47(1):55–60.
49. Boulet LP, Turcotte H, Boulet G, Simard B, Robichaud P. Deep inspiration avoidance and airway response to methacholine: influence of body mass index. Can Respir J. 2005;12(7):371–6.
50. Skloot G, Togias A. Bronchodilation and bronchoprotection by deep inspiration and their relationship to bronchial hyperresponsiveness. Clin Rev Allergy Immunol. 2003;24(1):55–72.
51. Ofir D, Laveneziana P, Webb KA, O'Donnell DE. Ventilatory and perceptual responses to cycle exercise in obese women. J Appl Physiol. 2007;102(6):2217–26.
52. Romagnoli I, Laveneziana P, Clini EM, Palange P, Valli G, de Blasio F, et al. Role of hyperinflation vs. deflation on dyspnoea in severely to extremely obese subjects. Acta Physiol (Oxf). 2008;193(4):393–402.
53. Ferretti A, Giampiccolo P, Cavalli A, Milic-Emili J, Tantucci C. Expiratory flow limitation and orthopnea in massively obese subjects. Chest. 2001;119(5):1401–8.
54. Martin J, Powell E, Shore S, Emrich J, Engel LA. The role of respiratory muscles in the hyperinflation of bronchial asthma. Am Rev Respir Dis. 1980;121(3):441–7.

55. Farah CS, Kermode JA, Downie SR, Brown NJ, Hardaker KM, Berend N, et al. Obesity is a determinant of asthma control, independent of inflammation and lung mechanics. Chest. 2011;140(3):659–66.
56. Zeyda M, Farmer D, Todoric J, Aszmann O, Speiser M, Gyori G, et al. Human adipose tissue macrophages are of an anti-inflammatory phenotype but capable of excessive pro-inflammatory mediator production. Int J Obes (Lond). 2007;31(9):1420–8.
57. Lumeng CN, Bodzin JL, Saltiel AR. Obesity induces a phenotypic switch in adipose tissue macrophage polarization. J Clin Invest. 2007;117(1):175–84.
58. Weisberg SP, McCann D, Desai M, Rosenbaum M, Leibel RL, Ferrante Jr AW. Obesity is associated with macrophage accumulation in adipose tissue. J Clin Invest. 2003;112(12):1796–808.
59. Strissel KJ, Stancheva Z, Miyoshi H, Perfield 2nd JW, DeFuria J, Jick Z, et al. Adipocyte death, adipose tissue remodeling, and obesity complications. Diabetes. 2007;56(12):2910–8.
60. Rausch ME, Weisberg S, Vardhana P, Tortoriello DV. Obesity in C57BL/6 J mice is characterized by adipose tissue hypoxia and cytotoxic T-cell infiltration. Int J Obes (Lond). 2008;32(3):451–63.
61. Ye J, Gao Z, Yin J, He Q. Hypoxia is a potential risk factor for chronic inflammation and adiponectin reduction in adipose tissue of ob/ob and dietary obese mice. Am J Physiol Endocrinol Metab. 2007;293(4):E1118–28.
62. Hosogai N, Fukuhara A, Oshima K, Miyata Y, Tanaka S, Segawa K, et al. Adipose tissue hypoxia in obesity and its impact on adipocytokine dysregulation. Diabetes. 2007;56(4): 901–11.
63. Nguyen MT, Favelyukis S, Nguyen AK, Reichart D, Scott PA, Jenn A, et al. A subpopulation of macrophages infiltrates hypertrophic adipose tissue and is activated by free fatty acids via Toll-like receptors 2 and 4 and JNK-dependent pathways. J Biol Chem. 2007;282(48): 35279–92.
64. Anderson EK, Gutierrez DA, Hasty AH. Adipose tissue recruitment of leukocytes. Curr Opin Lipidol. 2010;21(3):172–7.
65. Xu H, Barnes GT, Yang Q, Tan G, Yang D, Chou CJ, et al. Chronic inflammation in fat plays a crucial role in the development of obesity-related insulin resistance. J Clin Invest. 2003;112(12):1821–30.
66. Kintscher U, Hartge M, Hess K, Foryst-Ludwig A, Clemenz M, Wabitsch M, et al. T-lymphocyte infiltration in visceral adipose tissue: a primary event in adipose tissue inflammation and the development of obesity-mediated insulin resistance. Arterioscler Thromb Vasc Biol. 2008;28(7):1304–10.
67. Nishimura S, Manabe I, Nagasaki M, Eto K, Yamashita H, Ohsugi M, et al. CD8+ effector T cells contribute to macrophage recruitment and adipose tissue inflammation in obesity. Nat Med. 2009;15(8):914–20.
68. Winer S, Chan Y, Paltser G, Truong D, Tsui H, Bahrami J, et al. Normalization of obesity-associated insulin resistance through immunotherapy. Nat Med. 2009;15(8):921–9.
69. Feuerer M, Herrero L, Cipolletta D, Naaz A, Wong J, Nayer A, et al. Lean, but not obese, fat is enriched for a unique population of regulatory T cells that affect metabolic parameters. Nat Med. 2009;15(8):930–9.
70. Ohmura K, Ishimori N, Ohmura Y, Tokuhara S, Nozawa A, Horii S, et al. Natural killer T cells are involved in adipose tissues inflammation and glucose intolerance in diet-induced obese mice. Arterioscler Thromb Vasc Biol. 2010;30(2):193–9.
71. Caspar-Bauguil S, Cousin B, Andre M, Nibbelink M, Galinier A, Periquet B, et al. Weight-dependent changes of immune system in adipose tissue: importance of leptin. Exp Cell Res. 2006;312(12):2195–202.
72. Zuniga LA, Shen WJ, Joyce-Shaikh B, Pyatnova EA, Richards AG, Thom C, et al. IL-17 regulates adipogenesis, glucose homeostasis, and obesity. J Immunol. 2010;185(11):6947–59.
73. Liu J, Divoux A, Sun J, Zhang J, Clement K, Glickman JN, et al. Genetic deficiency and pharmacological stabilization of mast cells reduce diet-induced obesity and diabetes in mice. Nat Med. 2009;15(8):940–5.

74. Wu D, Molofsky AB, Liang HE, Ricardo-Gonzalez RR, Jouihan HA, Bando JK, et al. Eosinophils sustain adipose alternatively activated macrophages associated with glucose homeostasis. Science. 2011;332(6026):243–7.
75. Kang K, Reilly SM, Karabacak V, Gangl MR, Fitzgerald K, Hatano B, et al. Adipocyte-derived Th2 cytokines and myeloid PPARdelta regulate macrophage polarization and insulin sensitivity. Cell Metab. 2008;7(6):485–95.
76. Bastard JP, Jardel C, Bruckert E, Blondy P, Capeau J, Laville M, et al. Elevated levels of interleukin 6 are reduced in serum and subcutaneous adipose tissue of obese women after weight loss. J Clin Endocrinol Metab. 2000;85(9):3338–42.
77. Bastard JP, Jardel C, Bruckert E, Vidal H, Hainque B. Variations in plasma soluble tumour necrosis factor receptors after diet-induced weight loss in obesity. Diabetes Obes Metab. 2000;2(5):323–5.
78. Katsuki A, Sumida Y, Murashima S, Murata K, Takarada Y, Ito K, et al. Serum levels of tumor necrosis factor-alpha are increased in obese patients with noninsulin-dependent diabetes mellitus. J Clin Endocrinol Metab. 1998;83(3):859–62.
79. Roth CL, Kratz M, Ralston MM, Reinehr T. Changes in adipose-derived inflammatory cytokines and chemokines after successful lifestyle intervention in obese children. Metabolism. 2011;60(4):445–52.
80. Zaldivar F, McMurray RG, Nemet D, Galassetti P, Mills PJ, Cooper DM. Body fat and circulating leukocytes in children. Int J Obes (Lond). 2006;30(6):906–11.
81. Nijhuis J, Rensen SS, Slaats Y, van Dielen FM, Buurman WA, Greve JW. Neutrophil activation in morbid obesity, chronic activation of acute inflammation. Obesity (Silver Spring). 2009;17(11):2014–8.
82. Atabek ME, Vatansev H, Erkul I. Oxidative stress in childhood obesity. J Pediatr Endocrinol Metab. 2004;17(8):1063–8.
83. Bakker SJ, IJzerman RG, Teerlink T, Westerhoff HV, Gans RO, Heine RJ. Cytosolic triglycerides and oxidative stress in central obesity: the missing link between excessive atherosclerosis, endothelial dysfunction, and beta-cell failure? Atherosclerosis. 2000;148(1):17–21.
84. Keaney Jr JF, Larson MG, Vasan RS, Wilson PW, Lipinska I, Corey D, et al. Obesity and systemic oxidative stress: clinical correlates of oxidative stress in the Framingham Study. Arterioscler Thromb Vasc Biol. 2003;23(3):434–9.
85. Furukawa S, Fujita T, Shimabukuro M, Iwaki M, Yamada Y, Nakajima Y, et al. Increased oxidative stress in obesity and its impact on metabolic syndrome. J Clin Invest. 2004;114(12): 1752–61.
86. Lee YS, Kim AY, Choi JW, Kim M, Yasue S, Son HJ, et al. Dysregulation of adipose glutathione peroxidase 3 in obesity contributes to local and systemic oxidative stress. Mol Endocrinol. 2008;22(9):2176–89.
87. Johnson JB, Summer W, Cutler RG, Martin B, Hyun DH, Dixit VD, et al. Alternate day calorie restriction improves clinical findings and reduces markers of oxidative stress and inflammation in overweight adults with moderate asthma. Free Radic Biol Med. 2007;42(5): 665–74.
88. de Mello VD, Kolehmainen M, Schwab U, Mager U, Laaksonen DE, Pulkkinen L, et al. Effect of weight loss on cytokine messenger RNA expression in peripheral blood mononuclear cells of obese subjects with the metabolic syndrome. Metabolism. 2008;57(2):192–9.
89. Traupe T, D'Uscio LV, Muenter K, Morawietz H, Vetter W, Barton M. Effects of obesity on endothelium-dependent reactivity during acute nitric oxide synthase inhibition: modulatory role of endothelin. Clin Sci (Lond). 2002;103(Suppl 48):13S–5.
90. Fantuzzi G. Adipose tissue, adipokines, and inflammation. J Allergy Clin Immunol. 2005;115(5):911–9.
91. Scherer PE. Adipose tissue: from lipid storage compartment to endocrine organ. Diabetes. 2006;55(6):1537–45.
92. Arkan MC, Hevener AL, Greten FR, Maeda S, Li ZW, Long JM, et al. IKK-beta links inflammation to obesity-induced insulin resistance. Nat Med. 2005;11(2):191–8.

93. Uysal KT, Wiesbrock SM, Marino MW, Hotamisligil GS. Protection from obesity-induced insulin resistance in mice lacking TNF-alpha function. Nature. 1997;389(6651):610–4.
94. Hotamisligil GS, Shargill NS, Spiegelman BM. Adipose expression of tumor necrosis factor-alpha: direct role in obesity-linked insulin resistance. Science. 1993;259(5091):87–91.
95. Park EJ, Lee JH, Yu GY, He G, Ali SR, Holzer RG, et al. Dietary and genetic obesity promote liver inflammation and tumorigenesis by enhancing IL-6 and TNF expression. Cell. 2010;140(2):197–208.
96. Chow FY, Nikolic-Paterson DJ, Ma FY, Ozols E, Rollins BJ, Tesch GH. Monocyte chemoattractant protein-1-induced tissue inflammation is critical for the development of renal injury but not type 2 diabetes in obese db/db mice. Diabetologia. 2007;50(2):471–80.
97. Tamura Y, Sugimoto M, Murayama T, Minami M, Nishikaze Y, Ariyasu H, et al. C-C chemokine receptor 2 inhibitor improves diet-induced development of insulin resistance and hepatic steatosis in mice. J Atheroscler Thromb. 2010;17(3):219–28.
98. Burgess A, Li M, Vanella L, Kim DH, Rezzani R, Rodella L, et al. Adipocyte heme oxygenase-1 induction attenuates metabolic syndrome in both male and female obese mice. Hypertension. 2010;56(6):1124–30.
99. Haldar P, Pavord ID, Shaw DE, Berry MA, Thomas M, Brightling CE, et al. Cluster analysis and clinical asthma phenotypes. Am J Respir Crit Care Med. 2008;178(3):218–24.
100. van Veen IH, Ten Brinke A, Sterk PJ, Rabe KF, Bel EH. Airway inflammation in obese and nonobese patients with difficult-to-treat asthma. Allergy. 2008;63(5):570–4.
101. Berg CM, Thelle DS, Rosengren A, Lissner L, Toren K, Olin AC. Decreased fraction of exhaled nitric oxide in obese subjects with asthma symptoms: data from the population study INTERGENE/ADONIX. Chest. 2011;139(5):1109–16.
102. Komakula S, Khatri S, Mermis J, Savill S, Haque S, Rojas M, et al. Body mass index is associated with reduced exhaled nitric oxide and higher exhaled 8-isoprostanes in asthmatics. Respir Res. 2007;8:32.
103. Scott HA, Gibson PG, Garg ML, Wood LG. Airway inflammation is augmented by obesity and fatty acids in asthma. Eur Respir J. 2011;38(3):594–602.
104. Lessard A, Turcotte H, Cormier Y, Boulet LP. Obesity and asthma: a specific phenotype? Chest. 2008;134(2):317–23.
105. Todd DC, Armstrong S, D'Silva L, Allen CJ, Hargreave FE, Parameswaran K. Effect of obesity on airway inflammation: a cross-sectional analysis of body mass index and sputum cell counts. Clin Exp Allergy. 2007;37(7):1049–54.
106. Sutherland TJ, Cowan JO, Young S, Goulding A, Grant AM, Williamson A, et al. The association between obesity and asthma: interactions between systemic and airway inflammation. Am J Respir Crit Care Med. 2008;178(5):469–75.
107. de Vries A, Hazlewood L, Fitch PM, Seckl JR, Foster P, Howie SE. High-fat feeding redirects cytokine responses and decreases allergic airway eosinophilia. Clin Exp Allergy. 2009;39(5):731–9.
108. Calixto MC, Lintomen L, Schenka A, Saad MJ, Zanesco A, Antunes E. Obesity enhances eosinophilic inflammation in a murine model of allergic asthma. Br J Pharmacol. 2010;159(3):617–25.
109. Giouleka P, Papatheodorou G, Lyberopoulos P, Karakatsani A, Alchanatis M, Roussos C, et al. Body mass index is associated with leukotriene inflammation in asthmatics. Eur J Clin Invest. 2011;41(1):30–8.
110. Mancuso P, Canetti C, Gottschalk A, Tithof PK, Peters-Golden M. Leptin augments alveolar macrophage leukotriene synthesis by increasing phospholipase activity and enhancing group IVC iPLA2 (cPLA2gamma) protein expression. Am J Physiol Lung Cell Mol Physiol. 2004;287(3):L497–502.
111. Holguin F, Rojas M, Brown LA, Fitzpatrick AM. Airway and plasma leptin and adiponectin in lean and obese asthmatics and controls. J Asthma. 2011;48(3):217–23.
112. Lessard A, St-Laurent J, Turcotte H, Boulet LP. Leptin and adiponectin in obese and non-obese subjects with asthma. Biomarkers. 2011;16(3):271–3.

113. Zhu M, Hug C, Kasahara DI, Johnston RA, Williams AS, Verbout NG, et al. Impact of adiponectin deficiency on pulmonary responses to acute ozone exposure in mice. Am J Respir Cell Mol Biol. 2010;43(4):487–97.
114. Shore SA. Obesity and asthma: implications for treatment. Curr Opin Pulm Med. 2007;13(1):56–62.
115. Shore SA. Obesity and asthma: possible mechanisms. J Allergy Clin Immunol. 2008; 121(5):1087–93.
116. Shore SA, Schwartzman IN, Mellema MS, Flynt L, Imrich A, Johnston RA. Effect of leptin on allergic airway responses in mice. J Allergy Clin Immunol. 2005;115(1):103–9.
117. Shore SA, Terry RD, Flynt L, Xu A, Hug C. Adiponectin attenuates allergen-induced airway inflammation and hyperresponsiveness in mice. J Allergy Clin Immunol. 2006;118(2): 389–95.
118. Ferri C, Bellini C, Desideri G, Baldoncini R, Properzi G, Santucci A, et al. Circulating endothelin-1 levels in obese patients with the metabolic syndrome. Exp Clin Endocrinol Diabetes. 1997;105(Suppl 2):38–40.
119. Maeda S, Jesmin S, Iemitsu M, Otsuki T, Matsuo T, Ohkawara K, et al. Weight loss reduces plasma endothelin-1 concentration in obese men. Exp Biol Med (Maywood). 2006;231(6): 1044–7.
120. Cardillo C, Campia U, Iantorno M, Panza JA. Enhanced vascular activity of endogenous endothelin-1 in obese hypertensive patients. Hypertension. 2004;43(1):36–40.
121. Mather KJ, Mirzamohammadi B, Lteif A, Steinberg HO, Baron AD. Endothelin contributes to basal vascular tone and endothelial dysfunction in human obesity and type 2 diabetes. Diabetes. 2002;51(12):3517–23.
122. Macquin-Mavier I, Levame M, Istin N, Harf A. Mechanisms of endothelin-mediated bronchoconstriction in the guinea pig. J Pharmacol Exp Ther. 1989;250(2):740–5.
123. Uchida Y, Ninomiya H, Saotome M, Nomura A, Ohtsuka M, Yanagisawa M, et al. Endothelin, a novel vasoconstrictor peptide, as potent bronchoconstrictor. Eur J Pharmacol. 1988; 154(2):227–8.
124. D'Agostino B, Filippelli A, Falciani M, Rossi F. Endothelin-1 and bronchial hyperresponsiveness in the rabbit. Naunyn Schmiedebergs Arch Pharmacol. 1998;358(5):561–6.
125. Noguchi K, Ishikawa K, Yano M, Ahmed A, Cortes A, Abraham WM. Endothelin-1 contributes to antigen-induced airway hyperresponsiveness. J Appl Physiol. 1995;79(3):700–5.
126. Sumarac-Dumanovic M, Stevanovic D, Ljubic A, Jorga J, Simic M, Stamenkovic-Pejkovic D, et al. Increased activity of interleukin-23/interleukin-17 proinflammatory axis in obese women. Int J Obes (Lond). 2009;33(1):151–6.
127. Agache I, Ciobanu C, Agache C, Anghel M. Increased serum IL-17 is an independent risk factor for severe asthma. Respir Med. 2010;104(8):1131–7.
128. Winer S, Paltser G, Chan Y, Tsui H, Engleman E, Winer D, et al. Obesity predisposes to Th17 bias. Eur J Immunol. 2009;39(9):2629–35.
129. Lyons JA, Haring JS, Biga PR. Myostatin expression, lymphocyte population, and potential cytokine production correlate with predisposition to high-fat diet induced obesity in mice. PLoS One. 2010;5(9):e12928.
130. Pini M, Fantuzzi G. Enhanced production of IL-17A during zymosan-induced peritonitis in obese mice. J Leukoc Biol. 2010;87(1):51–8.
131. Finkelman FD, Hogan SP, Hershey GK, Rothenberg ME, Wills-Karp M. Importance of cytokines in murine allergic airway disease and human asthma. J Immunol. 2010;184(4): 1663–74.
132. Pichavant M, Goya S, Meyer EH, Johnston RA, Kim HY, Matangkasombut P, et al. Ozone exposure in a mouse model induces airway hyperreactivity that requires the presence of natural killer T cells and IL-17. J Exp Med. 2008;205(2):385–93.
133. Tantisira KG, Weiss ST. Complex interactions in complex traits: obesity and asthma. Thorax. 2001;56(Suppl 2):ii64–73.
134. Weiss ST. Obesity: insight into the origins of asthma. Nat Immunol. 2005;6(6):537–9.

135. Soutar A, Seaton A, Brown K. Bronchial reactivity and dietary antioxidants. Thorax. 1997; 52(2):166–70.
136. Shi H, Kokoeva MV, Inouye K, Tzameli I, Yin H, Flier JS. TLR4 links innate immunity and fatty acid-induced insulin resistance. J Clin Invest. 2006;116(11):3015–25.
137. Blackburn P, Despres JP, Lamarche B, Tremblay A, Bergeron J, Lemieux I, et al. Postprandial variations of plasma inflammatory markers in abdominally obese men. Obesity (Silver Spring). 2006;14(10):1747–54.
138. Ghanim H, Sia CL, Upadhyay M, Korzeniewski K, Viswanathan P, Abuaysheh S, et al. Orange juice neutralizes the proinflammatory effect of a high-fat, high-carbohydrate meal and prevents endotoxin increase and Toll-like receptor expression. Am J Clin Nutr. 2010;91(4):940–9.
139. Ghanim H, Sia CL, Korzeniewski K, Lohano T, Abuaysheh S, Marumganti A, et al. A resveratrol and polyphenol preparation suppresses oxidative and inflammatory stress response to a high-fat, high-carbohydrate meal. J Clin Endocrinol Metab. 2011;96(5):1409–14.
140. Wood LG, Garg ML, Gibson PG. A high-fat challenge increases airway inflammation and impairs bronchodilator recovery in asthma. J Allergy Clin Immunol. 2011;127(5):1133–40.
141. Ghanim H, Abuaysheh S, Sia CL, Korzeniewski K, Chaudhuri A, Fernandez-Real JM, et al. Increase in plasma endotoxin concentrations and the expression of Toll-like receptors and suppressor of cytokine signaling-3 in mononuclear cells after a high-fat, high-carbohydrate meal: implications for insulin resistance. Diabetes Care. 2009;32(12):2281–7.
142. Cani PD, Bibiloni R, Knauf C, Waget A, Neyrinck AM, Delzenne NM, et al. Changes in gut microbiota control metabolic endotoxemia-induced inflammation in high-fat diet-induced obesity and diabetes in mice. Diabetes. 2008;57(6):1470–81.
143. Cani PD, Neyrinck AM, Fava F, Knauf C, Burcelin RG, Tuohy KM, et al. Selective increases of bifidobacteria in gut microflora improve high-fat-diet-induced diabetes in mice through a mechanism associated with endotoxaemia. Diabetologia. 2007;50(11):2374–83.
144. Turnbaugh PJ, Ley RE, Mahowald MA, Magrini V, Mardis ER, Gordon JI. An obesity-associated gut microbiome with increased capacity for energy harvest. Nature. 2006; 444(7122): 1027–31.
145. Hilty M, Burke C, Pedro H, Cardenas P, Bush A, Bossley C, et al. Disordered microbial communities in asthmatic airways. PLoS One. 2010;5(1):e8578.
146. Maslowski KM, Vieira AT, Ng A, Kranich J, Sierro F, Yu D, et al. Regulation of inflammatory responses by gut microbiota and chemoattractant receptor GPR43. Nature. 2009;461(7268): 1282–6.
147. Shore SA. Environmental perturbations: obesity. Compr Physiol. 2010. doi:10.1002/cphy.c100017.

Chapter 3
The Effects of Obesity on Immune Function and Pulmonary Host Defense

Peter Mancuso

Abstract Obesity is a common condition in developed nations known to increase the risk of cardiometabolic disease and is now implicated as a contributing factor to ailments of the lung. Once thought of as a passive vessel for the storage of excess lipids, adipose tissue is now appreciated for its role as an endocrine gland that secretes adipocyte-derived factors or adipokines known to regulate numerous physiologic functions. Leptin is the best characterized adipokine, and it has been shown to play a profound role in the regulation of innate and adaptive immunity in respiratory infections. The accumulation of excess adipose tissue in the obese has dramatic effects on the systemic immune response by contributing to a chronic state of low-grade inflammation and altering the host response to infection. Recent epidemiologic evidence and carefully controlled animal studies have demonstrated that excess adiposity impairs the host response against influenza infection. Whether or not obesity contributes to the risk of community-acquired or nosocomial pneumonia is not clear and requires further examination. Future elucidation of the mechanisms by which excess adiposity impairs immune function is warranted and would foster development of novel therapeutic strategies to treat pulmonary infections in obese patients.

Keywords Obesity • Pneumonia • Influenza • Adipokines • Leptin • Adiponectin • Inflammation • Macrophage • Infection • Host defense

P. Mancuso, M.S., Ph.D. (✉)
Environmental Health Sciences and Graduate Program in Immunology,
109 S. Observatory, Ann Arbor, MI 48109, USA
e-mail: pmancuso@umich.edu

A.E. Dixon and E.M. Clerisme-Beaty (eds.), *Obesity and Lung Disease: A Guide to Management*, Respiratory Medicine, DOI 10.1007/978-1-62703-053-3_3,

Objectives

- Understand how excess adipose tissue contributes to a chronic state of low-grade systemic inflammation.
- Examine the influence of obesity on leukocyte function.
- Evaluate the evidence that obesity and comorbid conditions increase the risk respiratory infections.
- Illustrate the importance of leptin in host defense against infection in humans and animals.

Introduction

The prevalence of obesity and overweight among adults living in the USA has increased to alarming levels with 34% obese (BMI $\geq$ 30) and 68% overweight (BMI = 25–29.9) adults [1]. Moreover, 46–54% of hospitalized patients are overweight, 32% are obese, and 5% are extremely obese with a BMI of $\geq$40 [2]. Similar trends have been observed in other developed nations raising global concerns about the long-term health consequences of obesity [3]. While type II diabetes, cardiovascular disease, and nonalcoholic fatty liver disease are well-known comorbid conditions associated with obesity, the evidence that excess white adipose tissue suppresses host defense against infections of the lung is emerging [4–7]. Obesity is said to contribute to a "chronic state of systemic inflammation" that not only alters glucose and lipid metabolism but also has profound effects on immune cell function [8, 9]. The recent observation that the obese were uniquely susceptible to and suffered more severe outcomes from the 2009 H1N1 influenza pandemic underscores the need to elucidate the effects of obesity on innate and adaptive immune responses against respiratory infections [10]. This chapter will examine the evidence that obesity contributes to greater susceptibility to respiratory infections in humans and in animal models of obesity and will also discuss the mechanisms underlying these responses.

Adipose Tissue Is an Energy Storage Depot and Endocrine Gland that Influences the Immune System

Adipose Tissue Structure. Adipose tissue is a complex network of mature adipocytes, preadipocytes, mesenchymal cells, stromal cells, vascular endothelial cells, macrophages, and fibroblasts mainly found in subcutaneous and visceral regions. It serves as a storage depot that buffers the influx of dietary lipids by clearing triacylglycerol (TAG) and inhibiting the release of free fatty acids (FFA) into the systemic circulation. In addition to storing TAG, white adipose tissue also functions as an endocrine organ by elaborating adipokines (adipocyte-derived hormones that are structurally similar to cytokines), cytokines, acute-phase reactants, prostaglandins, and other hormones that participate in local and distal physiologic processes.

The levels of adipokines influence glucose homeostasis and inform the host, via the central nervous system, regarding lipid energy storage. Under conditions of a positive energy balance, adipose tissue expands not only in subcutaneous and visceral depots but also throughout the body in association with the heart, kidneys, bone marrow, adventitia of major blood vessels [11], and lungs [12]. While the significance of these organ-specific adipose tissue depots is unclear, the expansion of these depots under the influence of excess caloric intake can alter adipokine secretion, promoting a proinflammatory state ultimately influencing organ function [11, 12].

Adipose Tissue Inflammation. During the development of obesity, individual adipocytes undergo hypertrophy, and the vascular supply fails to adequately perfuse the expansion of adipose tissue resulting in tissue hypoxia and apoptotic cell death [13, 14]. This process is thought to initiate the proinflammatory condition of visceral adipose tissue and promote the development of type II diabetes and metabolic syndrome [15]. The cellular debris left behind from apoptotic adipocytes induces the elaboration of chemokines such as CCL2, which recruits peripheral blood monocytes and T cells [16, 17]. The accumulation of adipose tissue macrophages is proportional to total adiposity, and the monocytes recruited to adipose tissue differentiate into macrophages which exhibit a classically activated or M1 phenotype [14, 18, 19]. In contrast, M2 or alternatively activated macrophages found in adipose tissues of lean animals produce anti-inflammatory mediators known to resolve inflammation and protect against obesity-induced insulin resistance [20]. Recent reports have described an important role for regulatory CD4+ T cells and CD8+ effector T cells in promoting the polarization of adipose tissue macrophages toward the M1 phenotype which express inducible nitric oxide synthase and many proinflammatory factors known to contribute to insulin resistance [21]. In addition to these recruited leukocytes, mast cells have also been shown to increase in adipose tissue in murine models of diet-induced obesity, and these cells may contribute to glucose intolerance and inflammation [22]. Finally, a recent report by Stienstra and coworkers demonstrated an important role for NOD-, LRR-, and pyrin domain-containing 3 (NALP3) inflammasome, an innate immune receptor, in adipose tissue inflammation, MCP-1 expression, and macrophage recruitment into adipose tissue in mice [23]. NALP3-deficient mice were protected against diet-induced obesity and insulin resistance, and detailed metabolic and molecular phenotyping indicated an important role for the inflammasome in energy expenditure and adipogenic gene expression [23].

Pro- and Anti-inflammatory Adipokines in Obesity. The production of proinflammatory adipokines in white adipose tissue (WAT) such as leptin, resistin, retinol-binding protein 4 (RBP4), TNF-α, IL-6, lipocalin-2, IL-18, CXCL5, and nicotinamide phosphoribosyltransferase (NAMPT) increases during obesity [12]. In addition to these, acute-phase reactants, C-reactive protein (CRP), serum amyloid A (SAA), complement fragment C3, and other immune-modulating mediators are produced in WAT as well [24]. In contrast, the production of anti-inflammatory adipokines such as adiponectin and secreted frizzled-related protein 5 (SFRP5) is downregulated [25, 26]. These proinflammatory mediators spill over into the peripheral circulation and contribute to a low-grade state of chronic systemic inflammation that may ultimately influence the pulmonary immune response against infection [24, 27].

Although yet to be determined, the production of these adipocyte-derived mediators from local adipose tissue (e.g., adipocytes in the mediastinum) could potentially contribute to pulmonary inflammation.

Leptin and Inflammation. Of these proinflammatory systemic mediators that are increased during obesity, leptin is the best characterized. It was originally described as a satiety hormone that regulates energy homeostasis and informs the host, via the central nervous system, regarding peripheral lipid energy storage [28]. Obese individuals, who possess high serum leptin levels since this adipokine is positively correlated with total body fat mass, are said to be in a state of leptin resistance without the anorexic effects of this hormone [12, 29]. The long (LepRb) and short (LepRa-d) isoforms of the leptin receptor are expressed by bronchial and alveolar epithelial cells and alveolar macrophages [30–33], and all cells of the immune system express these receptors [34]. The LepRb signals via the Janus kinase (JAK2) and signal transducer and activator (STAT3) pathway, and the LepRa has been shown to activate the extracellular-regulated kinase pathways (ERK1/2) and phosphatidylinositol kinase (PI3K) pathways [35, 36]. Collectively, these intracellular signals regulate the immunostimulatory effects of leptin in myeloid cells such as the production of reactive oxygen intermediates and upregulation of phagocytic receptor expression in monocytes [37] and neutrophils [38–40]. These leptin-mediated signaling events also promote a T_H1 response through the enhanced production of IL-2 and IFN-γ as well as stimulating the proliferation and activation of T cells in response to mitogen activation [41]. Leptin can also prime leukocytes for increased IL-6, TNF-α, and leukotriene synthesis [38, 42–44] and enhance nitric oxide production in leukocytes in vitro [45]. Leptin also plays a critical role in B cell generation and development [46] and licenses DCs for priming T_H1 responses, promoting their survival and capacity to activate CD8+ T cells [47, 48]. Finally, leptin plays a critical role in the development and activation of natural killer cells [49].

Inflammatory Effects of Leptin in the Obese Host. In total, the increased synthesis of leptin in the obese appears to promote proinflammatory responses systemically and in the lung. While there is evidence that cells in the lung are capable of producing low levels of leptin [32, 50–52], the physiologic significance of this is not clear. Much higher levels of leptin appear in the peripheral blood during infection [33, 43, 53] and other systemic inflammatory responses, suggesting that it leaks in to the respiratory tract due to increases in microvascular permeability as a consequence of pulmonary inflammation [54, 55]. Within the lungs of obese patients, leptin may prolong the lifespan of leukocytes, provoking greater inflammation in the setting of pneumonia and chronic bronchitis [50, 53, 56]. However, relatively little is known regarding the influence of leptin in immune cells in the obese leptin-resistant host.

Anti-inflammatory Adipokines. In contrast to leptin, the synthesis of the anti-inflammatory adipokine, adiponectin, declines with increased adiposity, during an inflammatory response, or from tobacco smoke exposures [57, 58]. All three of the known adiponectin receptors (AdipoR1, AdipoR2, and T-cadherin) are expressed in the lungs, and low, medium, and high molecular weight forms of adiponectin have been isolated from bronchoalveolar lavage fluid [59, 60]. Adiponectin receptors mediate anti-inflammatory signals via the adenosine monophosphate (AMP)-activated kinase (AMPK) pathway and by inhibiting Toll-like receptor-mediated nuclear factor kappa B (NF-κB) activation in macrophages [61]. Adiponectin has been shown to increase prostaglandin synthesis in stromal cells [62] and IL-10 production in human macrophages [63]. In addition, exogenously administered adiponectin suppresses leukocyte recruitment, T_H2 cytokine production, and airway inflammation in a murine model of allergen-induced asthma [59]. Interestingly, the lungs of adiponectin-deficient mice exhibit an emphysema-like phenotype that is associated with activated alveolar macrophages that spontaneously elaborate TNF-α and matrix metalloproteinase-12 MMP-12 [64]. Adiponectin levels are reduced in smokers and increased in former smokers with COPD [65]. Adiponectin deficiency has also been shown to be associated with pulmonary inflammation and remodeling of the lung in a model of allergen-induced chronic asthma. Thus, reduced levels of adiponectin, the most abundant adipokine in peripheral blood (approximately 10 μg/ml) [66], may be an important mechanistic link between obesity and pulmonary inflammatory responses. Interestingly, a recent study by Uji et al. showed that adiponectin-knockout mice exhibit greater mortality and that pharmacologically induced increases in serum adiponectin improves survival in a murine model of polymicrobial sepsis [67]. Adiponectin also facilitates the uptake of apoptotic cells [68] by macrophages, and this response is critical for reducing inflammation in the lungs [66, 69, 70]. At present, there are no studies that have evaluated the role of adiponectin in pulmonary host defense against infection, and the physiologic significance of reduced adiponectin in obese humans warrants further investigation.

Antimicrobial Protein, Lipocalin-2. Lipocalin-2 is produced by adipose tissue and is abundant in the serum of obese mice and humans [71, 72]. The endogenous ligand for this transporter of lipophilic substances has not been identified. However, lipocalin-2, which is also produced by neutrophils and bronchial epithelial cells, is a siderophore (an iron-chelating molecule produced by bacteria)-binding antimicrobial protein that is required for host defense against *Klebsiella* pneumonia [73] and plays a protective role against murine *Escherichia coli* pneumonia [74]. Based on this evidence, it would appear that obese humans would be protected against bacterial pneumonia due to the abundance of leptin and lipocalin-2. While some have reported a protective effect of obesity in community-acquired pneumonia [75], other reports have demonstrated an increased risk for lower respiratory tract infections [76]. Clearly, future studies are needed to evaluate the contribution of these and other adipokines to immune dysfunction in the obese.

Alteration in Leukocyte Counts and Function in Obese Human Subjects

Obesity and Leukocytosis. A number of publications have attempted to define the effects of obesity on host defense by simply harvesting peripheral blood cells of obese individuals and studying their responses to various stimuli and pathogens in vitro. While this seems like a very logical approach, it assumes that human obesity is a signal phenotype that can be categorized solely on BMI. Human obesity is a

Table 3.1 Effects of obesity on human leukocyte function

Cell type	Effects of obesity (reference)
PMNs	Increased phagocytosis and ROS production [81]; defective bacterial killing [86, 87]
Macrophages/monocytes	Increased phagocytosis and ROS production [81]; enhanced proinflammatory cytokine production [12]
CD4+ T cells	T_H1 polarization [21]
CD8+ T cells	Diminished proliferative response to mitogen activation [81]
B cells	Reduced proliferation in response to mitogen activation [81]
NK cells	Impaired cytotoxic function [84, 85]

PMN neutrophils, *ROS* reactive oxygen intermediates, *NK* natural killer

complex multifactor syndrome that is caused by many different genetic and environmental influences and may be accompanied by comorbid conditions known to impair immune function such as type II diabetes. As a consequence, these factors may explain why investigators have not always reported consistent results regarding the function and number of immune cells harvested from obese humans. For example, Womack et al. [77] observed that CD4+ and CD8+ T cells were elevated in obese women compared with those with a BMI<25 kg/m^2. Likewise, O'Rourke [78] observed an increased frequency of these cells in obese human subjects. In contrast, Tanaka et al. [79] reported that the numbers of both CD4+ and CD8+ T cells were reduced in obese compared with nonobese subjects. In addition, Kim and Park [80] reported that lymphocyte counts in adolescent obese females were negatively correlated with BMI.

Affect of Obesity on Leukocyte Function. With regard to leukocyte function in obese subjects, Nieman et al. [81] reported that CD8+ T cell and B cell proliferation in response to exogenous stimuli was diminished. In another report from the same group of investigators, mild to moderate obesity was not associated with impairments in T cell, B cell, monocyte, and granulocyte functions [82]. While obesity has been reported to increase naïve T cell populations in humans and DIO mice, it has also been shown to restrict T cell diversity and accelerate thymic involution [83]. There is agreement, however, that obesity reduces NK cell populations and impairs the function of these cells [84, 85]. Interestingly, a study by Nieman et al. demonstrated that monocytes and neutrophils (PMNs) obtained from obese human subjects exhibited modest increases in the ability to phagocytose opsonized bacteria and generate a respiratory burst [81]. However, others have reported that PMNs recovered from obese patients exhibit defective bactericidal function [86, 87]. Elevated populations of these cells have also been reported in obese adults and children [80, 81, 88]. Surprisingly, there are no studies that have evaluated the impact of obesity on dendritic cell function. Taken together, obesity, in humans, is associated with selective impairment of cells that play a principle role in nosocomial infections (PMNs), adaptive immunity (CD4+ and CD8+ T cells and B cells), and host defense against viral infections (NK cells and CD8+ T cells). This may explain why obese individuals exhibit greater susceptibility to hospital-acquired infections [89], influenza [90], and impaired vaccine responsiveness [91–93]. A summary of the effects of obesity on immune cell function is provided in Table 3.1.

Obesity Is a Risk Factor for Susceptibility and Severity of Illness from H1N1 Pandemic Influenza

The H1N1 influenza pandemic of 2009 provides cogent evidence that the obese exhibit greater susceptibility to pulmonary viral infections [5, 94]. Individuals with known risk factors for influenza such as pregnancy, chronic heart and lung disease, neurologic disease, and diabetes were frequently reported as being among those with confirmed H1N1 infections and who experienced a more severe illness [90, 94–97]. Surprisingly, a number of reports indicated that the obese and morbidly obese also appeared to be more susceptible to pandemic H1N1 influenza and exhibited greater severity of illness [5, 94, 98, 99]. Additional studies confirmed these associations indicating that obesity and morbid obesity were independent risk factors for hospitalization [90], admission to an intensive care unit [100], and critical illness and death [94, 101] associated with H1N1 infection in the USA [102]. Similar reports from many other countries also indicate a greater severity of illness and death from pandemic H1N1 in obese patients [103–108]. Table 3.2 summarizes some of the studies demonstrating that obesity is associated with a higher risk and greater severity of illness from H1N1 pandemic influenza. Finally, obesity may also impair host defense against other types of viral infections of the respiratory tract since obesity was associated with a worse clinical course during respiratory syncytial virus (RSV) infection in a cohort of Chilean children [109]. Since mortality resulting from influenza is often associated with secondary bacterial pneumonia, future studies should investigate the association between obesity and the possibility that these individuals may be more likely to develop secondary bacterial pneumonia.

Does Obesity Increase the Risk of Community-Acquired or Nosocomial Pneumonia?

Obesity and Risk of Community-Acquired Pneumonia. While there is ample evidence that shows an increased risk of bacterial infections of the feet, surgical and catheter sites, gingival and periodontal tissues, gastrointestinal tract, and skin in obese patients, the impact of obesity on bacterial pneumonia is less certain [110]. Community-acquired pneumonia is most frequently caused by bacterial pathogens. Paradoxically, three studies have demonstrated a protective association between obesity and mortality from pneumonia [75, 111, 112]. Corrales-Medina et al. [75] demonstrated that increasing BMI was negatively correlated with 30-day mortality in patients with proven pneumococcal or *Haemophilus* community-acquired pneumonia. Similarly, LaCroix et al. [111] reported a negative relationship between mortality from pneumonia and BMI with increased mortality in men in the lowest BMI quartile compared with the highest BMI quartile. This study also suggests that the obese were protected from pneumonia as a cause of death. In a study that evaluated protective factors against death from pneumonia in 110,000 Japanese subjects, Inoue et al. [112] reported that low BMI (<18) was associated with an increased risk

Table 3.2 Obesity and H1N1 influenza pandemic of 2009

Reference	Number of subjects	Comparisons	Odds ratios (95% confidence interval)	Association
MMWR [5]	10 patients, 3 deaths	None	NA	9 of 10 ICU patients admitted for severe H1N1 infection were obese
Vaillant [94]	574 deaths	None	NA	Metabolic condition (including obesity), a risk factor for death
Jain [90]	272	None	NA	Obesity was an independent risk factor for hospitalization
Hanslik [96]	1,266	General population versus obese	3.8 (3.0–4.9)	Obesity associated with increased risk of death in patients with H1N1
Fuhrman [103]	758 patients hospitalized with H1N1	Severe disease versus nonsevere hospitalized adult cases	9.1 (4.4–18.7)	Obesity associated with severe disease
Morgan [126]	565 patients hospitalized with pandemic H1N1 influenza	Normal weight (BMI 18.5–24.9) versus overweight (25–29.9), obese (30–39.9), and morbidly obese (>40)	[a]4.9, (2.4–9.9) [b]4.7 (1.3–17.2) [c]3.1 (1.5–6.6) [d]7.6 (2.1–27.9)	Odds ratio for morbid obesity[a,b] and obesity[c,d] association with hospitalization[a,c] and death[b,d] in patients with[a] and without[b] ACIP[e], compared with normal weight group

NA not applicable

[e]Chronic medical conditions considered by the Advisory Committee on Immunization Practices (ACIP) to increase the risk of influenza-related complications

of death, while the opposite was true for subjects with a high BMI (25–30.9). The reported associations between lower BMI and an increased risk of death from pneumonia [75, 111, 112] probably reflects the greater frequency of chronic disease-associated malnutrition, e.g., emphysema, known to increase one's susceptibility to pneumonia. In contrast to these, a study by Baik et al., which included 26,429 men aged 44–79 years from the Health Professionals Follow-up Study and 78,062 women aged 27–44 years from the Nurses' Health Study II, demonstrated a significant association between a 40-lb weight gain and a twofold increased risk of community-acquired pneumonia [76]. Only one study, at the time that this chapter was written, has demonstrated an association between childhood obesity and respiratory infections [113]. In this study, the authors reported that overweight children (BMI in the 90th percentile) experienced twice as high a risk for acute respiratory infections than children with a low BMI. At present, the effect of obesity on susceptibility to community-acquired bacterial pneumonia is not clear, and additional studies are needed to evaluate this potential relationship.

Obesity and Risk of Nosocomial Pneumonia. Obese patients experience more complications while hospitalized for critical illness and after surgery, requiring greater hospital and ICU lengths of stay. Although there are numerous studies demonstrating that obesity is associated with a greater risk of surgical site infections [114], wound infections, catheter and blood stream infections [89], and infections of the urinary tract [115], the data on the association between obesity and the risk of nosocomial pneumonia, which is most often caused by bacteria, are mixed. For example, a prospective study by Bochicchio et al. involving 1,167 critically ill trauma patients demonstrated that obesity was associated with increased hospital and ICU lengths of stay and a twofold increased risk of urinary tract and blood stream infections and pneumonia [4]. Similarly, Newell also observed an increase in hospital and ICU lengths of stay, increased urinary tract infections, a longer period of ventilator support, as well as an increased risk of pneumonia in obese and severely obese critically injured blunt trauma patients [6]. A retrospective chart review of patients admitted to the medical ICU conducted by Yaegashi et al. [7] revealed that morbidly obese patients, defined as BMI ≥40, had higher rates of mortality, acute respiratory distress syndrome, catheter infections, acute renal failure, nosocomial pneumonia, and sepsis than obese patients with a BMI in the range of 30–39.9. The morbidly obese also required a longer period of time on ventilatory support. In contrast to the studies mentioned above, studies by Brant et al. [116] and Moulton [117] did not find a significant association between obesity and an increased risk of nosocomial pneumonia in patients undergoing heart surgery. Finally, Dossett et al. did not find a significant association of BMI with pulmonary complications (such as pneumonia) in a cohort study of critically injured adults [118]. Based on available evidence, an association between obesity and community-acquired or nosocomial pneumonia is not clear, and additional research is needed. Future studies should employ the use of viral and bacterial microbial DNA arrays for the identification of the causative agent and diagnosis of infectious pneumonia[119]. Since it is likely that obesity selectively alters the immune response, this type of identification would be very useful in understanding the mechanisms by which excess adiposity suppresses host defense against pathogens known to more frequently infect obese patients. Table 3.3 provides a summary of some of the studies mentioned above.

Table 3.3 Association between obesity and community-acquired and nosocomial pneumonia

Reference	Number of patients	Comparisons	Odds ratios (95% confidence interval) or other	Association
Baik [76]	26,429 men 78,062 women	WT maintained versus 40-lb WT gain	M 1.46 (1.00–2.14) W 1.55 (1.15–2.10)	Increased risk of community-acquired pneumonia
Jedrychowski [113]	1,129 children	Low BMI with BMI ≥ 20 (overweight children)	2.02 (1.13–3.59)	Increased risk of acute respiratory infection
Bochicchio [4]	1,167	Nonobese versus obese	2.0 (1.02–3.76)	Increased risk of nosocomial pneumonia
Newell [6]	1,543	BMI 18.5–24.9 versus 30–39.9, and ≥ 40	1.7 (1.21–2.44) 2.5 (1.48–4.30)	Increased risk of nosocomial pneumonia
Yaegashi [7]	63	BMI 30–39.9 versus BMI ≥ 40	3% versus 33%	Increased risk of nosocomial pneumonia for BMI > 40
Brant [116]	500	Normal BMI 18.5–25 versus BMI ≥ 30	3% versus 5%	No differences in risk of nosocomial pneumonia
Moulton [117]	2,299	BMI	NA	No differences in risk of nosocomial pneumonia
Dossett [118]	1,291	Normal BMI versus BMI 25–29.9, 30–39.9, and ≥ 40	Obese 0.96 (0.64–1.4) Severely obese 0.89 (0.46–1.7)	No differences in risk of nosocomial pneumonia

M men, *W* women, *NA* not applicable, *WT* weight

Comorbid Conditions Associated with Obesity Known to Affect Pulmonary Host Defense

Obesity is a complex multifactorial disease that is characterized by excess adiposity and is often accompanied by other comorbid conditions known to compromise immune function such as type II diabetes and gastroesophageal reflux disease (GERD) [120]. It is well established that diabetes delays wound healing, impairs host defense against skin and subcutaneous infections, and is associated with nosocomial infections and infectious complications of surgery [121]. It is also an important risk factor for pneumonia and influenza [122] and contributes to a higher risk of death from community-acquired pneumonia [123]. Since obese patients often have gastroesophageal reflux disease and are at a greater risk for aspiration pneumonia [124], care should be taken to position these patients in a semiupright position during hospitalization [110, 125]. While type II diabetes and GERD are known risk factors for pneumonia, less is known about the risk of respiratory infection in the absence of comorbid conditions. However, the greater severity of illness from H1N1 influenza in obese patients without comorbid disturbances suggests that increased adiposity may render individuals more susceptible to viral and possibly other types of infections [126]. Another important mechanism by which obesity might alter host defense is through metabolic disturbances induced by type II diabetes that often accompanies obesity. In this condition, endoplasmic reticulum stress, lipotoxicity, oxidative stress, and glucotoxicity are known to contribute to insulin resistance [15]. These same mechanisms may alter the metabolic activity of immune cells ultimately affecting their ability to respond to infection [127]. For example, quiescent naïve and memory T cells have lower energy demands and rely on aerobic phosphorylation for ATP generation required for their survival and migration. In contrast, the expansion quiescent T cells into cytotoxic CD8+ T cells that play a critical role in clearing virus-infected cells from the lung switch to anaerobic glycolysis to support their rapid proliferation and effector functions [128]. Metabolic disturbances in the obese may compromise this transition and impair the cytotoxic T cell response to infection. The effects of obesity on pulmonary host defense are summarized in Fig. 3.1.

Effect of Leptin and Leptin Receptor Deficiency on Susceptibility to Infection in Mice and Humans

Leptin and Leptin Receptor Deficiency Impairs Host Defense Against Pulmonary Bacterial Infections. There are relatively few studies that have evaluated the effects of obesity on host defense against pulmonary infections. Most of these have been conducted using obese leptin-deficient *ob/ob* mice which not only are obese but also exhibit many immune and endocrine abnormalities that are caused by both leptin deficiency and obesity, which complicates the interpretation of

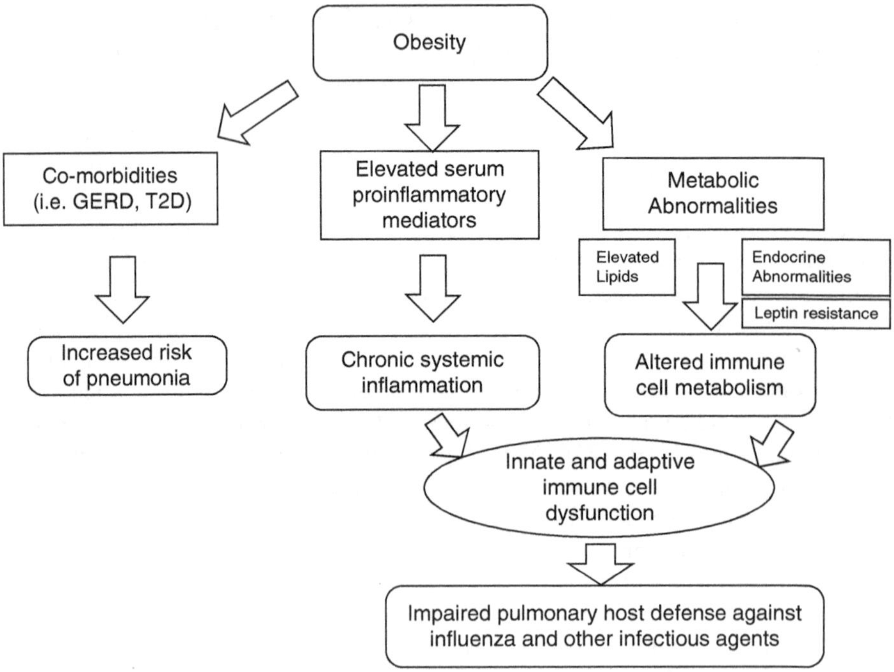

Fig. 3.1 Obesity-induced immune dysfunction that contributes to impaired pulmonary host defense

these studies [43, 129–131]. Leptin is essential for normal development and function of cells of the myeloid and lymphoid linage, affecting both innate and adaptive immune responses, and the absence of this hormone or its receptor results in severe immune abnormalities[132]. Studies conducted in our laboratory have shown that *ob/ob* mice exhibit increased pulmonary bacterial burdens and reduced survival following an intratracheal challenge with either *Klebsiella pneumoniae* or *Streptococcus pneumoniae* [43, 129]. The host defense impairment in these animals was related to defective alveolar macrophage and neutrophil phagocytosis and killing of bacteria in vitro. We also reported that leptin deficiency was associated with reduced leukotriene synthesis which is also known to contribute to impaired pulmonary host defense against bacterial pneumonia [43,44,53,133,134]. Likewise, Wieland et al. reported higher lung *Mycobacterium tuberculosis* counts in *ob/ob* compared with WT mice that was associated with reduced levels of IFN-γ in a murine model of tuberculosis [131]. Ordway reported similar results in that IFN-γ+CD4+ T cell recruitment to the lungs was delayed in *ob/ob* compared with WT mice challenged with *M. abscessus* [130]. Lung *Mycobacterium abscessus* burdens were higher, and mycobacterial clearance was delayed in *ob/ob* mice.

Leptin and Leptin Receptor Deficiency Impairs Host Defense Against Bacterial, Fungal, and Viral Infections. In addition to pulmonary infections, leptin- and leptin receptor-deficient (*db/db*) obese mice exhibit increased susceptibility to subcutaneous *Listeria monocytogenes* infection despite a more robust and persistent inflammatory response [135]. In another study by Conge [136], the immune response against *K. pneumoniae* and *Salmonella typhimurium* was also impaired in *ob/ob* and *db/db* mice. A recent study by Tschop et al. [137] demonstrated that *ob/ob* mice exhibited greater mortality and more severe organ damage following cecal ligation and puncture-induced polymicrobial sepsis. *Db/db* mice have also been shown to exhibit greater susceptibility to *Staphylococcus aureus* [138] and *Helicobacter pylori* [139] infections. Leptin also appears to play an important role in viral infections since *ob/ob* mice have been shown to exhibit greater susceptibility to encephalomyocarditis virus [140] and group B coxsackie virus infections [141]. Finally, leptin receptor mutant obese (*fa/fa*) rats have also been shown to exhibit impaired host defense against *Candida albicans* [142]. Only one study failed to show differences between WT and *ob/ob* mice following bacterial infection [143]. Based on these studies, leptin appears to play a critical role in the host defense against bacterial, viral, and fungal infections of the lung and other tissues. While human leptin deficiency is rare, individuals with this genetic defect are known to exhibit greater susceptibility to respiratory infections, indicating an important role for leptin in the human immune response to infectious disease as well [144].

Effects of Leptin Receptor Signaling and Leptin Resistance in Infection. While there is disagreement in the literature regarding the susceptibility of the obese to community-acquired and nosocomial pneumonia, obesity appears to be a risk factor for influenza and possibly other viral infections. As mentioned above, obesity is associated with a chronic state of systemic inflammation, and one might infer that this condition would lead to a heightened state of host defense. However, there is more agreement that obesity impairs host defense against influenza infection, and this may occur via leptin resistance and metabolic dysfunction. Leptin resistance is a condition by which cells become insensitive to leptin as a consequence of prolonged exposure to elevated levels of this adipokine [29]. This effect is mediated through the downregulation of LepRb in immune cells and through the prolonged activation of STAT3 signaling and accumulation of intracellular SOCS3 which inhibits leptin receptor activation [145]. Leptin resistance has been demonstrated in NK cells [146], T cells [147], and peripheral blood monocytes [148], and this might contribute to suboptimal responses in the obese during influenza infection. Lastly, it is interesting to note that polymorphisms in the human leptin receptor gene have been associated not only with obesity but also with susceptibility to infectious disease as well [149, 150]. It is envisioned that leptin receptor mutations in humans may be related to impairments in pulmonary host defense that may or may not be associated with an obese phenotype. Alternatively, leptin receptor mutations can lead to obesity and a protective immune phenotype against pulmonary infections [33]. In total, more research is needed to determine the role of leptin receptor dysfunction in infectious disease.

Diet-Induced Obesity Impairs Host Defense against Murine Influenza A Infection

The recent obesity epidemic in developed nations is most likely due to environmental, dietary, and polygenetic influences that ultimately contribute to a positive energy balance which most commonly occurs as a consequence of an energy-rich diet. Many investigators have taken a similar approach in producing obese mice by feeding these animals diets consisting of 40–60% fat, usually in the form of saturated fatty acids, to induce obesity within a relatively short period of time (100–120 days) [151]. While this approach mimics human obesity, the high saturated fat content in these diets may also differentially regulate the immune response [152]. Although there are relatively few studies that have examined the effects of diet-induced obesity (DIO) on host defense against influenza infection, the use of this approach has provided very useful information on the influence of obesity on influenza infection [153–156]. Compared to their lean counterparts, DIO mice exhibit greater mortality and increased lung pathology following infection with a mouse-adapted influenza virus (influenza A/PR/8/34) [153]. This impairment in host defense in DIO mice was associated with a decrease in type I IFNs (IFN-α and IFN-β), a delay in the expression of IL-6 and TNF-α that eventually increased to levels greater than that observed in lean animals, and impaired natural killer (NK) cell cytotoxicity. In addition, DIO also impairs host defense against influenza A by reducing dendritic cell antigen presentation to T cells, attenuating monocyte and CD8+ T cell recruitment, and diminishing IL-2 and IL-12 production [154]. Following a primary challenge with nonlethal influenza H3N2, Karlsson et al. demonstrated that DIO mice exhibited increased morbidity and mortality following a secondary infection with influenza A/PR/8 that was associated with reduced CD8+ T cell and IFN-γ production and defective antigen presentation by dendritic cells [155, 157]. This impairment was due to an inability of DIO mice to generate and maintain functional antigen-specific memory CD8+ T cells. Finally, a recent study by Easterbrook et al. showed that DIO mice experience greater mortality despite similar viral loads following infection with 2009 pandemic H1N1 influenza virus [156]. In this report, the authors observed that pulmonary IFN-β and proinflammatory cytokine production were lower in DIO than lean control mice. Interestingly, serum cytokine levels were elevated in DIO, and this response did not occur after influenza infection in lean mice. The results of these studies provide valuable insights into mechanisms by which obesity may impair host defense against influenza infections that may be relevant to human disease. Future studies should explore mechanisms by which obesity, and potentially alterations in the metabolic state of the host, may dysregulate immune cell function during viral infection [157]. Although DIO mice have been shown to have increased susceptibility to *S. aureus*-induced sepsis [158] and *P. gingivalis* [159] infections, there are no studies that have demonstrated that DIO, using animal models, impairs pulmonary host defense against bacterial or fungal infections of the lung, and investigators should explore this possibility.

Conclusions

Health care professionals are well acquainted with the association between obesity, type II diabetes, atherosclerosis, and ischemic heart disease. However, overweight and obese adults and children may also be especially susceptible to respiratory infections, and this was evident during the recent H1N1 influenza pandemic of 2009. Since the prevalence of obesity is likely to be stable within the foreseeable future, this condition should be recognized as a chronic medical condition known to increase the risk of influenza-related complications requiring vaccination against seasonal influenza. Only a small number of studies have characterized the mechanisms by which obesity increases the risk of influenza in animal models, and this research should be expanded to increase our understanding of the mechanistic underpinnings of this association. Even less is known regarding the susceptibility of the obese to bacteria and other respiratory pathogens, and this warrants further investigation. Finally, future studies should also determine if therapeutic strategies employed to prevent obesity-related metabolic and cardiovascular disease would also improve immune function against respiratory infections.

References

1. Flegal KM, Carroll MD, Ogden CL, Curtin LR. Prevalence and trends in obesity among US adults, 1999–2008. JAMA. 2010;303(3):235–41.
2. Doyle SL, Lysaght J, Reynolds JV. Obesity and post-operative complications in patients undergoing non-bariatric surgery. Obes Rev. 2010;11(12):875–86.
3. Finucane MM, Stevens GA, Cowan MJ, Danaei G, Lin JK, Paciorek CJ, et al. National, regional, and global trends in body-mass index since 1980: systematic analysis of health examination surveys and epidemiological studies with 960 country-years and 9.1 million participants. Lancet. 2011;377(9765):557–67.
4. Bochicchio GV, Joshi M, Bochicchio K, Nehman S, Tracy JK, Scalea TM. Impact of obesity in the critically ill trauma patient: a prospective study. J Am Coll Surg. 2006;203(4):533–8.
5. Intensive-care patients with severe novel influenza A (H1N1) virus infection – Michigan, June 2009. MMWR Morb Mortal Wkly Rep. 2009;58(27):749–52.
6. Newell MA, Bard MR, Goettler CE, Toschlog EA, Schenarts PJ, Sagraves SG, et al. Body mass index and outcomes in critically injured blunt trauma patients: weighing the impact. J Am Coll Surg. 2007;204(5):1056–61. discussion 62–4.
7. Yaegashi M, Jean R, Zuriqat M, Noack S, Homel P. Outcome of morbid obesity in the intensive care unit. J Intensive Care Med. 2005;20(3):147–54.
8. Bullo M, Garcia-Lorda P, Megias I, Salas-Salvado J. Systemic inflammation, adipose tissue tumor necrosis factor, and leptin expression. Obes Res. 2003;11(4):525–31.
9. Lumeng CN, Saltiel AR. Inflammatory links between obesity and metabolic disease. J Clin Invest. 2011;121(6):2111–7.
10. Fuhrman C, Bonmarin I, Bitar D, Cardoso T, Duport N, Herida M, et al. Adult intensive-care patients with 2009 pandemic influenza A (H1N1) infection. Epidemiol Infect. 2010;26:1–8.
11. Chatterjee TK, Stoll LL, Denning GM, Harrelson A, Blomkalns AL, Idelman G, et al. Proinflammatory phenotype of perivascular adipocytes. Circ Res. 2009;104(4):541–9.
12. Ouchi N, Parker JL, Lugus JJ, Walsh K. Adipokines in inflammation and metabolic disease. Nat Rev Immunol. 2011;11(2):85–97.

13. Cinti S, Mitchell G, Barbatelli G, Murano I, Ceresi E, Faloia E, et al. Adipocyte death defines macrophage localization and function in adipose tissue of obese mice and humans. J Lipid Res. 2005;46(11):2347–55.
14. Weisberg SP, McCann D, Desai M, Rosenbaum M, Leibel RL, Ferrante Jr AW. Obesity is associated with macrophage accumulation in adipose tissue. J Clin Invest. 2003;112(12): 1796–808.
15. Donath MY, Shoelson SE. Type 2 diabetes as an inflammatory disease. Nat Rev Immunol. 2011;11(2):98–107.
16. Rausch ME, Weisberg S, Vardhana P, Tortoriello DV. Obesity in C57BL/6 J mice is characterized by adipose tissue hypoxia and cytotoxic T-cell infiltration. Int J Obes (Lond). 2008;32(3):451–63.
17. Kim JY, van de Wall E, Laplante M, Azzara A, Trujillo ME, Hofmann SM, et al. Obesity-associated improvements in metabolic profile through expansion of adipose tissue. J Clin Invest. 2007;117(9):2621–37.
18. Xu H, Barnes GT, Yang Q, Tan G, Yang D, Chou CJ, et al. Chronic inflammation in fat plays a crucial role in the development of obesity-related insulin resistance. J Clin Invest. 2003;112(12):1821–30.
19. Lumeng CN, Bodzin JL, Saltiel AR. Obesity induces a phenotypic switch in adipose tissue macrophage polarization. J Clin Invest. 2007;117(1):175–84.
20. Odegaard JI, Chawla A. Alternative macrophage activation and metabolism. Annu Rev Pathol. 2011;6:275–97.
21. Nishimura S, Manabe I, Nagasaki M, Eto K, Yamashita H, Ohsugi M, et al. CD8+ effector T cells contribute to macrophage recruitment and adipose tissue inflammation in obesity. Nat Med. 2009;15(8):914–20.
22. Liu J, Divoux A, Sun J, Zhang J, Clement K, Glickman JN, et al. Genetic deficiency and pharmacological stabilization of mast cells reduce diet-induced obesity and diabetes in mice. Nat Med. 2009;15(8):940–5.
23. Stienstra R, van Diepen JA, Tack CJ, Zaki MH, van de Veerdonk FL, Perera D, et al. Inflammasome is a central player in the induction of obesity and insulin resistance. Proc Natl Acad Sci. 2011;108(37):15324–9.
24. Tilg H, Moschen AR. Role of adiponectin and PBEF/visfatin as regulators of inflammation: involvement in obesity-associated diseases. Clin Sci (Lond). 2008;114(4):275–88.
25. Hu E, Liang P, Spiegelman BM. AdipoQ is a novel adipose-specific gene dysregulated in obesity. J Biol Chem. 1996;271(18):10697–703.
26. Ouchi N, Higuchi A, Ohashi K, Oshima Y, Gokce N, Shibata R, et al. Sfrp5 is an anti-inflammatory adipokine that modulates metabolic dysfunction in obesity. Science. 2010;329(5990):454–7.
27. Sethi JK, Vidal-Puig AJ. Thematic review series: adipocyte biology. Adipose tissue function and plasticity orchestrate nutritional adaptation. J Lipid Res. 2007;48(6):1253–62.
28. Zhang Y, Proenca R, Maffei M, Barone M, Leopold L, Friedman J. Positional cloning of the mouse obese gene and its human homologue. Nature. 1994;372:425–32.
29. Friedman JM, Halaas JL. Leptin and the regulation of body weight in mammals. Nature. 1998;395(6704):763–70.
30. Bergen HT, Cherlet TC, Manuel P, Scott JE. Identification of leptin receptors in lung and isolated fetal type II cells. Am J Respir Cell Mol Biol. 2002;27(1):71–7.
31. Bellmeyer A, Martino JM, Chandel NS, Scott Budinger GR, Dean DA, Mutlu GM. Leptin resistance protects mice from hyperoxia-induced acute lung injury. Am J Respir Crit Care Med. 2007;175(6):587–94.
32. Bruno A, Pace E, Chanez P, Gras D, Vachier I, Chiappara G, et al. Leptin and leptin receptor expression in asthma. J Allergy Clin Immunol. 2009;124(2):230–7.
33. Mancuso P, Peters-Golden M, Goel D, Goldberg J, Brock TG, Greenwald-Yarnell M, et al. Disruption of leptin receptor-stat3 signaling enhances leukotriene production and pulmonary host defense against pneumococcal pneumonia. J Immunol. 2011;186(2):1081–90.

34. La Cava A, Matarese G. The weight of leptin in immunity. Nat Rev Immunol. 2004;4: 371–9.
35. Tilg H, Moschen AR. Adipocytokines: mediators linking adipose tissue, inflammation and immunity. Nat Rev Immunol. 2006;6(10):772–83.
36. Bruno A, Conus S, Schmid I, Simon HU. Apoptotic pathways are inhibited by leptin receptor activation in neutrophils. J Immunol. 2005;174(12):8090–6.
37. Santos-Alvarez J, Goberna R, Sanchez-Margalet V. Human leptin stimulates proliferation and activation of human circulating monocytes. Cell Immunol. 1999;194:6–11.
38. Zarkesh-Esfahani H, Pockley AG, Wu Z, Hellewell PG, Weetman AP, Ross RJM. Leptin indirectly activates human neutrophils via induction of TNF-α. J Immunol. 2004;172(3): 1809–14.
39. Caldefie-Chezet F, Poulin A, Tridon A, Sion B, Vasson MP. Leptin: a potential regulator of polymorphonuclear neutrophil bactericidal action? J Leukoc Biol. 2001;69(3):414–8.
40. Moore SI, Huffnagle GB, Chen GH, White ES, Mancuso P. Leptin modulates neutrophil phagocytosis of *Klebsiella pneumoniae*. Infect Immun. 2003;71(7):4182–5.
41. Lord GM, Matarese G, Howard JK, Baker RJ, Bloom SR, Lechler RI. Leptin modulates the T- cell immune response and reverses starvation-induced immunosuppression. Nature. 1998;394:897–901.
42. Gainsford T, Willson TA, Metcalf D, Handman E, McFarlane C, Ng A, et al. Leptin can induce proliferation, differentiation, and functional activation of hemopoietic cells. Proc Natl Acad Sci USA. 1996;93(25):14564–8.
43. Mancuso P, Gottschalk A, Phare SM, Peters-Golden M, Lukacs NW, Huffnagle GB. Leptin-deficient mice exhibit impaired host defense in gram-negative pneumonia. J Immunol. 2002;168(8):4018–24.
44. Mancuso P, Canetti C, Gottschalk A, Tithof PK, Peters-Golden M. Leptin augments alveolar macrophage leukotriene synthesis by increasing phospholipase activity and enhancing group IVC iPLA$_2$ (cPLA$_2\gamma$) protein expression. Am J Physiol Lung Cell Mol Physiol. 2004;287:L497–502.
45. Raso GM, Pacilio M, Esposito E, Coppola A, Di Carlo R, Meli R. Leptin potentiates IFN-gamma-induced expression of nitric oxide synthase and cyclo-oxygenase-2 in murine macrophage J774A.1. Br J Pharmacol. 2002;137(6):799–804.
46. Claycombe K, King LE, Fraker PJ. A role for leptin in sustaining lymphopoiesis and myelopoiesis. Proc Natl Acad Sci USA. 2008;105(6):2017–21.
47. Mattioli B, Straface E, Quaranta MG, Giordani L, Viora M. Leptin promotes differentiation and survival of human dendritic cells and licenses them for Th1 priming. J Immunol. 2005;174(11):6820–8.
48. Mattioli B, Straface E, Matarrese P, Quaranta MG, Giordani L, Malorni W, et al. Leptin as an immunological adjuvant: enhanced migratory and CD8+ T cell stimulatory capacity of human dendritic cells exposed to leptin. FASEB J. 2008;22(6):2012–22.
49. Tian Z, Sun R, Wei H, Gao B. Impaired natural killer (NK) cell activity in leptin receptor deficient mice: leptin as a critical regulator in NK cell development and activation. Biochem Biophys Res Commun. 2002;298(3):297–302.
50. Bruno A, Chanez P, Chiappara G, Siena L, Giammanco S, Gjomarkaj M, et al. Does leptin play a cytokine-like role within the airways of COPD patients? Eur Respir J. 2005;26(3): 398–405.
51. Vernooy JH, Drummen NE, van Suylen RJ, Cloots RH, Moller GM, Bracke KR, et al. Enhanced pulmonary leptin expression in patients with severe COPD and asymptomatic smokers. Thorax. 2009;64(1):26–32.
52. Broekhuizen R, Vernooy JH, Schols AM, Dentener MA, Wouters EF. Leptin as local inflammatory marker in COPD. Respir Med. 2005;99(1):70–4.
53. Mancuso P, Huffnagle GB, Olszewski MA, Phipps J, Peters-Golden M. Leptin corrects host defense defects following acute starvation in murine pneumococcal pneumonia. Am J Respir Crit Care Med. 2006;173(Jan 15):212–8.

54. Faggioni R, Fantuzzi G, Fuller J, Dinarello CA, Feingold KR, Grunfeld C. IL-1 beta mediates leptin induction during inflammation. Am J Physiol. 1998;274(1 Pt 2):R204–8.
55. Shore S, Schwartzman I, Mellema M, Flynt L, Imrich A, Johnston R. Effect of leptin on allergic airway responses in mice. J Allergy Clin Immunol. 2005;115:103–9.
56. Shore SA. Obesity and asthma: possible mechanisms. J Allergy Clin Immunol. 2008;121(5):1087–93. quiz 94–5.
57. Koerner A, Kratzsch J, Kiess W. Adipocytokines: leptin–the classical, resistin–the controversical, adiponectin–the promising, and more to come. Best Pract Res. 2005;19(4):525–46.
58. Kawamoto R, Tabara Y, Kohara K, Miki T, Ohtsuka N, Kusunoki T, et al. Smoking status is associated with serum high molecular adiponectin levels in community-dwelling Japanese men. J Atheroscler Thromb. 2010;17(4):423–30.
59. Shore SA, Terry RD, Flynt L, Xu A, Hug C. Adiponectin attenuates allergen-induced airway inflammation and hyperresponsiveness in mice. J Allergy Clin Immunol. 2006;118(2): 389–95.
60. Medoff BD, Okamoto Y, Leyton P, Weng M, Sandall BP, Raher MJ, et al. Adiponectin-deficiency Increases allergic airway inflammation and pulmonary vascular remodeling. Am J Respir Cell Mol Biol. 2009;41(4):397–406.
61. Yamaguchi N, Argueta JG, Masuhiro Y, Kagishita M, Nonaka K, Saito T, et al. Adiponectin inhibits Toll-like receptor family-induced signaling. FEBS Lett. 2005;579(30):6821–6.
62. Yokota T, Meka CSR, Medina KL, Igarashi H, Comp PC, Takahashi M, et al. Paracrine regulation of fat cell formation in bone marrow cultures via adiponectin and prostaglandins. J Clin Invest. 2002;109(10):1303–10.
63. Yokota T, Oritani K, Takahashi I, Ishikawa J, Matsuyama A, Ouchi N, et al. Adiponectin, a new member of the family of soluble defense collagens, negatively regulates the growth of myelomonocytic progenitors and the functions of macrophages. Blood. 2000;96(5): 1723–32.
64. Summer R, Little FF, Ouchi N, Takemura Y, Aprahamian T, Dwyer D, et al. Alveolar macrophage activation and an emphysema-like phenotype in adiponectin-deficient mice. Am J Physiol Lung Cell Mol Physiol. 2008;294(6):L1035–42.
65. Miller M, Cho JY, Pham A, Ramsdell J, Broide DH. Adiponectin and functional adiponectin receptor 1 are expressed by airway epithelial cells in chronic obstructive pulmonary disease. J Immunol. 2009;182(1):684–91.
66. Sowers MR, Wildman RP, Mancuso P, Eyvazzadeh AD, Karvonen-Gutierrez CA, Rillamas-Sun E, et al. Change in adipocytokines and ghrelin with menopause. Maturitas. 2008;59(2):149–57.
67. Uji Y, Yamamoto H, Tsuchihashi H, Maeda K, Funahashi T, Shimomura I, et al. Adiponectin deficiency is associated with severe polymicrobial sepsis, high inflammatory cytokine levels, and high mortality. Surgery. 2009;145(5):550–7.
68. Takemura Y, Ouchi N, Shibata R, Aprahamian T, Kirber MT, Summer RS, et al. Adiponectin modulates inflammatory reactions via calreticulin receptor-dependent clearance of early apoptotic bodies. J Clin Invest. 2007;117(2):375–86.
69. Saijo S, Nagata K, Nakano Y, Tobe T, Kobayashi Y. Inhibition by adiponectin of IL-8 production by human macrophages upon coculturing with late apoptotic cells. Biochem Biophys Res Commun. 2005;334(4):1180–3.
70. Nakanishi K, Takeda Y, Tetsumoto S, Iwasaki T, Tsujino K, Kuhara H, et al. Involvement of endothelial apoptosis underlying chronic obstructive pulmonary disease-like phenotype in adiponectin-null mice: implications for therapy. Am J Respir Crit Care Med. 2011;183(9): 1164–75.
71. Wang Y, Lam KS, Kraegen EW, Sweeney G, Zhang J, Tso AW, et al. Lipocalin-2 is an inflammatory marker closely associated with obesity, insulin resistance, and hyperglycemia in humans. Clin Chem. 2007;53(1):34–41.
72. Catalán V, Gómez-Ambrosi J, Rodríguez A, Ramírez B, Silva C, Rotellar F, et al. Increased adipose tissue expression of lipocalin-2 in obesity is related to inflammation and matrix metalloproteinase-2 and metalloproteinase-9 activities in humans. J Mol Med. 2009;87(8): 803–13.

73. Chan YR, Liu JS, Pociask DA, Zheng M, Mietzner TA, Berger T, et al. Lipocalin 2 is required for pulmonary host defense against Klebsiella infection. J Immunol. 2009;182(8):4947–56.
74. Wu H, Santoni-Rugiu E, Ralfkiaer E, Porse B, Moser C, Hoiby N, et al. Lipocalin 2 is protective against *E. coli* pneumonia. Respir Res. 2010;11(1):96.
75. Corrales-Medina VF, Valayam J, Serpa JA, Rueda AM, Musher DM. The obesity paradox in community-acquired bacterial pneumonia. Int J Infect Dis. 2011;15(1):e54–7.
76. Baik I, Curhan GC, Rimm EB, Bendich A, Willett WC, Fawzi WW. A prospective study of age and lifestyle factors in relation to community-acquired pneumonia in US men and women. Arch Intern Med. 2000;160(20):3082–8.
77. Womack J, Tien PC, Feldman J, Shin JH, Fennie K, Anastos K, et al. Obesity and immune cell counts in women. Metabolism. 2007;56(7):998–1004.
78. O'Rourke R, Kay T, Scholz M, Diggs B, Jobe B, Lewinsohn D, et al. Alterations in T-cell subset frequency in peripheral blood in obesity. Obes Surg. 2005;15(10):1463–8.
79. Tanaka S, Isoda F, Ishihara Y, Kimura M, Yamakawa T. T lymphopaenia in relation to body mass index and TNF-alpha in human obesity: adequate weight reduction can be corrective. Clin Endocrinol (Oxf). 2001;54(3):347–54.
80. Kim JA, Park HS. White blood cell count and abdominal fat distribution in female obese adolescents. Metabolism. 2008;57(10):1375–9.
81. Nieman DC, Henson DA, Nehlsen-Cannarella SL, Ekkens M, Utter AC, Butterworth DE, et al. Influence of obesity on immune function. J Am Diet Assoc. 1999;99:294–9.
82. Nieman DC, Nehlsen-Cannarella SI, Henson DA, Butterworth DE, Fagoaga OR, Warren BJ, et al. Immune response to obesity and moderate weight loss. Int J Obes Relat Metab Disord. 1996;20(4):353–60.
83. Yang H, Youm YH, Vandanmagsar B, Rood J, Kumar KG, Butler AA, et al. Obesity accelerates thymic aging. Blood. 2009;114(18):3803–12.
84. Lynch LA, O'Connell JM, Kwasnik AK, Cawood TJ, O'Farrelly C, O'Shea DB. Are natural killer cells protecting the metabolically healthy obese patient? Obesity (Silver Spring). 2009;17(3):601–5.
85. O'Shea D, Cawood TJ, O'Farrelly C, Lynch L. Natural killer cells in obesity: impaired function and increased susceptibility to the effects of cigarette smoke. PLoS One. 2010; 5(1):e8660.
86. Chandra RK, Kutty KM. Immunocompetence in obesity. Acta Paediatr Scand. 1980;69(1): 25–30.
87. Palmblad J, Hallberg D, Engstedt L. Polymorphonuclear (PMN) function after small intestinal shunt operation for morbid obesity. Br J Haematol. 1980;44(1):101–8.
88. Zaldivar F, McMurray RG, Nemet D, Galassetti P, Mills PJ, Cooper DM. Body fat and circulating leukocytes in children. Int J Obes (Lond). 2006;30(6):906–11.
89. Dossett LA, Dageforde LA, Swenson BR, Metzger R, Bonatti H, Sawyer RG, et al. Obesity and site-specific nosocomial infection risk in the intensive care unit. Surg Infect (Larchmt). 2009;10(2):137–42.
90. Jain S, Kamimoto L, Bramley AM, Schmitz AM, Benoit SR, Louie J, et al. Hospitalized patients with 2009 H1N1 influenza in the United States, April–June 2009. N Engl J Med. 2009;361(20):1935–44.
91. Weber DJ, Rutala WA, Samsa GP, Santimaw JE, Lemon SM. Obesity as a predictor of poor antibody response to hepatitis B plasma vaccine. JAMA. 1985;254(22):3187–9.
92. Weber DJ, Rutala WA, Samsa GP, Bradshaw SE, Lemon SM. Impaired immunogenicity of hepatitis B vaccine in obese persons. N Engl J Med. 1986;314(21):1393.
93. Sheridan PA, Paich HA, Handy J, Karlsson EA, Hudgens MG, Sammon AB, et al. Obesity is associated with impaired immune response to influenza vaccination in humans. Int J Obes (Lond). 2011;1–6.
94. Vaillant L, La Ruche G, Tarantola A, Barboza P. Epidemiology of fatal cases associated with pandemic H1N1 influenza 2009. Euro Surveill. 2009;14(33):1–6.
95. Jamieson D, Honein M, Rasmussen S, Williams J, Swerdlow D, Biggerstaff M, et al. H1N1 2009 influenza virus infection during pregnancy in the USA. Lancet. 2009;374:451–8.

96. Hanslik T, Boelle PY, Flahault A. Preliminary estimation of risk factors for admission to intensive care units and for death in patients infected with A(H1N1)2009 influenza virus, France, 2009–2010. PLoS Curr. 2010; 2:RRN1150.
97. Naseem A, Satti S, Khan MA, Saeed W. A clinical account of hospitalized 2009 pandemic influenza A (H1N1) cases. J Coll Physicians Surg Pak. 2011;21(2):97–102.
98. La Ruche G, Tarantola A, Barboza P, Vaillant L, Gueguen J, Gastellu-Etchegorry M. The 2009 pandemic H1N1 influenza and indigenous populations of the Americas and the Pacific. Euro Surveill 2009;14(42):1–6.
99. Gill JR, Sheng ZM, Ely SF, Guinee DG, Beasley MB, Suh J, et al. Pulmonary pathologic findings of fatal 2009 pandemic influenza A/H1N1 viral infections. Arch Pathol Lab Med. 2010;134(2):235–43.
100. Fezeu L, Julia C, Henegar A, Bitu J, Hu FB, Grobbee DE, et al. Obesity is associated with higher risk of intensive care unit admission and death in influenza A (H1N1) patients: a systematic review and meta-analysis. Obes Rev. 2011;12:653–659.
101. Dominguez-Cherit G, Lapinsky SE, Macias AE, Pinto R, Espinosa-Perez L, de la Torre A, et al. Critically Ill patients with 2009 influenza A(H1N1) in Mexico. JAMA. 2009;302(17):1880–7.
102. Jhung MA, Swerdlow D, Olsen SJ, Jernigan D, Biggerstaff M, Kamimoto L, et al. Epidemiology of 2009 pandemic influenza A (H1N1) in the United States. Clin Infect Dis. 2011;52(suppl 1):S13–26.
103. Fuhrman C, Bonmarin I, Paty AC, Duport N, Chiron E, Lucas E, et al. Severe hospitalised 2009 pandemic influenza A(H1N1) cases in France, 1 July-15 November 2009. Euro Surveill. 2010;15(2):17–21.
104. Sigurdsson GH, Moller AD, Kristinsson B, Gudlaugsson O, Karason S, Sigurdsson SE, et al. Intensive care patients with influenza A (H1N1) infection in Iceland 2009. Laeknabladid. 2010;96(2):83–90.
105. Mayoral Cortes JM, Ruiz Fernandez J, Pachon Diaz J, Navarro Mari JM, Puell Gomez L, Perez Morilla E, et al. Infection by the pandemic virus (H1N1) 2009 in Andalusia. Rev Esp Salud Publica. 2010;84(5):517–28.
106. Dee S, Jayathissa S. Clinical and epidemiological characteristics of the hospitalised patients due to pandemic H1N1 2009 viral infection: experience at Hutt Hospital, New Zealand. N Z Med J. 2010;123(1312):45–53.
107. Gauzere BA, Bussienne F, Bouchet B, Jabot J, Roussiaux A, Drouet D, et al. Severe cases of A (H1N1)v2009 infection in Reunion Island in 2009 and 2010. Bull Soc Pathol Exot. 2011;104(2):97–104.
108. Cardenosa N, Rodes A, Follia N, Plasencia E, Lafuente S, Arias C, et al. Epidemiological analysis of severe hospitalized 2009 pandemic influenza A (H1N1) cases in Catalonia, Spain. Hum Vaccin. 2011;7:226–9.
109. Rivera Claros R, Marin V, Castillo-Duran C, Jara L, Guardia S, Diaz N. Nutritional status and clinical evolution of hospitalized Chilean infants with infection by respiratory syncytial virus (RSV). Arch Latinoam Nutr. 1999;49(4):326–32.
110. Falagas ME, Kompoti M. Obesity and infection. Lancet Infect Dis. 2006;6(7):438–46.
111. LaCroix AZ, Lipson S, Miles TP, White L. Prospective study of pneumonia hospitalizations and mortality of U.S. older people: the role of chronic conditions, health behaviors, and nutritional status. Public Health Rep. 1989;104(4):350–60.
112. Inoue Y, Koizumi A, Wada Y, Iso H, Watanabe Y, Date C, et al. Risk and protective factors related to mortality from pneumonia among middleaged and elderly community residents: the JACC Study. J Epidemiol. 2007;17(6):194–202.
113. Jedrychowski W, Maugeri U, Flak E, Mroz E, Bianchi I. Predisposition to acute respiratory infections among overweight preadolescent children: an epidemiologic study in Poland. Public Health. 1998;112(3):189–95.
114. Choban PS, Heckler R, Burge JC, Flancbaum L. Increased incidence of nosocomial infections in obese surgical patients. Am Surg. 1995;61(11):1001–5.

115. Canturk Z, Canturk NZ, Cetinarslan B, Utkan NZ, Tarkun I. Nosocomial infections and obesity in surgical patients. Obes Res. 2003;11(6):769–75.
116. Brandt M, Harder K, Walluscheck KP, Schottler J, Rahimi A, Moller F, et al. Severe obesity does not adversely affect perioperative mortality and morbidity in coronary artery bypass surgery. Eur J Cardiothorac Surg. 2001;19(5):662–6.
117. Moulton MJ, Creswell LL, Mackey ME, Cox JL, Rosenbloom M. Obesity is not a risk factor for significant adverse outcomes after cardiac surgery. Circulation. 1996;94(9):II87–92.
118. Dossett LA, Heffernan D, Lightfoot M, Collier B, Diaz JJ, Sawyer RG, et al. Obesity and pulmonary complications in critically injured adults. Chest. 2008;134(5):974–80.
119. Gardner S, Jaing C, McLoughlin K, Slezak T. A microbial detection array (MDA) for viral and bacterial detection. BMC Genomics. 2010;11(1):668.
120. Ahima RS. Digging deeper into obesity. J Clin Invest. 2011;121(6):2076–9.
121. Shah BR, Hux JE. Quantifying the risk of infectious diseases for people with diabetes. Diabetes Care. 2003;26(2):510–3.
122. Valdez R, Narayan KM, Geiss LS, Engelgau MM. Impact of diabetes mellitus on mortality associated with pneumonia and influenza among non-Hispanic black and white US adults. Am J Public Health. 1999;89(11):1715–21.
123. Yende S, van der Poll T, Lee M, Huang DT, Newman AB, Kong L, et al. The influence of pre-existing diabetes mellitus on the host immune response and outcome of pneumonia: analysis of two multicentre cohort studies. Thorax. 2010;65(10):870–7.
124. Koenig SM. Pulmonary complications of obesity. Am J Med Sci. 2001;321(4):249–79.
125. Marik P, Varon J. The obese patient in the ICU. Chest. 1998;113:492–8.
126. Morgan OW, Bramley A, Fowlkes A, Freedman DS, Taylor TH, Gargiullo P, et al. Morbid obesity as a risk factor for hospitalization and death due to 2009 pandemic influenza A(H1N1) disease. PLoS One. 2010;5(3):e9694.
127. Karlsson EA, Beck MA. The burden of obesity on infectious disease. Exp Biol Med (Maywood). 2010;235(12):1412–24.
128. Finlay D, Cantrell DA. Metabolism, migration and memory in cytotoxic T cells. Nat Rev Immunol. 2011;11(2):109–17.
129. Hsu A, Aronoff DM, Phipps J, Goel D, Mancuso P. Leptin improves pulmonary bacterial clearance and survival in ob/ob mice during pneumococcal pneumonia. Clin Exp Immunol. 2007;150(2):332–9.
130. Ordway D, Henao-Tamayo M, Smith E, Shanley C, Harton M, Troudt J, et al. Animal model of *Mycobacterium abscessus* lung infection. J Leukoc Biol. 2008;83(6):1502–11.
131. Wieland CW, Florquin S, Chan ED, Leemans JC, Weijer S, Verbon A, et al. Pulmonary *Mycobacterium tuberculosis* infection in leptin-deficient *ob/ob* mice. Int Immunol. 2005;17(11):1399–408.
132. Fernandez-Riejos P, Najib S, Santos-Alvarez J, Martin-Romero C, Perez-Perez A, Gonzalez-Yanes C, et al. Role of leptin in the activation of immune cells. Mediators Inflamm. 2010;2010:568343.
133. Bailie MB, Standiford TJ, Laichalk LL, Coffey MJ, Strieter RM, Peters-Golden M. Leukotriene-deficient mice manifest enhanced lethality from *Klebsiella pneumonia* in association with decreased alveolar macrophage phagocytic and bactericidal activities. J Immunol. 1996;157:5221–4.
134. Mancuso P, Lewis C, Serezani CH, Goel D, Peters-Golden M. Intrapulmonary administration of leukotriene B4 enhances pulmonary host defense against pneumococcal pneumonia. Infect Immun. 2010;78(5):2264–71.
135. Ikejima S, Sasaki S, Sashinami H, Mori F, Ogawa Y, Nakamura T, et al. Impairment of host resistance to *Listeria monocytogenes* infection in liver of *db/db* and *ob/ob* mice. Diabetes. 2005;54(1):182–9.
136. Conge GA, Gouache P, Joyeux Y, Goichot J, Fournier JM. Influence of different types of experimental obesity on resistance of the mouse to infection by *Salmonella typhimurium* and *Klebsiella pneumoniae*. Ann Nutr Metab. 1988;32(3):113–20.

137. Tschop J, Nogueiras R, Haas-Lockie S, Kasten KR, Castaneda TR, Huber N, et al. CNS leptin action modulates immune response and survival in sepsis. J Neurosci. 2010;30(17):6036–47.
138. Park S, Rich J, Hanses F, Lee JC. Defects in innate immunity predispose C57BL/6 J- Leprdb/ Leprdb mice to infection by *Staphylococcus aureus*. Infect Immun. 2009;77(3):1008–14.
139. Wehrens A, Aebischer T, Meyer TF, Walduck AK. Leptin receptor signaling is required for vaccine-induced protection against *Helicobacter pylori*. Helicobacter. 2008;13(2):94–102.
140. D'Andrea BJ, Wilson GL, Craighead JE. Effect of genetic obesity in mice on the induction of diabetes by encephalomyocarditis virus. Diabetes. 1981;30(5):451–4.
141. Webb SR, Loria RM, Madge GE, Kibrick S. Susceptibility of mice to group B coxsackie virus is influenced by the diabetic gene. J Exp Med. 1976;143(5):1239–48.
142. Plotkin BJ, Paulson D, Chelich A, Jurak D, Cole J, Kasimos J, et al. Immune responsiveness in a rat model for type II diabetes (Zucker rat, fa/fa): susceptibility to *Candida albicans* infection and leucocyte function. J Med Microbiol. 1996;44:277–83.
143. Wieland CW, Stegenga ME, Florquin S, Fantuzzi G, van der Poll T. Leptin and host defense against gram-positive and gram-negative pneumonia in mice. Shock. 2006;25(4):414–9.
144. Ozata M, Ozdemir IC, Licinio J. Human leptin deficiency caused by a missense mutation: multiple endocrine defects, decreased sympathetic tone, and immune system dysfunction indicate new targets for leptin action, greater central than peripheral resistance to the effects of leptin, and spontaneous correction of leptin-mediated defects. J Clin Endocrinol Metab. 1999;84(10):3686–95.
145. Reed AS, Unger EK, Olofsson LE, Piper ML, Myers Jr MG, Xu AW. Functional role of suppressor of cytokine signaling 3 upregulation in hypothalamic leptin resistance and long- term energy homeostasis. Diabetes. 2010;59(4):894–906.
146. Nave H, Mueller G, Siegmund B, Jacobs R, Stroh T, Schueler U, et al. Resistance of Janus kinase-2 dependent leptin signaling in natural killer (NK) cells: a novel mechanism of NK cell dysfunction in diet-induced obesity. Endocrinology. 2008;149(7):3370–8.
147. Papathanassoglou E, El-Haschimi K, Li XC, Matarese G, Strom T, Mantzoros C. Leptin receptor expression and signaling in lymphocytes: kinetics during lymphocyte activation, role in lymphocyte survival, and response to high fat diet in mice. J Immunol. 2006;176(12):7745–52.
148. Tsiotra PC, Pappa V, Raptis SA, Tsigos C. Expression of the long and short leptin receptor isoforms in peripheral blood mononuclear cells: implications for leptin's actions. Metabolism. 2000;49(12):1537–41.
149. Farooqi IS, Bullmore E, Keogh J, Gillard J, O'Rahilly S, Fletcher PC. Leptin regulates striatal regions and human eating behavior. Science. 2007;317(5843):1355.
150. Duggal P, Guo X, Haque R, Peterson KM, Ricklefs S, Mondal D, et al. A mutation in the leptin receptor is associated with *Entamoeba histolytica* infection in children. J Clin Invest. 2011;121(3):1191–8.
151. Buettner R, Scholmerich J, Bollheimer LC. High-fat diets: modeling the metabolic disorders of human obesity in rodents[ast]. Obesity. 2007;15(4):798–808.
152. Shi H, Kokoeva MV, Inouye K, Tzameli I, Yin H, Flier JS. TLR4 links innate immunity and fatty acid-induced insulin resistance. J Clin Invest. 2006;116(11):3015–25.
153. Smith AG, Sheridan PA, Harp JB, Beck MA. Diet-induced obese mice have increased mortality and altered immune responses when infected with influenza virus. J Nutr. 2007;137(5):1236–43.
154. Smith AG, Sheridan PA, Tseng RJ, Sheridan JF, Beck MA. Selective impairment in dendritic cell function and altered antigen-specific CD8+ T-cell responses in diet-induced obese mice infected with influenza virus. Immunology. 2009;126(2):268–79.
155. Karlsson EA, Sheridan PA, Beck MA. Diet-induced obesity in mice reduces the maintenance of influenza-specific CD8+ memory T cells. J Nutr. 2010;140(9):1691–7.
156. Easterbrook JD, Dunfee RL, Schwartzman LM, Jagger BW, Sandouk A, Kash JC, et al. Obese mice have increased morbidity and mortality compared to non-obese mice during infection with the 2009 pandemic H1N1 influenza virus. Influenza Other Respi Viruses. 2011;5(6):418–25.

157. Karlsson EA, Sheridan PA, Beck MA. Diet-induced obesity impairs the T cell memory response to influenza virus infection. J Immunol. 2010;184(6):3127–33.
158. Strandberg L, Verdrengh M, Enge M, Andersson N, Amu S, Önnheim K, et al. Mice chronically fed high-fat diet have increased mortality and disturbed immune response in sepsis. PLoS One. 2009;4(10):e7605.
159. Amar S, Zhou Q, Shaik-Dasthagirisaheb Y, Leeman S. Diet-induced obesity in mice causes changes in immune responses and bone loss manifested by bacterial challenge. Proc Natl Acad Sci USA. 2007;104(51):20466–71.

Chapter 4
Pathogenesis of Obstructive Sleep Apnea in Obesity

Jason Paul Kirkness and Susheel P. Patil

Abstract Obstructive sleep apnea is a sleep-related breathing disorder characterized by repetitive upper airway obstruction and is associated with significant morbidity and mortality. Obesity is one of the primary modifiable risk factors for the management of patients with sleep apnea as there is a positive association between the increasing obesity prevalence and sleep apnea prevalence. Several mechanisms link obesity and sleep apnea pathogenesis, including the potential increase in additional mechanical load on the upper and lower respiratory systems from regional adiposity, possible effects of obesity-related inflammation on neuromuscular and neuroventilatory function of the upper airway, or a combination of these effects. By examining the relationship between obesity and obstructive sleep apnea as well as the mechanisms by which obesity may contribute to the development of sleep apnea and its related comorbidities, we can evaluate the effect of weight reduction on the management of sleep apnea.

Keywords Sleep apnea risk factors • Regional adiposity • Upper airway pathophysiology • Pharynx • Weight loss • Sleep-disordered breathing treatments • Constant positive air pressure • Bariatric surgery

J.P. Kirkness, Ph.D. (✉)
Division of Pulmonary and Critical Care Medicine, Johns Hopkins School of Medicine, 5501 Hopkins Bayview Circle, Baltimore, MD 21224, USA
e-mail: Jason.Kirkness@jhmi.edu

S.P. Patil, M.D., Ph.D.
Division of Pulmonary and Critical Care Medicine, Johns Hopkins School of Medicine, 5501 Hopkins Bayview Circle, Room 4B.41, Baltimore, MD 21224, USA
e-mail: spatil@jhmi.edu

A.E. Dixon and E.M. Clerisme-Beaty (eds.), *Obesity and Lung Disease: A Guide to Management*, Respiratory Medicine, DOI 10.1007/978-1-62703-053-3_4,

Objectives

- Review the epidemiology of obesity prevalence and OSA risk.
- Examine the association between obesity and OSA-related morbidity.
- Understand the mechanisms by which obesity may contribute to the development of sleep apnea.
- Illustrate the effect of weight loss on OSA risk.

Introduction

Obstructive sleep apnea is a sleep-related breathing disorder characterized by repetitive upper airway obstruction during sleep which results in recurrent oxyhemoglobin desaturations and arousals. Sleep apnea is associated with significant morbidity and mortality, including increased risk of all-cause mortality [1], cardiovascular disease [2], and lower quality of life [3]. Although there are several approved treatments for obstructive sleep apnea, such as positive-pressure ventilation, oral devices, and oral-facial surgery, one of the mainstays of the management of patients with sleep apnea involves addressing modifiable risk factors such as obesity.

Obesity remains the most important determinant associated with the development of the sleep apnea syndrome [4–6]. Several epidemiologic studies have reported a positive association between the increasing obesity prevalence and sleep apnea prevalence. The effect of obesity on sleep apnea risk appears to be dependent on body fat distribution, with central obesity being a better predictor of sleep apnea severity than body mass index [7]. Although not completely understood, several mechanisms have been proposed to explain the link between regional adipose tissue deposits and sleep apnea. These include the potential increase in additional mechanical load on the upper and lower respiratory systems from regional adiposity, possible effects of obesity-related inflammation on neuromuscular and neuroventilatory function of the upper airway, or a combination of these effects.

This chapter will focus on the relationship between obesity and obstructive sleep apnea by examining the mechanisms by which obesity may contribute to the development of sleep apnea and its related comorbidities. In addition, we will also evaluate the effect of weight reduction on sleep apnea pathophysiology and related morbidity.

Obstructive Sleep Apnea: Diagnosis, Definitions, and Nomenclature

Obstructive sleep apnea syndrome is defined as an apnea-hypopnea index (AHI) >5 events/hour associated with excessive sleepiness. Obstructive apneas are defined as ≥90% reduction in airflow for ≥10 s with continued or increased effort during this period [8]. The recommended hypopnea definition is a >30% decline in airflow for ≥10 s in association with a >4% oxyhemoglobin desaturation. An alternative hypopnea definition which incorporates arousals from sleep is also acceptable and is defined as a >50% decline in airflow with a >3% oxyhemoglobin desaturation or an arousal. The severity of sleep apnea is determined based on the frequency of AHI per hour of sleep with 5.0–14.9 events/hour, 15.0–29.9 events/hour, and >30 events/hour, being classified as mild, moderate, and severe sleep apnea, respectively. However, even though the AHI reflects the frequency of collapse, it does not provide information on the severity of the neuromechanical properties that predispose the upper airway to collapse.

Clinical Characteristics of Obstructive Sleep Apnea

Frequent snoring is one of the most frequently noted nocturnal symptoms in sleep apnea. Snoring is either an early symptom of upper airway airflow limitation or a contributor to the development of airway obstruction by causing local tissue damage and inflammation. Other symptoms include feeling of choking or breathlessness at night [9], restlessness or other types of body movements during sleep, and nocturia. Obstructive sleep apnea is associated with suppression of stage 3 and 4 sleep or REM sleep, secondary to sleep-related breathing problems [10, 11] from high frequency bursts of EEG activity, which leads to multiple arousals from sleep and sleep fragmentation. The incidence of sleep fragmentation is a critical factor contributing to daytime sleepiness [12, 13]. In addition, patients with sleep apnea also have daytime symptoms, such as morning headaches, dry sore throat, lethargy, and excessive daytime sleepiness. Sleep apnea is also associated with cognitive and functional impairments including memory loss, impaired concentration, hypnagogic hallucinations, depression, irritability, and sexual dysfunction [14–16].

Several modifiable risk factors have been identified to contribute to obstructive sleep apnea. Lifestyle factors such as diet, alcohol consumption, smoking, and use of central nervous system depressants have been shown to contribute to the incidence of apnea frequency and duration [17]. Sleep deprivation, irregular sleep patterns [18], and allergic rhinitis are also potential contributory factors to worsening sleep apnea [19]. However, as mentioned above, obesity is the most prevalent independent and confounding risk factor for determining the prevalence of obstructive sleep apnea.

Epidemiology of Obesity and Obstructive Sleep Apnea

Prevalence

The most accepted sleep apnea prevalence data comes from the Wisconsin Sleep Cohort, a random sample of Wisconsin state employees between the ages of 30 and 60 years old [4]. In this study, the prevalence of obstructive sleep apnea ranged from

2% to 9% in women and 4% to 24% in men depending on whether the diagnosis of sleep apnea was based solely on AHI cut or the combination of AHI and significant self-reported sleepiness.

The prevalence of sleep apnea in severely obese individuals (mean BMI >40 kg/m^2) is exceedingly high, with rates of at least 40% [20–22]. In the landmark study by Young et al., a one standard deviation increase in body mass index was associated with a fourfold increase in risk for sleep apnea [4]. However, we have documented a prevalence of approximately 40% in an asymptomatic community cohort of overweight and obese but otherwise healthy men. Data from the US National Health and Nutrition Examination Survey show a dramatic rise in the prevalence of obesity, with prevalence estimates of approximately 60% overweight (BMI >25 kg/m^2) and 30% obese (BMI >30 kg/m^2) among US adults [23].

Mild to moderate obesity has been associated with markedly increased sleep apnea prevalence [24, 25], and severe obesity has been linked to sleep apnea of increased severity [20, 26]. Approximately 70% of those with sleep apnea are obese [27], while the prevalence of sleep apnea in obese men and women is about 40% [25]. There appears to be a progression in the association between obesity and sleep apnea, in that a higher body mass index is associated with higher prevalence of disease [28]. The specific mechanisms linking obesity and sleep apnea are discussed below.

Risk Factors for OSA

It is well recognized that male sex constitutes a significant risk factor for sleep apnea as evidenced by a two- to threefold increased risk of sleep apnea in men in the population at large [4]. The increased risk has been attributed to sex-related differences in body fat distribution. Men manifest a predominantly central pattern of fat distribution compared to women [29–32]. Direct mechanical effects of central adiposity on the upper airway predispose to upper airway narrowing [33–35], collapse [31, 36–41], and airflow obstruction during sleep. This may explain why men typically develop sleep apnea at a lower BMI than women.

The increased prevalence in the elderly has been recently confirmed in the Sleep Heart Health Study, a longitudinal study of the cardiovascular consequences of sleep apnea [25]. Throughout adult life, there is an inexorable decline in skeletal muscle mass and strength and a concurrent increase in total and percent body fat [42, 43]. Aging is associated with decrease in the circulating levels of several hormones including testosterone, DHEAS, estrogen, and growth hormone by 70% or more, which may contribute to the increased fat accumulation with age [44–46]. Indeed, while premenopausal women appear to be protected against sleep apnea [25], epidemiologic studies have demonstrated that menopause is a significant independent risk factor for the development of sleep apnea, suggesting that alterations in hormonal status also play a role in the disorder. Women experience a relatively defined period of rapid decline in estrogen, although most hormones in both genders gradually decline such that many older adults have levels that would be considered pathological in younger adults. Moreover, in a recent study, women developed adverse adipokine and inflammatory profiles during the menopausal transition as a consequence of increased central adiposity [47]. Studies have shown that women who are postmenopausal have higher total fat mass and a different distribution of body fat [48]. After menopause, body fat distribution tends to change from a high proportion of peripheral fat to a higher proportion of central fat, more closely resembling the body fat distribution of a male [49]. Restoration to "normal" levels does result in increased lean mass and decreased adiposity. Whether changes in body fat composition related to menopause contribute to this increased risk of sleep apnea is unknown. Ironically, both epidemiologic and small clinical studies of hormone replacement therapy administration have yielded conflicting results [50]. Studies examining the prevalence of sleep apnea in middle age and elderly populations [25] have shown that the prevalence of sleep apnea is significantly higher in the elderly compared to the middle-aged persons [51–53].

While these associations do not impute causality, changes or differences in hormonal status, metabolism, and body composition may represent intermediate or causal risk factors for the development of sleep apnea.

Regional Fat Distribution

Regional fat distribution is an important determinant of the impact of obesity on sleep apnea in individuals. Notably, male gender constitutes a particularly strong risk factor, conferring a two- to threefold increased risk of sleep apnea relative to females [25, 54]. Mechanistic studies of upper airway collapse have shown increasing obesity (BMI) to cause more upper airway collapse in men compared to women (Fig. 4.1) [55, 56].

Several other lines of evidence also suggest that obesity is associated with anatomic alterations that predispose to upper airway obstruction during sleep. First, obesity has been associated with increases in neck circumference and greater amounts of fat deposited around the upper airway [29, 57]. Second, upper airway collapsibility is greater in obese compared to nonobese individuals [26] and less amenable to treatment with anterior mandibular advancement during complete neuromuscular blockade [40]. Third, obesity, and in particular central obesity, reduces lung volume [58] that may increase upper airway collapsibility by decreasing longitudinal traction on the upper airway [59, 60].

The mechanistic role excessive deposition of adipose tissue plays in sleep apnea severity is described in brief. Adipose tissue in the peripharyngeal area of the neck is thought to apply pressure to the extraluminal tissue surrounding the upper airway [61]. Fat in the thoracic compartment compresses the rib cage reducing lung volume (see Chap. 1) [62]. Abdominal fat may result in cranial displacement of the diaphragm decreasing longitudinal tension on the upper airway, increasing upper airway collapsibility [63, 64]. Reduced prevalence and severity of sleep apnea in obese women are likely to be due to differential distribution of excess fat tending to deposit peripherally around the hips, buttocks, and thighs. In contrast, men tend to distribute excess fat more centrally on the abdomen and neck [65]. Consequently, even though women have a proportionally greater fat mass than men, they have reduced mechanical loads on their upper airway [65].

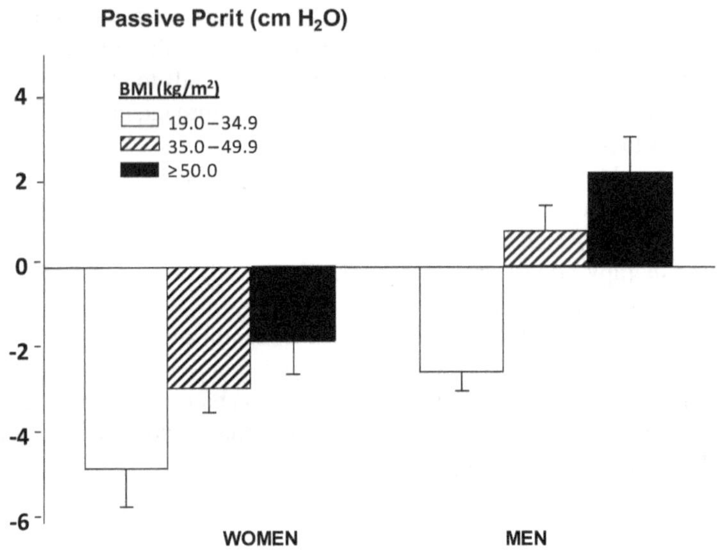

Fig. 4.1 In men and women, there is a significant correlation between the biomechanical upper airway collapsibility (passive P_{CRIT}) and body mass index (adjusted for age). Overall, the passive P_{CRIT} for each BMI tertile was lower in women compared to men. The magnitude of the change in P_{CRIT} per tertile of body mass index unit was almost double in men compared to women

Morbidity/Mortality

The main consequences of sleep apnea are increased cardiovascular morbidity and mortality [66–69], the metabolic sequelae [70–74], traffic or work-related accidents due to sleepiness [75, 76], and quality of life impairment [25, 77–79]. In addition, afflicted individuals may suffer from severe daytime sleepiness that can affect performance and cognitive function. In the Sleep Heart Health Study, a prospective cohort study of all-cause mortality in patients with untreated sleep apnea, participants with severe sleep-disordered breathing (an AHI of ≥30) were about one and a half times more likely to die from any cause than those without any sleep-disordered breathing after adjustment for potential confounding factors [1]. Given the concomitant effect of obesity on mortality and cardiovascular risk, it is unclear to what extent the morbidity and mortality associated with sleep apnea is due to obesity.

Cardiovascular Disease

Both obesity and sleep apnea have been associated with hypertension [24, 80, 81] and cardiovascular disease [82, 83]. The mechanisms through which obstructive sleep apnea promotes daytime hypertension have not been fully elucidated.

Several mechanisms have been proposed, including neural, humeral, and cellular factors. However, converging evidence from physiological studies in humans and animals points toward intermittent hypoxia and sympathetic nervous system activation as playing central roles. Repetitive episodes of obstructive apnea, hypoxia, and hypercapnia act through chemoreceptor reflexes and other mechanisms to increase sympathetic drive [84]. Remarkably, the high sympathetic drive is present even during daytime wakefulness when subjects are breathing normally and both arterial oxygen saturation and carbon dioxide levels are also normal. This is true whether these patients are newly diagnosed, never-treated sleep apnea patients on no medications, or whether they are on antihypertensive therapy [84–86]. Several neural and humeral mechanisms may contribute to maintenance of higher sympathetic activity and blood pressure during wakefulness including baroreflex dysfunction [86, 87], chemoreflex dysfunction [88, 89], vasoconstrictor effects of nocturnal endothelin release [90], and endothelial dysfunction [91]. Although obesity is a known risk factor for both obstructive sleep apnea and cardiovascular disease, little is known about the concomitant risk of developing these two conditions [92].

Metabolic Consequences

Obesity leads to extreme metabolic disturbances, which are related to alterations in signaling factors produced by adipose tissue [93, 94]. One of the key factors secreted by adipocytes is leptin that suppresses appetite, increases metabolic rate, and improves insulin sensitivity of peripheral tissues [95–102]. Fat accumulation leads to increases in leptin expression, secretion, and pronounced circulating concentrations [103, 104] and glucose intolerance [24, 105, 106].

Regional fat redistribution (lipodystrophy) has also been associated with hyperlipidemia, insulin resistance, and hypertension [107–110]. These clinical findings combine to form the metabolic syndrome [111], a disorder with convenient overlap between the development of central adiposity and disturbances in metabolism and cardiovascular control. Recent studies have shown that leptin replacement significantly reverses the metabolic abnormalities in patients with the metabolic syndrome and lipoatrophy due either to genetic mutation or medication-related leptin deficiency [112–114]. A true leptin deficiency per se is rare, whereas central leptin resistance with high levels of circulating leptin is common in obesity [115, 116]. Peripherally, redistribution of body fat due to changing leptin levels may alter upper airway mechanical loads and work of breathing. In obesity, serum leptin levels are more closely associated with hypoventilation than body mass index or fat mass; therefore, leptin resistance may reflect both a resistance to the satiety effects of leptin and a resistance to the respiratory stimulatory effects. On the other hand, increased leptin levels in obesity hypoventilation syndrome may reflect neuroventilatory compensatory response to counteract a sleep-associated rise in CO_2 [117, 118]. The controversy of the role of leptin in sleep apnea may be attributed to the conflicting mechanisms of action in peripherally versus centrally located fat.

Sleep apnea may contribute to both metabolic dysregulation and systemic inflammation in patients with metabolic syndrome, regardless of symptoms of daytime sleepiness [119]. Sleep apnea severity is also linked with alterations in glucose homeostasis in severely obese men and women across a range of glucose tolerances [73, 120, 121]. Moreover, the level of increased basal pancreatic beta-cell function is associated with severity of sleep apnea in those with normal but not those with impaired glucose metabolism. It has been shown that sleep apnea is associated with increased triglycerides and glucose concentrations as well as levels of cholesterol/HDL ratio, uric acid, and C-reactive protein [122]. Obesity and insulin resistance also lead to liver steatosis, but causes of progression of hepatic steatosis to nonalcoholic steatohepatitis are not known [123, 124]. The impact of hypoxic stress of sleep apnea may be implicated in the development of insulin resistance and nonalcoholic steatohepatitis in severe obesity, although more evidence is required.

Sleepiness, Neurocognitive Dysfunction, and Quality of Life

Polysomnographic evidence of sleep disruption due to sleep apnea has been associated with daytime sleepiness [125], mood and neurocognitive dysfunction [126, 127], and substantially increased risk of motor vehicle and workplace accidents [76, 128, 129].

Sleep apnea is also associated with a range of defects in neurocognitive function [3]. Both sleep fragmentation and hypoxemia are thought to contribute [127, 130]. The predominant cognitive defects associated with sleep apnea relate to difficulties in maintaining attention and alertness and impairments in memory and executive function [131]. Sleep apnea patients regularly report deficits in quality of life in various domains, including work performance, relationships, and fatigue [130]. CPAP use has been related to improvements in quality of life in sleep apnea patients [132]. However, this finding is not always consistent [133], likely due to lack of treatment efficacy related to suboptimal adherence [134].

Obesity also has a major negative impact on both physical and mental components of health-related quality of life [135, 136]. Several studies have now clearly demonstrated that, in the absence of sleep apnea, obese patients commonly report symptoms of poor sleep quality and excessive daytime sleepiness [137], but the cause in the absence of sleep apnea remains unclear. Obesity is associated with other conditions that may disrupt sleep such as asthma, gastroesophageal reflux, osteoarthritis, and nocturia. Thus, the combination of obesity and moderate to severe sleep apnea is formidable in its impairment of quality of life.

Pathophysiology of Obstructive Sleep Apnea

The number of investigations of the mechanical properties of the upper airway, principally attempting to understand the pathophysiology of the sleep apnea, has rapidly increased in the preceding 20–30 years. Studies evaluating airway pressure and airflow measurements have revealed that the upper airway in sleep apnea is more collapsible than that of normal healthy subjects [138, 139]. The relationship between the structurally smaller airway and the reductions in upper airway function as measured by pressure and airflow highlights the role of the upper airway collapsibility in sleep apnea.

Mechanical, nonmechanical, and genetic factors are involved in the development of sleep apnea. Mechanical factors include upper airway anatomy, neck and jaw posture, surface adhesive forces, tracheal tug, and gravity. Any anatomic feature that decreases the size of the upper airway increases the risk of sleep apnea. During sleep, supine positioning and gravitational forces allow the retroposition of the tongue and soft palate reducing the cross-sectional area of the upper airway. Nonmechanical factors largely consist of pharyngeal dilator muscles and neuroventilatory modulators (such as pharmaceutical or biochemical stimulants or suppressants). Genetic factors affecting sleep apnea and its risk factors are burgeoning area of discovery.

Upper Airway Imaging

High positive predictive value for presence of sleep apnea can be obtained by direct linear measurements of the oral cavity, BMI, and neck circumference [140]. Cephalometric measurements identified that retrognathia, elongated soft palate, narrow posterior airway space, and inferiorly positioned hyoid bone are characteristics of sleep apnea [141]. Measurements revealed that the mandible is both small and repositioned [142] and the hyoid bone more inferiorly positioned in sleep apnea [143]. More recently, three-dimensional upper airway CT in sleep apnea clearly showed dynamic airway obstruction in sleep apnea; however, this is not strongly correlated with disease severity [144]. Results from CT imaging studies have demonstrated lateral wall folding in the upper airway [145] leading to decrease airway caliber during sleep in both normal subjects and sleep apnea patients [34, 146], with increased lateral airway dimensions with the application of CPAP [147].

The lateral pharyngeal walls are a complex structure made up of a number of muscles, lymphoid tissue, and pharyngeal mucosa. Although the mechanisms that control the dimensions of the lateral walls remain undefined, deposition of adipose tissue due to increasing obesity is likely to change the upper airway properties. Increased edema and possibly increased fat content of the tongue muscles in sleep apnea have also been investigated using MRI [148].

Thus, findings from various imaging studies have revealed that the upper airway in sleep apnea is anatomically smaller and more elliptical in shape than in normal healthy subjects. These factors predispose the upper airway of sleep apnea patients to collapse particularly during sleep and are significantly compromised in obesity.

Regional Obesity and Upper Airway Function

Truncal obesity has two potential impacts on upper airway collapsibility. Firstly, its effects may be mediated through direct compression of the upper airway from

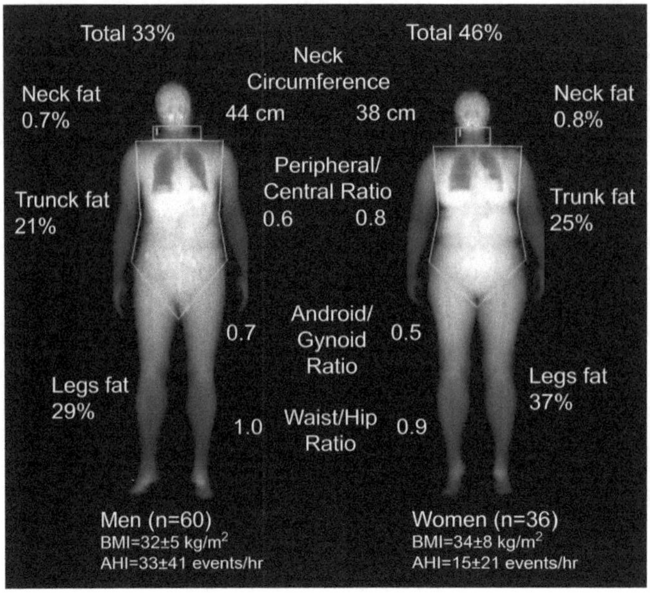

Fig. 4.2 Sex difference in regional body fat distribution contributes to altered mechanical loads. When matched for BMI, the severity of sleep-disordered breathing events is high in men, whereas the percentage of total body fat is greater in women

peripharyngeal fat deposition. Secondly, truncal obesity-associated reductions in lung volume [58] may increase upper airway collapsibility by decreasing longitudinal traction on the upper airway [59, 60]. In recent studies, it has been demonstrated that decreases in lung volume were associated with substantial worsening of upper airway collapsibility with P_{CRIT} increasing by ~11 cmH_2O L^{-1} [64].

There is an association of traditional anthropometric measures and DXA-measured mass with each other and with sleep apnea severity in a case series of men and women [149]. When considered separately, DXA measures of fat mass were more predictive of sleep apnea severity than anthropometric measures in women. The men and women in this series had comparable BMI, but the men had a lower ratio of fat to lean body mass in all body regions, and neck circumference and weight were as predictive of disease severity as DXA-measured fat mass in men (Fig. 4.2). In both men and women, however, a combination of anthropometric measurements and DXA-measured mass improved this predictive capacity. DXA measures may therefore have clinical and epidemiological utility.

In both men and women, centrally located rather than peripherally located fat contributes to the pathogenesis and severity of sleep apnea. However, there are substantial gender-based differences in the association between fat distribution and severity of sleep apnea. Neck fat is associated with disease severity in women but not in men, while neck circumference was associated with disease severity in both genders. In men, lean tissue is a substantial contributor to neck circumference; however, in women, an increased neck circumference is more likely to be associated with an increase in fat. This suggests that the male preponderance of sleep apnea is likely to be related to more than simply the direct compressive effect of neck fat on the airway.

The relative amount of abdominal fat is associated with sleep apnea severity in men, and visceral adipose tissue in the abdomen has been found to correlate with AHI [32]. The role of abdominal fat in upper airway instability is increasingly recognized when recumbent abdominal obesity is likely to be associated with increased cranial displacement of the diaphragm, decreasing longitudinal tracheal tension, and increasing upper airway collapse [63]. Accumulation of fat in the chest wall (abdominal and thoracic) also decreases functional residual capacity, particularly when recumbent and asleep, increasing intrathoracic pressure and thereby extramural tissue pressure at the thoracic inlet, further increasing upper airway collapsibility [150].

In studies examining the predictive value of regional obesity measures on the severity of sleep apnea over traditional surrogate measures of obesity such as neck and waist circumference and BMI, most [151–153], but not all [154, 155], concluded abdominal fat measures to be a better predictor of metabolic risk factors than anthropometric surrogates. Clinical epidemiological studies often rely upon BMI or waist circumference to control for the confounding influence of obesity when investigating risk factors. However, men and women who are similar with respect to both BMI and waist circumference were found to have differences in fat and lean mass in the whole body and regionally. Therefore, reliance upon BMI or waist circumference alone to measure obesity, which confounds the relationship between almost all cardiovascular and metabolic risk factors, is likely to misrepresent the potentially important influence of regional obesity.

Nonmechanical Factors

Sleep apnea is due to a deficit of both the mechanical properties of the upper airway and the ability to adequately activate neuroventilatory and neuromuscular responses during obstructed breathing. Neuroventilatory factors such as proinflammatory cytokines can modulate upper airway muscle activity. A loss of neuromuscular compensatory activity during sleep prevents dilating forces from providing stability to a collapsible airway. Some circulating factors that suppress upper airway stability during sleep have familial aggregation and are thus also likely to have inherited genetic basis. While not an exhaustive review of the nonmechanical characteristics attributable to obstructive sleep apnea or obesity, the predominant nonmechanical factors that link pathogenesis of obesity and obstructive sleep apnea are discussed below.

Neuroventilatory and Humeral Factors

Obesity generates a proinflammatory condition [156–158] due to the abundant sources of cytokines in adipose tissue [159–167]. Some of these cytokines including tumor necrosis factor-α (TNF-α), TNF-α receptor 1 (TNF-αR1), interleukin-6 (IL-6), and interleukin-1β (IL-1β) have neuroventilatory modulating properties during sleep [168–175]. In particular, TNF-α and its soluble receptor, TNF-αR1, markedly increase due to sleep deprivation [176] and help to mediate the somnogenic effect of TNF-α centrally [171, 173, 174, 177]. Moreover, TNF-α activity [168–172, 177] can increase sleep apnea susceptibility and severity [175]. Its depressant effects on the central nervous system can account for defects in upper airway neuroventilatory control in normal men compared to women [178–182]. Progression of obesity and sleep apnea severity propagate sleep fragmentation and hypoxia-induced free radicals that trigger additional elevations in inflammatory cytokines [116, 164, 165, 183–195], suppressing pharyngeal neuromuscular activity [116, 164, 188, 191–195]. Nevertheless, the impact of sleep apnea on inflammatory cytokines remains unclear in view of recent evidence demonstrating no change [196] or reductions [165] in cytokines with standard CPAP treatment for sleep apnea. Primary treatment of obesity may conservatively alter upper airway structural properties, as well as improve pharyngeal muscle activity via suppression of proinflammatory conditions.

Pharyngeal Muscle Activity

Sleep has a differential effect on the basal activity of tonic versus phasic upper airway muscles [197] in that with sleep onset, there is a decrement in upper airway dilator muscle activity that may attribute to a decrease in airway caliber [198]. It is unclear as to whether the decreased upper airway muscle activity varies with different sleep stages.

In sleep apnea patients, abnormal neuromuscular control of pharyngeal dilating muscles in conjunction with a mechanically disadvantaged airway leads to reduced airflow during sleep. There are likely multiple reasons for this, including defects in ventilatory control, defects in arousal mechanisms, and diminished responses to negative upper airway pressure during sleep [199]. Thus, the loss of augmented dilator muscle activity may predispose sleep apnea patients to airway obstruction, with passive airway occlusion in response to negative airway pressures.

Obesity and fatty deposit in the upper airway tissues may decrease the mechanical advantage and likely reduce the efficiency of upper airway dilator muscles during sleep during obstruction (Fig. 4.3). The collapsibility of the upper airway can be described by two functional components [139]: (1) the anatomical and passive mechanical properties (passive P_{CRIT} as described above) and (2) the neuromuscular compensatory responses to upper airway obstruction (Δactive responses). The combination of the passive P_{CRIT} and the compensatory responses is known as the active P_{CRIT} and quantifies an individual's ability to maintain airway patency during sleep. Figure 4.3 quantifies the relative contribution of mechanical and nonmechanical factors to weight-loss-related decreases in upper airway collapsibility.

Hereditary and Genetic Factors

Familial factors also play a role in the expression of sleep apnea as relatives of patients with sleep apnea have a two- to fourfold increased risk of sleep apnea

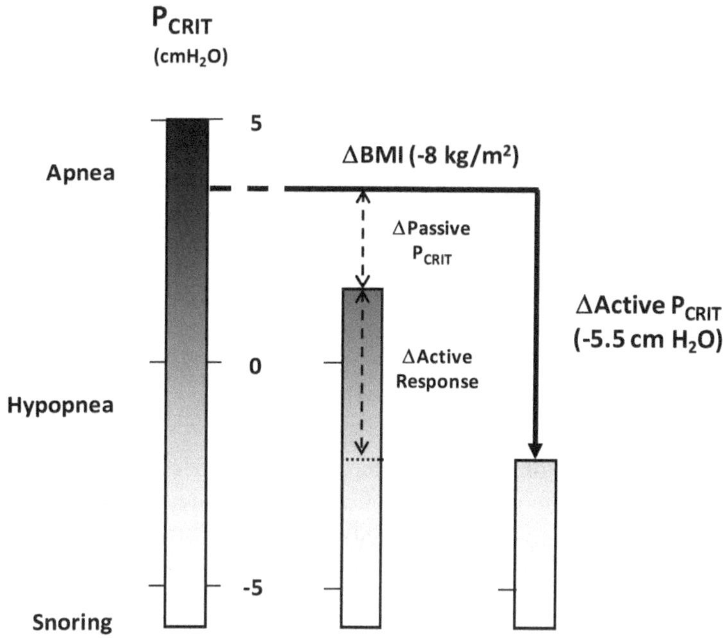

Fig. 4.3 *Extrapolation of P_{CRIT} versus BMI cross-sectional data to longitudinal weight-loss-mediated decrease in P_{CRIT}.* Upper airway collapsibility (P_{CRIT}) is a marker of sleep apnea severity where increased P_{CRIT} is characteristic of more obstructed airway (*left bar*). A previous study demonstrated a 5.5-cmH_2O decrease in the active P_{CRIT} [26], which represents the combined mechanical (passive P_{CRIT}) and nonmechanical (Δactive response) factors of upper airway collapsibility associated with weight loss of ~8 kg/m^2 [244]. Approximately 2 cmH_2O can be attributed to change in the passive P_{CRIT}, with the remainder being attributable to increases in active responses with weight loss

compared with non-apneic subjects. Several case series and familial aggregation studies have demonstrated heritability of factors associated with sleep apnea [200–208]. Subjective excessive daytime sleepiness and self-reported snoring have been demonstrated to have inherited or shared environmental factors that contribute to the development of sleep apnea [209]. Studies also show that sleep apnea and obesity share substantial genetic basis but have underscored the potential importance of genetic factors unrelated to obesity that may determine sleep apnea susceptibility [204, 208]. Anatomical factors of the upper airway, such as the lateral pharyngeal walls and tongue volume, are partially determined by genetic factors [205, 207]. For example, in African Americans, the serotonin receptor 2a gene was associated with an increased odds ratio for risk of sleep apnea. Serotonin effects sleep-wake cycles, in particular, the amount of rapid eye movement (REM) sleep and regulation of upper airway dilator muscle through an excitatory influence on hypoglossal motor output. Serotonin is involved in appetite regulation, thus playing a role in obesity.

Both obesity and sleep apnea are complex disorders, which interact in an intricate manner. Obesity has a strong genetic basis, as has sleep apnea, which is likely due to the effects of small to moderate contributions from multiple genetic loci.

As previously mentioned above, obesity is a strong risk factor for sleep apnea, and it is likely that sleep apnea contributes to obesity. It is possible that many susceptibility genes for obesity and sleep apnea are therefore shared. Reports demonstrate that approximately half of the genetic variance in AHI is shared with obesity. Genetic factors that increase obesity are likely to be risk factors for apnea. Intermediate phenotypes for sleep apnea are upper airway collapsibility, ventilatory control, upper airway muscle function, and sleep quality. On the other hand, environmental factors that are produced by sleep apnea such as intermittent hypoxia and sleep fragmentation may interact with obesity.

Treatment of Obstructive Sleep Apnea

Current management regimes for long-term control of sleep apnea are aimed at providing pneumatic (continuous positive airway pressure, CPAP) or mechanical (various dental devices, e.g., mandibular advancement splints) support for the upper airway during sleep and need to be applied nightly. Although cumbersome, these therapies can be very successful (especially CPAP) at reducing sleep-disordered breathing but suffer from significant patient compliance, acceptance, and resource-allocation issues. There is a growing need to develop less invasive, more sophisticated, and more patient-"friendly" adjunct therapies, especially preventive therapies that could be applied widely to combat disease progression. Positional therapy can be implemented in mild disease, but not usually for severe sleep-disordered breathing. Other novel treatment modalities include neuromuscular stimulation of upper airway dilator muscles, high-flow nasal insufflations, and expiratory nasal splints.

In addition to these therapeutic interventions, treatment of obesity using behavioral and lifestyle modifications or surgery may be an important initial approach to affect both mechanical and neuroventilatory factors.

Weight Loss and Improved Upper Airway Function During Sleep

Lifestyle changes such as losing weight have been shown to improve sleep apnea severity. In a longitudinal cohort study, a 10% weight loss was associated with a 26% decrease in AHI [5]. It has been speculated that sleep apnea itself may modulate secretion of hormones and other biological mediators which promote obesity or preferential abdominal fat accumulation, thus further engaging sleep apnea and metabolic dysfunction in a vicious cycle [210, 211]. However, to date, there is no strong evidence to show that control of sleep apnea per se affects fat accumulation or its distribution. Studies have reported that a decrease in the visceral fat is concomitant with a decrease in leptin levels with CPAP treatment of sleep apnea [212, 213]. Alternatively, weight loss may lead to complete resolution of sleep apnea, especially in patients with mild to moderate AHI range [214]. Thus, a combination of CPAP and behavioral modification is more effective for weight reduction than behavioral modification alone, suggesting a contributory effect of CPAP treatment toward weight control [215].

Weight reduction is best achieved through behavioral changes aimed at reducing energy intake via dietary modifications and increasing energy expenditure using physical activity. For those with morbid obesity, bariatric surgery has been used and shown to improve the individual's metabolic profile as well as their sleep-disordered breathing [216–218]. Reduction of adiposity will not only decrease the severity of sleep apnea but also directly mitigate cardiometabolic derangements and disease outcomes. Hence, active measures targeted at weight control should be considered an integral part of sleep apnea management.

Longitudinal Post-Bariatric Surgery Weight Loss

Weight loss remains highly effective in treating sleep apnea [26, 214, 219–226]. In early studies, we demonstrated that a 10–15% reduction in body weight leads to an approximately 50% reduction in sleep apnea severity (apnea-hypopnea index) in moderately obese male patients [26, 223]. Marked weight loss can be achieved with bariatric surgery, which combines gastric restriction and/or intestinal bypass to induce early satiety and nutrient malabsorption [227–231], and leads to an approximately 60% loss in excess body weight [218, 232–243]. Weight loss following bariatric surgery leads to reductions in upper airway mechanical loads and improvements in pharyngeal neuromuscular control [244], which are likely related to improvements in lung volume and systemic inflammation [245–249].

Although there have only been a limited number of studies that have evaluated the effect of substantial weight loss on polysomnography, all have shown polysomnographic evidence of significant improvements or resolution of sleep apnea [250, 251]. In a recent meta-analysis, bariatric surgery has been documented to produce dramatic improvements in sleep apnea with reductions in apnea-hypopnea index of 33.9 episodes/hour (95% CI, 17.5–50.2 episodes/hour) and sleep apnea resolution in 85.7% (95% CI, 79.2–92.2%) of patients [252]. It has previously been demonstrated that these improvements are due to a decrease in upper airway collapsibility (P_{CRIT}) [26, 223], although the mechanism for this reduction was not known. Changes in upper airway collapsibility as obesity and regional fat distribution change postoperatively suggest a pathogenic link between obesity and upper airway dysfunction in sleep apnea. However, it is still unknown how to predict which patients will have improved upper airway function during sleep following weight loss interventions.

Conclusion

Obesity is the main risk factor for the development of sleep apnea. Current evidence suggests that obesity and central adiposity lead to alterations in pharyngeal neural and mechanical control that increase collapsibility and sleep apnea susceptibility.

In addition, systemic and local (pharyngeal) inflammatory mechanisms related to obesity may further compromise neuromuscular control mechanisms in obesity and lead to a worsening of sleep apnea over time. A combined therapeutic approach of sleep apnea treatment and weight loss may lead to improved clinical outcome.

References

1. Punjabi NM, Caffo BS, Goodwin JL, Gottlieb DJ, Newman AB, O'Connor GT, et al. Sleep-disordered breathing and mortality: a prospective cohort study. PLoS Med. 2009;6: e1000132.
2. Punjabi NM. Do sleep disorders and associated treatments impact glucose metabolism? Drugs. 2009;69(Suppl 2):13–27.
3. Quan SF, Wright R, Baldwin CM, Kaemingk KL, Goodwin JL, Kuo TF, et al. Obstructive sleep apnea-hypopnea and neurocognitive functioning in the Sleep Heart Health Study. Sleep Med. 2006;7(6):498–507.
4. Young T, Palta M, Dempsey J, Skatrud J, Weber S, Badr S. The occurrence of sleep-disordered breathing among middle-aged adults. N Engl J Med. 1993;328:1230–5.
5. Peppard PE, Young T, Palta M, Dempsey J, Skatrud J. Longitudinal study of moderate weight change and sleep-disordered breathing. JAMA. 2000;284:3015–21.
6. Hiestand DM, Britz P, Goldman M, Phillips B. Prevalence of symptoms and risk of sleep apnea in the US population: results from the national sleep foundation sleep in America 2005 poll. Chest. 2006;130:780–6.
7. Kyzer S, Charuzi I. Obstructive sleep apnea in the obese. World J Surg. 1998;22:998–1001.
8. Iber C, Ancoli-Israel S, Chesson AL, Quan SF. The AASM manual for the scoring of sleep and associated events: rules, terminology and technical specifications. 1st ed. Westchester: American Academy of Sleep Medicine; 2007.
9. Olsen KD, Suh KW, Staats BA. Surgically correctable causes of sleep apnea syndrome. Otolaryngol Head Neck Surg. 1981;89:726–31.
10. Svanborg E, Guilleminault C. EEG frequency changes during sleep apneas. Sleep. 1996;19: 248–54.
11. Smurra MV, Dury M, Aubert G, Rodenstein DO, Liistro G. Sleep fragmentation: comparison of two definitions of short arousals during sleep in OSAS patients. Eur Respir J. 2001;17: 723–7.
12. Martin SE, Engleman HM, Deary IJ, Douglas NJ. The effect of sleep fragmentation on daytime function. Am J Respir Crit Care Med. 1996;153:1328–32.
13. Redline S, Strohl KP. Recognition and consequences of obstructive sleep apnea hypopnea syndrome. Clin Chest Med. 1998;19:1–19.
14. Bearpark H, Grunstein R, Touyz S. Cognitive and psychological dysfunction in sleep apnea before and after treatment with CPAP. Sleep Res. 1987;16:303.
15. Sforza E, Roche F, Thomas-Anterion C, Kerleroux J, Beauchet O, Celle S, et al. Cognitive function and sleep related breathing disorders in a healthy elderly population: the SYNAPSE study. Sleep. 2010;33:515–21.
16. Canet E, Castronovo V, Capp SF, Aloia MS, Marelli S, Falini A. Obstructive sleep apnea: brain structural changes and neurocognitive function before and after treatment. Am J Respir Crit Care Med. 2011;183(10):1419–26.
17. Roth T, Roehrs T, Zorick F, Conway W. Pharmacological effects of sedative-hypnotics, narcotic analgesics, and alcohol during sleep. Med Clin North Am. 1985;69:1281–8.
18. Hack MA, Choi SJ, Vijayapalan P, Davies RJ, Stradling JR. Comparison of the effects of sleep deprivation, alcohol and obstructive sleep apnoea (OSA) on simulated steering performance. Respir Med. 2001;95:594–601.

19. McNicholas WT, Tarlo S, Cole P, Zamel N, Rutherford R, Griffin D, et al. Obstructive apneas during sleep in patients with seasonal allergic rhinitis. Am Rev Respir Dis. 1982;126:625–8.
20. Rajala R, Partinen M, Sane T, Pelkonen R, Huikuri K, Seppalainen AM. Obstructive sleep apnoea syndrome in morbidly obese patients. J Intern Med. 1991;230:125–9.
21. Richman RM, Elliott LM, Burns CM, Bearpark HM, Steinbeck KS, Caterson ID. The prevalence of obstructive sleep apnoea in an obese female population. Int J Obes Relat Metab Disord. 1994;18:173–7.
22. Vgontzas AN, Tan TL, Bixler EO, Martin LF, Shubert D, Kales A. Sleep apnea and sleep disruption in obese patients. Arch Intern Med. 1994;154:1705–11.
23. Flegal KM, Carroll MD, Ogden CL, Johnson CL. Prevalence and trends in obesity among US adults, 1999–2000. JAMA. 2002;288:1723–7.
24. Punjabi NM, Sorkin JD, Katzel LI, Goldberg AP, Schwartz AR, Smith PL. Sleep-disordered breathing and insulin resistance in middle-aged and overweight men. Am J Respir Crit Care Med. 2002;165:677–82.
25. Young T, Peppard PE, Gottlieb DJ. Epidemiology of obstructive sleep apnea: a population health perspective. Am J Respir Crit Care Med. 2002;165:1217–39.
26. Schwartz AR, Gold AR, Schubert N, Stryzak A, Wise RA, Permutt S, et al. Effect of weight loss on upper airway collapsibility in obstructive sleep apnea. Am Rev Respir Dis. 1991;144:494–8.
27. Malhotra A, White DP. Obstructive sleep apnoea. Lancet. 2002;360:237–45.
28. Valencia-Flores M, Orea A, Castano VA, Resendiz M, Rosales M, Rebollar V, et al. Prevalence of sleep apnea and electrocardiographic disturbances in morbidly obese patients. Obes Res. 2000;8:262–9.
29. Katz I, Stradling J, Slutsky AS, Zamel N, Hoffstein V. Do patients with obstructive sleep apnea have thick necks? Am Rev Respir Dis. 1990;141:1228–31.
30. Legato MJ. Gender-specific aspects of obesity. Int J Fertil Womens Med. 1997;42:184–97.
31. Millman RP, Carlisle CC, McGarvey ST, Eveloff SE, Levinson PD. Body fat distribution and sleep apnea severity in women. Chest. 1995;107:362–6.
32. Shinohara E, Kihara S, Yamashita S, Yamane M, Nishida M, Arai T, et al. Visceral fat accumulation as an important risk factor for obstructive sleep apnoea syndrome in obese subjects. J Intern Med. 1997;241:11–8.
33. Haponik EF, Smith PL, Bohlman ME, Allen RP, Goldman SM, Bleecker ER. Computerized tomography in obstructive sleep apnea. Correlation of airway size with physiology during sleep and wakefulness. Am Rev Respir Dis. 1983;127:221–6.
34. Schwab RJ, Gupta KB, Gefter WB, Metzger LJ, Hoffman EA, Pack AI. Upper airway and soft tissue anatomy in normal subjects and patients with sleep-disordered breathing. Significance of the lateral pharyngeal walls. Am J Respir Crit Care Med. 1995;152:1673–89.
35. Suratt PM, Dee P, Atkinson RL, Armstrong P, Wilhoit SC. Fluoroscopic and computed tomographic features of the pharyngeal airway in obstructive sleep apnea. Am Rev Respir Dis. 1983;127:487–92.
36. Gleadhill IC, Schwartz AR, Schubert N, Wise RA, Permutt S, Smith PL. Upper airway collapsibility in snorers and in patients with obstructive hypopnea and apnea. Am Rev Respir Dis. 1991;143:1300–3.
37. Isono S, Remmers JE, Tanaka A, Sho Y, Sato J, Nishino T. Anatomy of the pharynx in patients with obstructive sleep apnea and in normal subjects. J Appl Physiol. 1997;82:1319–26.
38. Isono S, Tanaka A, Tagaito Y, Sho Y, Nishino T. Respiratory stability in unconscious patients with OSA: a role of surface adhesive force. Am J Respir Crit Care Med. 1997;155(4):A413.
39. Isono S, Feroah TR, Hajduk EA, Brant R, Whitelaw WA, Remmers JE. Interaction of cross-sectional area, driving pressure, and airflow of passive velopharynx. J Appl Physiol. 1997;83:851–9.
40. Isono S, Tanaka A, Tagaito Y, Sho Y, Nishino T. Pharyngeal patency in response to advancement of the mandible in obese anesthetized persons. Anesthesiology. 1997;87:1055–62.

41. Smith PL, Wise RA, Gold AR, Schwartz AR, Permutt S. Upper airway pressure-flow relationships in obstructive sleep apnea. J Appl Physiol. 1988;64:789–95.
42. Hughes VA, Frontera WR, Roubenoff R, Evans WJ, Singh MA. Longitudinal changes in body composition in older men and women: role of body weight change and physical activity. Am J Clin Nutr. 2002;76:473–81.
43. Pierson Jr RN, Lin DH, Phillips RA. Total-body potassium in health: effects of age, sex, height, and fat. Am J Physiol. 1974;226:206–12.
44. Harman SM, Metter EJ, Tobin JD, Pearson J, Blackman MR. Longitudinal effects of aging on serum total and free testosterone levels in healthy men. Baltimore Longitudinal Study of Aging. J Clin Endocrinol Metab. 2001;86:724–31.
45. Labrie F, Belanger A, Cusan L, Gomez JL, Candas B. Marked decline in serum concentrations of adrenal C19 sex steroid precursors and conjugated androgen metabolites during aging. J Clin Endocrinol Metab. 1997;82:2396–402.
46. Muniyappa R, Wong KA, Baldwin HL, Sorkin JD, Johnson ML, Bhasin S, et al. Dehydroepiandrosterone secretion in healthy older men and women: effects of testosterone and growth hormone administration in older men. J Clin Endocrinol Metab. 2006;91: 4445–52.
47. Lee CG, Carr MC, Murdoch SJ, Mitchell E, Woods NF, Wener MH, et al. Adipokines, inflammation, and visceral adiposity across the menopausal transition: a prospective study. J Clin Endocrinol Metab. 2009;94:1104–10.
48. Ley CJ, Lees B, Stevenson JC. Sex- and menopause-associated changes in body-fat distribution. Am J Clin Nutr. 1992;55:950–4.
49. Zamboni M, Armellini F, Milani MP, De MM, Todesco T, Robbi R, et al. Body fat distribution in pre- and post-menopausal women: metabolic and anthropometric variables and their inter-relationships. Int J Obes Relat Metab Disord. 1992;16:495–504.
50. Young T. Menopause, hormone replacement therapy, and sleep-disordered breathing: are we ready for the heat? Am J Respir Crit Care Med. 2001;163:597–8.
51. Ancoli-Israel S, Kripke DF, Klauber MR, Mason WJ, Fell R, Kaplan O. Sleep-disordered breathing in community-dwelling elderly. Sleep. 1991;14:486–95.
52. Bixler EO, Vgontzas AN, Ten Have T, Tyson K, Kales A. Effects of age on sleep apnea in men: I. Prevalence and severity. Am J Respir Crit Care Med. 1998;157:144–8.
53. Bliwise DL, Bliwise NG, Partinen M, Pursley AM, Dement WC. Sleep apnea and mortality in an aged cohort. Am J Public Health. 1988;78:544–7.
54. Strohl KP, Redline S. Recognition of obstructive sleep apnea. Am J Respir Crit Care Med. 1996;154:279–89.
55. Kirkness JP, Schwartz AR, Schneider H, Punjabi NM, Maly JJ, Laffan AM, et al. Contribution of male sex, age, and obesity to mechanical instability of the upper airway during sleep. J Appl Physiol. 2008;104:1618–24.
56. Jordan AS, Wellman A, Edwards JK, Schory K, Dover L, MacDonald M, et al. Respiratory control stability and upper airway collapsibility in men and women with obstructive sleep apnea. J Appl Physiol. 2005;99:2020–7.
57. Davies RJ, Stradling JR. The relationship between neck circumference, radiographic pharyngeal anatomy, and the obstructive sleep apnoea syndrome. Eur Respir J. 1990;3:509–14.
58. Sharp JT, Henry JP, Sweany SK, Meadows WR, Pietras RJ. Effects of mass loading the respiratory system in man. J Appl Physiol. 1964;19:959–66.
59. Heinzer RC, Stanchina ML, Malhotra A, Fogel RB, Patel SR, Jordan AS, et al. Lung volume and continuous positive airway pressure requirements in obstructive sleep apnea. Am J Respir Crit Care Med. 2005;172:114–7.
60. Heinzer RC, Stanchina ML, Malhotra A, Jordan AS, Patel SR, Lo YL, et al. Effect of increased lung volume on sleep disordered breathing in sleep apnoea patients. Thorax. 2006;61:435–9.
61. Kairaitis K, Byth K, Parikh R, Stavrinou R, Wheatley JR, Amis TC. Tracheal traction effects on upper airway patency in rabbits: the role of tissue pressure. Sleep. 2007;30:179–86.

62. Babb TG, Wyrick BL, Delorey DS, Chase PJ, Feng MY. Fat distribution and end-expiratory lung volume in lean and obese men and women. Chest. 2008;134:704–11.
63. Rowley JA, Permutt S, Willey S, Smith PL, Schwartz AR. Effect of tracheal and tongue displacement on upper airway airflow dynamics. J Appl Physiol. 1996;80:2171–8.
64. Squier SB, Patil SP, Schneider H, Kirkness JP, Smith PL, Schwartz AR. Effect of end-expiratory lung volume on upper airway collapsibility in sleeping men and women. J Appl Physiol. 2010;109:977–85.
65. Whittle AT, Marshall I, Mortimore IL, Wraith PK, Sellar RJ, Douglas NJ. Neck soft tissue and fat distribution: comparison between normal men and women by magnetic resonance imaging. Thorax. 1999;54:323–8.
66. Koskenvuo M, Kaprio J, Partinen M, Langinvainio H, Sarna S, Heikkila K. Snoring as a risk factor for hypertension and angina pectoris. Lancet. 1985;1:893–6.
67. He J, Kryger MH, Zorick FJ, Conway W, Roth T. Mortality and apnea index in obstructive sleep apnea. Experience in 385 male patients. Chest. 1988;94:9–14.
68. Partinen M, Jamieson A, Guilleminault C. Long-term outcome for obstructive sleep apnea syndrome patients. Mortality. Chest. 1988;94:1200–4.
69. Hung J, Whitford EG, Parsons RW, Hillman DR. Association of sleep apnoea with myocardial infarction in men. Lancet. 1990;336:261–4.
70. Basta M, Vgontzas AN. Metabolic abnormalities in obesity and sleep apnea are in a continuum. Sleep Med. 2007;8:5–7.
71. Redline S, Storfer-Isser A, Rosen CL, Johnson NL, Kirchner HL, Emancipator J, et al. Association between metabolic syndrome and sleep-disordered breathing in adolescents. Am J Respir Crit Care Med. 2007;176:401–8.
72. Jean-Louis G, Zizi F, Clark LT, Brown CD, McFarlane SI. Obstructive sleep apnea and cardiovascular disease: role of the metabolic syndrome and its components. J Clin Sleep Med. 2008;4:261–72.
73. Attal P, Chanson P. Endocrine aspects of obstructive sleep apnea. J Clin Endocrinol Metab. 2010;95:483–95.
74. Chin K, Oga T, Takahashi K, Takegami M, Nakayama-Ashida Y, Wakamura T, et al. Associations between obstructive sleep apnea, metabolic syndrome, and sleep duration, as measured with an actigraph, in an urban male working population in Japan. Sleep. 2010;33:89–95.
75. Barbe F, Pericas J, Munoz A, Findley L, Anto JM, Agusti AG. Automobile accidents in patients with sleep apnea syndrome. An epidemiological and mechanistic study. Am J Respir Crit Care Med. 1998;158:18–22.
76. Teran-Santos J, Jimenez-Gomez A, Cordero-Guevara J. The association between sleep apnea and the risk of traffic accidents. Cooperative Group Burgos-Santander. N Engl J Med. 1999;340:847–51.
77. Chami HA, Baldwin CM, Silverman A, Zhang Y, Rapoport D, Punjabi NM, et al. Sleepiness, quality of life, and sleep maintenance in REM versus non-REM sleep-disordered breathing. Am J Respir Crit Care Med. 2010;181:997–1002.
78. Al Lawati NM, Patel SR, Ayas NT. Epidemiology, risk factors, and consequences of obstructive sleep apnea and short sleep duration. Prog Cardiovasc Dis. 2009;51:285–93.
79. Goncalves MA, Paiva T, Ramos E, Guilleminault C. Obstructive sleep apnea syndrome, sleepiness, and quality of life. Chest. 2004;125:2091–6.
80. Nieto FJ, Young TB, Lind BK, Shahar E, Samet JM, Redline S, et al. Association of sleep-disordered breathing, sleep apnea, and hypertension in a large community-based study. Sleep Heart Health Study. JAMA. 2000;283:1829–36.
81. Peppard PE, Young T, Palta M, Skatrud J. Prospective study of the association between sleep-disordered breathing and hypertension. N Engl J Med. 2000;342:1378–84.
82. Mooe T, Franklin KA, Holmstrom K, Rabben T, Wiklund U. Sleep-disordered breathing and coronary artery disease. Long-term prognosis. Am J Respir Crit Care Med. 2001;164:1910–3.

83. Shahar E, Whitney CW, Redline S, Lee ET, Newman AB, Javier NF, et al. Sleep-disordered breathing and cardiovascular disease: cross-sectional results of the Sleep Heart Health Study. Am J Respir Crit Care Med. 2001;163:19–25.
84. Somers VK, Dyken ME, Clary MP, Abboud FM. Sympathetic neural mechanisms in obstructive sleep apnea. J Clin Invest. 1995;96:1897–904.
85. Carlson JT, Hedner J, Elam M, Ejnell H, Sellgren J, Wallin BG. Augmented resting sympathetic activity in awake patients with obstructive sleep apnea. Chest. 1993;103:1763–8.
86. Narkiewicz K, Pesek CA, Kato M, Phillips BG, Davison DE, Somers VK. Baroreflex control of sympathetic nerve activity and heart rate in obstructive sleep apnea. Hypertension. 1998;32:1039–43.
87. Carlson JT, Hedner JA, Sellgren J, Elam M, Wallin BG. Depressed baroreflex sensitivity in patients with obstructive sleep apnea. Am J Respir Crit Care Med. 1996;154:1490–6.
88. Hedner JA, Wilcox I, Laks L, Grunstein RR, Sullivan CE. A specific and potent pressor effect of hypoxia in patients with sleep apnea. Am Rev Respir Dis. 1992;146:1240–5.
89. Narkiewicz K, van de Borne PJ, Pesek CA, Dyken ME, Montano N, Somers VK. Selective potentiation of peripheral chemoreflex sensitivity in obstructive sleep apnea. Circulation. 1999;99:1183–9.
90. Phillips BG, Narkiewicz K, Pesek CA, Haynes WG, Dyken ME, Somers VK. Effects of obstructive sleep apnea on endothelin-1 and blood pressure. J Hypertens. 1999;17:61–6.
91. Kato M, Roberts-Thomson P, Phillips BG, Haynes WG, Winnicki M, Accurso V, et al. Impairment of endothelium-dependent vasodilation of resistance vessels in patients with obstructive sleep apnea. Circulation. 2000;102:2607–10.
92. Narkiewicz K, van de Borne PJ, Cooley RL, Dyken ME, Somers VK. Sympathetic activity in obese subjects with and without obstructive sleep apnea. Circulation. 1998;98:772–6.
93. Rajala MW, Scherer PE. Minireview: the adipocyte–at the crossroads of energy homeostasis, inflammation, and atherosclerosis. Endocrinology. 2003;144:3765–73.
94. Fischer-Posovszky P, Wabitsch M, Hochberg Z. Endocrinology of adipose tissue – an update. Horm Metab Res. 2007;39:314–21.
95. Friedman JM. Leptin, leptin receptors, and the control of body weight. Nutr Rev. 1998;56: s38–46.
96. Zhang Y, Proenca R, Maffei M, Barone M, Leopold L, Friedman JM. Positional cloning of the mouse obese gene and its human homologue. Nature. 1994;372:425–32.
97. Considine RV, Sinha MK, Heiman ML, Kriauciunas A, Stephens TW, Nyce MR, et al. Serum immunoreactive-leptin concentrations in normal-weight and obese humans. N Engl J Med. 1996;334:292–5.
98. Maffei M, Halaas J, Ravussin E, Pratley RE, Lee GH, Zhang Y, et al. Leptin levels in human and rodent: measurement of plasma leptin and ob RNA in obese and weight-reduced subjects. Nat Med. 1995;1:1155–61.
99. Breslow MJ, Min-Lee K, Brown DR, Chacko VP, Palmer D, Berkowitz DE. Effect of leptin deficiency on metabolic rate in ob/ob mice. Am J Physiol. 1999;276:E443–9.
100. Montague CT, Farooqi IS, Whitehead JP, Soos MA, Rau H, Wareham NJ, et al. Congenital leptin deficiency is associated with severe early-onset obesity in humans. Nature. 1997;387:903–8.
101. Farooqi IS, Keogh JM, Kamath S, Jones S, Gibson WT, Trussell R, et al. Partial leptin deficiency and human adiposity. Nature. 2001;414:34–5.
102. Ravussin E, Pratley RE, Maffei M, Wang H, Friedman JM, Bennett PH, et al. Relatively low plasma leptin concentrations precede weight gain in Pima Indians. Nat Med. 1997;3: 238–40.
103. Fruhbeck G, Gomez-Ambrosi J, Muruzabal FJ, Burrell MA. The adipocyte: a model for integration of endocrine and metabolic signaling in energy metabolism regulation. Am J Physiol Endocrinol Metab. 2001;280:E827–47.
104. Zhang HH, Kumar S, Barnett AH, Eggo MC. Dexamethasone inhibits tumor necrosis factor-alpha-induced apoptosis and interleukin-1 beta release in human subcutaneous adipocytes and preadipocytes. J Clin Endocrinol Metab. 2001;86:2817–25.

105. Tasali E, Leproult R, Ehrmann DA, Van CE. Slow-wave sleep and the risk of type 2 diabetes in humans. Proc Natl Acad Sci USA. 2008;105:1044–9.
106. Spiegel K, Leproult R, Van Cauter E. Impact of sleep debt on metabolic and endocrine function. Lancet. 1999;354:1435–9.
107. Chow DC, Souza SA, Chen R, Richmond-Crum SM, Grandinetti A, Shikuma C. Elevated blood pressure in HIV-infected individuals receiving highly active antiretroviral therapy. HIV Clin Trials. 2003;4:411–6.
108. Carr A, Samaras K, Chisholm DJ, Cooper DA. Pathogenesis of HIV-1-protease inhibitor-associated peripheral lipodystrophy, hyperlipidaemia, and insulin resistance. Lancet. 1998;351:1881–3.
109. Carr A, Samaras K, Burton S, Law M, Freund J, Chisholm DJ, et al. A syndrome of peripheral lipodystrophy, hyperlipidaemia, and insulin resistance in patients receiving HIV protease inhibitors. AIDS. 1998;12:F51–8.
110. Roth VR, Kravcik S, Angel JB. Development of cervical fat pads following therapy with human immunodeficiency virus type 1 protease inhibitors. Clin Infect Dis. 1998;27:65–7.
111. Grundy SM, Brewer Jr HB, Cleeman JI, Smith Jr SC, Lenfant C. Definition of metabolic syndrome: report of the National Heart, Lung, and Blood Institute/American Heart Association conference on scientific issues related to definition. Circulation. 2004;109:433–8.
112. Oral EA, Simha V, Ruiz E, Andewelt A, Premkumar A, Snell P, et al. Leptin-replacement therapy for lipodystrophy. N Engl J Med. 2002;346:570–8.
113. Mulligan K, Khatami H, Schwarz JM, Sakkas GK, DePaoli AM, Tai VW, et al. The effects of recombinant human leptin on visceral fat, dyslipidemia, and insulin resistance in patients with human immunodeficiency virus-associated lipoatrophy and hypoleptinemia. J Clin Endocrinol Metab. 2009;94:1137–44.
114. Lee JH, Chan JL, Sourlas E, Raptopoulos V, Mantzoros CS. Recombinant methionyl human leptin therapy in replacement doses improves insulin resistance and metabolic profile in patients with lipoatrophy and metabolic syndrome induced by the highly active antiretroviral therapy. J Clin Endocrinol Metab. 2006;91:2605–11.
115. Yee BJ, Cheung J, Phipps P, Banerjee D, Piper AJ, Grunstein RR. Treatment of obesity hypoventilation syndrome and serum leptin. Respiration. 2006;73:209–12.
116. Phipps PR, Starritt E, Caterson I, Grunstein RR. Association of serum leptin with hypoventilation in human obesity. Thorax. 2002;57:75–6.
117. Piper AJ, Grunstein RR. Obesity hypoventilation syndrome: mechanisms and management. Am J Respir Crit Care Med. 2011;183:292–8.
118. Piper AJ, Grunstein RR. Big breathing: the complex interaction of obesity, hypoventilation, weight loss, and respiratory function. J Appl Physiol. 2010;108:199–205.
119. Romero-Corral A, Caples SM, Lopez-Jimenez F, Somers VK. Interactions between obesity and obstructive sleep apnea: implications for treatment. Chest. 2010;137:711–9.
120. Punjabi NM, Polotsky VY. Disorders of glucose metabolism in sleep apnea. J Appl Physiol. 2005;99:1998–2007.
121. Punjabi NM, Ahmed MM, Polotsky VY, Beamer BA, O'Donnell CP. Sleep-disordered breathing, glucose intolerance, and insulin resistance. Respir Physiol Neurobiol. 2003;136:167–78.
122. Lavie L. Oxidative stress – a unifying paradigm in obstructive sleep apnea and comorbidities. Prog Cardiovasc Dis. 2009;51:303–12.
123. Savransky V, Nanayakkara A, Vivero A, Li J, Bevans S, Smith PL, et al. Chronic intermittent hypoxia predisposes to liver injury. Hepatology. 2007;45:1007–13.
124. Tatsumi K, Saibara T. Effects of obstructive sleep apnea syndrome on hepatic steatosis and nonalcoholic steatohepatitis. Hepatol Res. 2005;33:100–4.
125. Punjabi NM, O'hearn DJ, Neubauer DN, Nieto FJ, Schwartz AR, Smith PL, et al. Modeling hypersomnolence in sleep-disordered breathing. A novel approach using survival analysis. Am J Respir Crit Care Med. 1999;159:1703–9.
126. Gooneratne NS, Weaver TE, Cater JR, Pack FM, Arner HM, Greenberg AS, et al. Functional outcomes of excessive daytime sleepiness in older adults. J Am Geriatr Soc. 2003;51: 642–9.

127. Bonnet MH, Arand DL. Clinical effects of sleep fragmentation versus sleep deprivation. Sleep Med Rev. 2003;7:297–310.
128. Mitler MM, Carskadon MA, Czeisler CA, Dement WC, Dinges DF, Graeber RC. Catastrophes, sleep, and public policy: consensus report. Sleep. 1988;11:100–9.
129. Young T, Blustein J, Finn L, Palta M. Sleep-disordered breathing and motor vehicle accidents in a population-based sample of employed adults. Sleep. 1997;20:608–13.
130. Engleman HM, Kingshott RN, Martin SE, Douglas NJ. Cognitive function in the sleep apnea/hypopnea syndrome (SAHS). Sleep. 2000;23(Suppl 4):S102–8.
131. Felver-Gant JC, Bruce AS, Zimmerman M, Sweet LH, Millman RP, Aloia MS. Working memory in obstructive sleep apnea: construct validity and treatment effects. J Clin Sleep Med. 2007;3:589–94.
132. Engleman HM, Martin SE, Deary IJ, Douglas NJ. Effect of continuous positive airway pressure treatment on daytime function in sleep apnoea/hypopnoea syndrome. Lancet. 1994;343:572–5.
133. Engleman HM, Martin SE, Kingshott RN, Mackay TW, Deary IJ, Douglas NJ. Randomised placebo controlled trial of daytime function after continuous positive airway pressure (CPAP) therapy for the sleep apnoea/hypopnoea syndrome. Thorax. 1998;53:341–5.
134. Haynes PL. The role of behavioral sleep medicine in the assessment and treatment of sleep disordered breathing. Clin Psychol Rev. 2005;25:673–705.
135. Dixon JB, Bhathal PS, O'Brien PE. Nonalcoholic fatty liver disease: predictors of nonalcoholic steatohepatitis and liver fibrosis in the severely obese. Gastroenterology. 2001;121:91–100.
136. Dixon JB, Schachter LM, O'Brien PE. Sleep disturbance and obesity: changes following surgically induced weight loss. Arch Intern Med. 2001;161:102–6.
137. Dixon JB, Dixon ME, Anderson ML, Schachter L, O'Brien PE. Daytime sleepiness in the obese: not as simple as obstructive sleep apnea. Obesity (Silver Spring). 2007;15:2504–11.
138. Schwartz AR, O'Donnell CP, Baron J, Schubert N, Alam D, Samadi SD, et al. The hypotonic upper airway in obstructive sleep apnea: role of structures and neuromuscular activity. Am J Respir Crit Care Med. 1998;157:1051–7.
139. Smith PL, Patil SP, Kirkness JP, Schneider H, Schwartz AR. Biomechanics of upper airway during sleep – sleep apnea: pathogenesis, diagnosis, and treatment. In: Pack AI, editor. Sleep apnea pathogenesis, diagnosis and treatment. New York: Marcel Dekker; 2011.
140. Kushida CA, Efron B, Guilleminault C. A predictive morphometric model for the obstructive sleep apnea syndrome. Ann Intern Med. 1997;127:581–7.
141. Riley R, Guilleminault C, Herran J, Powell N. Cephalometric analyses and flow-volume loops in obstructive sleep apnea patients. Sleep. 1983;6:303–11.
142. Rivlin J, Hoffstein V, Kalbfleisch J, McNicholas W, Zamel N, Bryan AC. Upper airway morphology in patients with idiopathic obstructive sleep apnea. Am Rev Respir Dis. 1984;129:355–60.
143. Lyberg T, Krogstad O, Djupesland G. Cephalometric analysis in patients with obstructive sleep apnoea syndrome. I. Skeletal morphology. J Laryngol Otol. 1989;103:287–92.
144. Bhattacharyya N, Blake SP, Fried MP. Assessment of the airway in obstructive sleep apnea syndrome with 3-dimensional airway computed tomography. Otolaryngol Head Neck Surg. 2000;123:444–9.
145. Kuna ST, Bedi DG, Ryckman C. Effect of nasal airway positive pressure on upper airway size and configuration. Am Rev Respir Dis. 1988;138:969–75.
146. Schwab RJ, Gupta KB, Metzger LJ, Pack AI, Gefter WB. State related changes in upper airway caliber and surrounding soft tissue structures in normals and apneics. Am J Respir Crit Care Med. 1995;151:A667.
147. Schwab RJ, Pack AI, Gupta KB, Metzger LJ, Oh E, Getsy JE, et al. Upper airway and soft tissue structural changes induced by CPAP in normal subjects. Am J Respir Crit Care Med. 1996;154:1106–16.
148. Schotland HM, Insko EK, Schwab RJ. Quantitative magnetic resonance imaging demonstrates alterations of the lingual musculature in obstructive sleep apnea. Sleep. 1999;22:605–13.

149. Simpson L, Mukherjee S, Cooper MN, Ward KL, Lee JD, Fedson AC, et al. Sex differences in the association of regional fat distribution with the severity of obstructive sleep apnea. Sleep. 2010;33:467–74.
150. Stanchina ML, Malhotra A, Fogel RB, Trinder J, Edwards JK, Schory K, et al. The influence of lung volume on pharyngeal mechanics, collapsibility, and genioglossus muscle activation during sleep. Sleep. 2003;26:851–6.
151. Carey DG, Jenkins AB, Campbell LV, Freund J, Chisholm DJ. Abdominal fat and insulin resistance in normal and overweight women: direct measurements reveal a strong relationship in subjects at both low and high risk of NIDDM. Diabetes. 1996;45:633–8.
152. Paradisi G, Smith L, Burtner C, Leaming R, Garvey WT, Hook G, et al. Dual energy X-ray absorptiometry assessment of fat mass distribution and its association with the insulin resistance syndrome. Diabetes Care. 1999;22:1310–7.
153. Rissanen P, Hamalainen P, Vanninen E, Tenhunen-Eskelinen M, Uusitupa M. Relationship of metabolic variables to abdominal adiposity measured by different anthropometric measurements and dual-energy X-ray absorptiometry in obese middle-aged women. Int J Obes Relat Metab Disord. 1997;21:367–71.
154. Lee K, Lee S, Kim YJ, Kim YJ. Waist circumference, dual-energy X-ray absortiometrically measured abdominal adiposity, and computed tomographically derived intra-abdominal fat area on detecting metabolic risk factors in obese women. Nutrition. 2008;24:625–31.
155. dos Santos RE, Aldrighi JM, Lanz JR, Ferezin PC, Marone MM. Relationship of body fat distribution by waist circumference, dual-energy X-ray absorptiometry and ultrasonography to insulin resistance by homeostasis model assessment and lipid profile in obese and non-obese postmenopausal women. Gynecol Endocrinol. 2005;21:295–301.
156. Bernstein LE, Berry J, Kim S, Canavan B, Grinspoon SK. Effects of etanercept in patients with the metabolic syndrome. Arch Intern Med. 2006;166:902–8.
157. Catalan V, Gomez-Ambrosi J, Ramirez B, Rotellar F, Pastor C, Silva C, et al. Proinflammatory cytokines in obesity: impact of type 2 diabetes mellitus and gastric bypass. Obes Surg. 2007;17:1464–74.
158. Pou KM, Massaro JM, Hoffmann U, Vasan RS, Maurovich-Horvat P, Larson MG, et al. Visceral and subcutaneous adipose tissue volumes are cross-sectionally related to markers of inflammation and oxidative stress: the Framingham Heart Study. Circulation. 2007;116:1234–41.
159. Yamamoto Y, Gaynor RB. IkappaB kinases: key regulators of the NF-kappaB pathway. Trends Biochem Sci. 2004;29:72–9.
160. Karin M, Lin A. NF-kappaB at the crossroads of life and death. Nat Immunol. 2002;3: 221–7.
161. Sen R, Baltimore D. Inducibility of kappa immunoglobulin enhancer-binding protein Nf-kappa B by a posttranslational mechanism. Cell. 1986;47:921–8.
162. Fried SK, Bunkin DA, Greenberg AS. Omental and subcutaneous adipose tissues of obese subjects release interleukin-6: depot difference and regulation by glucocorticoid. J Clin Endocrinol Metab. 1998;83:847–50.
163. Hotamisligil GS, Shargill NS, Spiegelman BM. Adipose expression of tumor necrosis factor-alpha: direct role in obesity-linked insulin resistance. Science. 1993;259:87–91.
164. Manzella D, Parillo M, Razzino T, Gnasso P, Buonanno S, Gargiulo A, et al. Soluble leptin receptor and insulin resistance as determinant of sleep apnea. Int J Obes Relat Metab Disord. 2002;26:370–5.
165. Arias MA, Garcia-Rio F, Onso-Fernandez A, Hernanz A, Hidalgo R, Martinez-Mateo V, et al. CPAP decreases plasma levels of soluble tumour necrosis factor-alpha receptor 1 in obstructive sleep apnoea. Eur Respir J. 2008;32:1009–15.
166. Arner P. Regional differences in protein production by human adipose tissue. Biochem Soc Trans. 2001;29:72–5.
167. Dusserre E, Moulin P, Vidal H. Differences in mRNA expression of the proteins secreted by the adipocytes in human subcutaneous and visceral adipose tissues. Biochim Biophys Acta. 2000;1500:88–96.

168. Fang J, Wang Y, Krueger JM. Effects of interleukin-1 beta on sleep are mediated by the type I receptor. Am J Physiol. 1998;274:R655–60.
169. Krueger JM, Fang J, Hansen MK, Zhang J, Obal Jr F. Humoral regulation of sleep. News Physiol Sci. 1998;13:189–94.
170. Krueger JM, Obal FJ, Fang J, Kubota T, Taishi P. The role of cytokines in physiological sleep regulation. Ann N Y Acad Sci. 2001;933:211–21.
171. Takahashi S, Kapas L, Fang J, Krueger JM. Somnogenic relationships between tumor necrosis factor and interleukin-1. Am J Physiol. 1999;276:R1132–40.
172. Opp MR. Cytokines and sleep. Sleep Med Rev. 2005;9:355–64.
173. Fang J, Wang Y, Krueger JM. Mice lacking the TNF 55 kDa receptor fail to sleep more after TNFalpha treatment. J Neurosci. 1997;17:5949–55.
174. Krueger JM, Fang J, Taishi P, Chen Z, Kushikata T, Gardi J. Sleep. A physiologic role for IL-1 beta and TNF-alpha. Ann N Y Acad Sci. 1998;856:148–59.
175. Vgontzas AN, Zoumakis E, Lin HM, Bixler EO, Trakada G, Chrousos GP. Marked decrease in sleepiness in patients with sleep apnea by etanercept, a tumor necrosis factor-alpha antagonist. J Clin Endocrinol Metab. 2004;89:4409–13.
176. Shearer WT, Reuben JM, Mullington JM, Price NJ, Lee BN, Smith EO, et al. Soluble TNF-alpha receptor 1 and IL-6 plasma levels in humans subjected to the sleep deprivation model of spaceflight. J Allergy Clin Immunol. 2001;107:165–70.
177. Churchill L, Rector DM, Yasuda K, Fix C, Rojas MJ, Yasuda T, et al. Tumor necrosis factor alpha: activity dependent expression and promotion of cortical column sleep in rats. Neuroscience. 2008;156:71–80.
178. O'Donnell CP, Schwartz AR, Smith PL. Upper airway collapsibility: the importance of gender and adiposity. Am J Respir Crit Care Med. 2000;162:1606–7.
179. Pillar G, Malhotra A, Fogel R, Beauregard J, Schnall R, White DP. Airway mechanics and ventilation in response to resistive loading during sleep: influence of gender. Am J Respir Crit Care Med. 2000;162:1627–32.
180. Leech JA, Onal E, Dulberg C, Lopata MA. A comparison of men and women with occlusive sleep apnea syndrome. Chest. 1988;94:983–8.
181. Mohsenin V. Gender differences in the expression of sleep-disordered breathing: role of upper airway dimensions. Chest. 2001;120:1442–7.
182. O'Connor C, Thornley KS, Hanly PJ. Gender differences in the polysomnographic features of obstructive sleep apnea. Am J Respir Crit Care Med. 2000;161:1465–72.
183. Ip MS, Lam KS, Ho C, Tsang KW, Lam W. Serum leptin and vascular risk factors in obstructive sleep apnea. Chest. 2000;118:580–6.
184. Shamsuzzaman AS, Winnicki M, Lanfranchi P, Wolk R, Kara T, Accurso V, et al. Elevated C-reactive protein in patients with obstructive sleep apnea. Circulation. 2002;105:2462–4.
185. Vgontzas AN, Papanicolaou DA, Bixler EO, Hopper K, Lotsikas A, Lin HM, et al. Sleep apnea and daytime sleepiness and fatigue: relation to visceral obesity, insulin resistance, and hypercytokinemia. J Clin Endocrinol Metab. 2000;85:1151–8.
186. Alberti A, Sarchielli P, Gallinella E, Floridi A, Floridi A, Mazzotta G, et al. Plasma cytokine levels in patients with obstructive sleep apnea syndrome: a preliminary study. J Sleep Res. 2003;12:305–11.
187. Kataoka T, Enomoto F, Kim R, Yokoi H, Fujimori M, Sakai Y, et al. The effect of surgical treatment of obstructive sleep apnea syndrome on the plasma TNF-alpha levels. Tohoku J Exp Med. 2004;204:267–72.
188. Punjabi NM, Beamer BA. C-reactive protein is associated with sleep disordered breathing independent of adiposity. Sleep. 2007;30:29–34.
189. Ryan S, Taylor CT, McNicholas WT. Predictors of elevated nuclear factor-{kappa} B-dependent genes in obstructive sleep apnea syndrome. Am J Respir Crit Care Med. 2006;174:824–30.
190. Yokoe T, Minoguchi K, Matsuo H, Oda N, Minoguchi H, Yoshino G, et al. Elevated levels of C-reactive protein and interleukin-6 in patients with obstructive sleep apnea syndrome are decreased by nasal continuous positive airway pressure. Circulation. 2003;107:1129–34.

191. Phillips BG, Kato M, Narkiewicz K, Choe I, Somers VK. Increases in leptin levels, sympathetic drive, and weight gain in obstructive sleep apnea. Am J Physiol Heart Circ Physiol. 2000;279:H234–7.
192. Ozturk L, Unal M, Tamer L, Celikoglu F. The association of the severity of obstructive sleep apnea with plasma leptin levels. Arch Otolaryngol Head Neck Surg. 2003;129:538–40.
193. Marik PE. Leptin, obesity, and obstructive sleep apnea. Chest. 2000;118:569–71.
194. Fitzpatrick M. Leptin and the obesity hypoventilation syndrome: a leap of faith? Thorax. 2002;57:1–2.
195. Chin K, Shimizu K, Nakamura T, Narai N, Masuzaki H, Ogawa Y, et al. Changes in intra-abdominal visceral fat and serum leptin levels in patients with obstructive sleep apnea syndrome following nasal continuous positive airway pressure therapy. Circulation. 1999;100:706–12.
196. Vgontzas AN, Zoumakis E, Bixler EO, Lin HM, Collins B, Basta M, et al. Selective effects of CPAP on sleep apnoea-associated manifestations. Eur J Clin Invest. 2008;38:585–95.
197. Tangel DJ, Mezzanotte WS, Sandberg EJ, White DP. Influences of NREM sleep on the activity of tonic vs. inspiratory phasic muscles in normal men. J Appl Physiol. 1992;73: 1058–66.
198. Henson LC, Ward DS. Effects of anaesthetics and sedatives on the control of breathing. Ann Acad Med Singapore. 1994;23:125–9.
199. Wheatley JR, Mezzanotte WS, Tangel DJ, White DP. Influence of sleep on genioglossus muscle activation by negative pressure in normal men. Am Rev Respir Dis. 1993;148:597–605.
200. Redline S, Tosteson T, Tishler PV, Carskadon MA, Millman RP, Milliman RP. Studies in the genetics of obstructive sleep apnea. Familial aggregation of symptoms associated with sleep-related breathing disturbances. Am Rev Respir Dis. 1992;145:440–4.
201. Pillar G, Lavie P. Assessment of the role of inheritance in sleep apnea syndrome. Am J Respir Crit Care Med. 1995;151:688–91.
202. Redline S, Tishler PV, Tosteson TD, Williamson J, Kump K, Browner I, et al. The familial aggregation of obstructive sleep apnea. Am J Respir Crit Care Med. 1995;151:682–7.
203. Carmelli D, Bliwise DL, Swan GE, Reed T. Genetic factors in self-reported snoring and excessive daytime sleepiness: a twin study. Am J Respir Crit Care Med. 2001;164:949–52.
204. Patel SR. Shared genetic risk factors for obstructive sleep apnea and obesity. J Appl Physiol. 2005;99:1600–6.
205. Schwab RJ. Genetic determinants of upper airway structure that predispose to obstructive sleep apnea. Respir Physiol Neurobiol. 2005;147:289–98.
206. Riha RL. Genetic aspects of the obstructive sleep apnoea-hypopnoea syndrome. Somnologie. 2006;10:101–12.
207. Schwab RJ, Pasirstein M, Kaplan L, Pierson R, Mackley A, Hachadoorian R, et al. Family aggregation of upper airway soft tissue structures in normal subjects and patients with sleep apnea. Am J Respir Crit Care Med. 2006;173:453–63.
208. Patel SR, Larkin EK, Redline S. Shared genetic basis for obstructive sleep apnea and adiposity measures. Int J Obes (Lond). 2008;32:795–800.
209. Holberg CJ, Natrajan S, Cline MG, Quan SF. Familial aggregation and segregation analysis of snoring and symptoms of obstructive sleep apnea. Sleep Breath. 2000;4:21–30.
210. Vgontzas AN, Bixler EO, Chrousos GP. Metabolic disturbances in obesity versus sleep apnoea: the importance of visceral obesity and insulin resistance. J Intern Med. 2003;254:32–44.
211. Vgontzas AN, Bixler EO, Chrousos GP. Sleep apnea is a manifestation of the metabolic syndrome. Sleep Med Rev. 2005;9:211–24.
212. Harsch IA, Konturek PC, Koebnick C, Kuehnlein PP, Fuchs FS, Schahin SP, et al. Leptin and ghrelin levels in patients with obstructive sleep apnoea: effect of CPAP treatment. Eur Respir J. 2003;22:251–7.
213. Takahashi K, Chin K, Akamizu T, Morita S, Sumi K, Oga T, et al. Acylated ghrelin level in patients with OSA before and after nasal CPAP treatment. Respirology. 2008;13:810–6.

214. Morgenthaler TI, Kapen S, Lee-Chiong T, Alessi C, Boehlecke B, Brown T, et al. Practice parameters for the medical therapy of obstructive sleep apnea. Sleep. 2006;29:1031–5.
215. Nerfeldt P, Nilsson BY, Mayor L, Udden J, Friberg D. A two-year weight reduction program in obese sleep apnea patients. J Clin Sleep Med. 2010;6:479–86.
216. Monteforte MJ, Turkelson CM. Bariatric surgery for morbid obesity. Obes Surg. 2000;10: 391–401.
217. Sugerman HJ. Bariatric surgery for severe obesity. J Assoc Acad Minor Phys. 2001;12: 129–36.
218. Charuzi I, Lavie P, Peiser J, Peled R. Bariatric surgery in morbidly obese sleep-apnea patients: short- and long-term follow-up. Am J Clin Nutr. 1992;55:594S–6.
219. Aubert-Tulkens G, Culee C, Rodenstein DO. Cure of sleep apnea syndrome after long-term nasal continuous positive airway pressure therapy and weight loss. Sleep. 1989;12:216–22.
220. Browman CP, Sampson MG, Yolles SF, Gujavarty KS, Weiler SJ, Walsleben JA, et al. Obstructive sleep apnea and body weight. Chest. 1984;85:435–8.
221. Dixon JB, Schachter LM, O'Brien PE. Polysomnography before and after weight loss in obese patients with severe sleep apnea. Int J Obes (Lond). 2005;29:1048–54.
222. Harman EM, Wynne JW, Block AJ. The effect of weight loss on sleep-disordered breathing and oxygen desaturation in morbidly obese men. Chest. 1982;82:291–4.
223. Smith PL, Gold AR, Meyers DA, Haponik EF, Bleecker ER. Weight loss in mildly to moderately obese patients with obstructive sleep apnea. Ann Intern Med. 1985;103:850–5.
224. Strobel RJ, Rosen RC. Obesity and weight loss in obstructive sleep apnea: a critical review. Sleep. 1996;19:104–15.
225. Suratt PM, McTier RF, Findley LJ, Pohl SL, Wilhoit SC. Changes in breathing and the pharynx after weight loss in obstructive sleep apnea. Chest. 1987;92:631–7.
226. Veasey SC, Guilleminault C, Strohl KP, Sanders MH, Ballard RD, Magalang UJ. Medical therapy for obstructive sleep apnea: a review by the medical therapy for obstructive sleep apnea task force of the Standards of practice committee of the American academy of sleep medicine. Sleep. 2006;29:1036–44.
227. Serafini FM, MacDowell AW, Rosemurgy AS, Strait T, Murr MM. Clinical predictors of sleep apnea in patients undergoing bariatric surgery. Obes Surg. 2001;11:28–31.
228. Busetto L, Tregnaghi A, Bussolotto M, Sergi G, Beninca P, Ceccon A, et al. Visceral fat loss evaluated by total body magnetic resonance imaging in obese women operated with laparoscopic adjustable silicone gastric banding. Int J Obes Relat Metab Disord. 2000;24:60–9.
229. Huerta S, DeShields S, Shpiner R, Li Z, Liu C, Sawicki M, et al. Safety and efficacy of postoperative continuous positive airway pressure to prevent pulmonary complications after Roux-en-Y gastric bypass. J Gastrointest Surg. 2002;6:354–8.
230. Cummings DE, Weigle DS, Frayo RS, Breen PA, Ma MK, Dellinger EP, et al. Plasma ghrelin levels after diet-induced weight loss or gastric bypass surgery. N Engl J Med. 2002;346: 1623–30.
231. Balsiger BM, Kennedy FP, Abu-Lebdeh HS, Collazo-Clavell M, Jensen MD, O'Brien T, et al. Prospective evaluation of Roux-en-Y gastric bypass as primary operation for medically complicated obesity. Mayo Clin Proc. 2000;75:673–80.
232. Bouldin MJ, Ross LA, Sumrall CD, Loustalot FV, Low AK, Land KK. The effect of obesity surgery on obesity comorbidity. Am J Med Sci. 2006;331:183–93.
233. Charuzi I, Fraser D, Peiser J, Ovnat A, Lavie P. Sleep apnea syndrome in the morbidly obese undergoing bariatric surgery. Gastroenterol Clin North Am. 1987;16:517–9.
234. Fritscher LG, Mottin CC, Canani S, Chatkin JM. Obesity and obstructive sleep apnea-hypopnea syndrome: the impact of bariatric surgery. Obes Surg. 2007;17:95–9.
235. Haines KL, Nelson LG, Gonzalez R, Torrella T, Martin T, Kandil A, et al. Objective evidence that bariatric surgery improves obesity-related obstructive sleep apnea. Surgery. 2007;141: 354–8.
236. Kalra M, Inge T. Effect of bariatric surgery on obstructive sleep apnoea in adolescents. Paediatr Respir Rev. 2006;7:260–7.

237. Kushner RF, Noble CA. Long-term outcome of bariatric surgery: an interim analysis. Mayo Clin Proc. 2006;81:S46–51.
238. Lankford DA, Proctor CD, Richard R. Continuous positive airway pressure (CPAP) changes in bariatric surgery patients undergoing rapid weight loss. Obes Surg. 2005;15:336–41.
239. Loube DI, Loube AA, Mitler MM. Weight loss for obstructive sleep apnea: the optimal therapy for obese patients. J Am Diet Assoc. 1994;94:1291–5.
240. Scheuller M, Weider D. Bariatric surgery for treatment of sleep apnea syndrome in 15 morbidly obese patients: long-term results. Otolaryngol Head Neck Surg. 2001;125:299–302.
241. Spivak H, Hewitt MF, Onn A, Half EE. Weight loss and improvement of obesity-related illness in 500 U.S. patients following laparoscopic adjustable gastric banding procedure. Am J Surg. 2005;189:27–32.
242. Valencia-Flores M, Orea A, Herrera M, Santiago V, Rebollar V, Castano VA, et al. Effect of bariatric surgery on obstructive sleep apnea and hypopnea syndrome, electrocardiogram, and pulmonary arterial pressure. Obes Surg. 2004;14:755–62.
243. Verse T. Bariatric surgery for obstructive sleep apnea. Chest. 2005;128:485–7.
244. Patil SP, Schneider H, Marx JJ, Gladmon E, Schwartz AR, Smith PL. Neuromechanical control of upper airway patency during sleep. J Appl Physiol. 2007;102:547–56.
245. Holdstock C, Engstrom BE, Ohrvall M, Lind L, Sundbom M, Karlsson FA. Ghrelin and adipose tissue regulatory peptides: effect of gastric bypass surgery in obese humans. J Clin Endocrinol Metab. 2003;88:3177–83.
246. Li C, Ioffe E, Fidahusein N, Connolly E, Friedman JM. Absence of soluble leptin receptor in plasma from dbPas/dbPas and other db/db mice. J Biol Chem. 1998;273:10078–82.
247. Faraj M, Havel PJ, Phelis S, Blank D, Sniderman AD, Cianflone K. Plasma acylation-stimulating protein, adiponectin, leptin, and ghrelin before and after weight loss induced by gastric bypass surgery in morbidly obese subjects. J Clin Endocrinol Metab. 2003;88:1594–602.
248. Ott V, Fasshauer M, Dalski A, Meier B, Perwitz N, Klein HH, et al. Direct peripheral effects of ghrelin include suppression of adiponectin expression. Horm Metab Res. 2002;34:640–5.
249. Whitson BA, Leslie DB, Kellogg TA, Maddaus MA, Buchwald H, Billington CJ, et al. Adipokine response in diabetics and nondiabetics following the roux-en-y gastric bypass: a preliminary study. J Surg Res. 2007;142:295–300.
250. Rasheid S, Banasiak M, Gallagher SF, Lipska A, Kaba S, Ventimiglia D, et al. Gastric bypass is an effective treatment for obstructive sleep apnea in patients with clinically significant obesity. Obes Surg. 2003;13:58–61.
251. Guardiano SA, Scott JA, Ware JC, Schechner SA. The long-term results of gastric bypass on indexes of sleep apnea. Chest. 2003;124:1615–9.
252. Buchwald H, Avidor Y, Braunwald E, Jensen MD, Pories W, Fahrbach K, et al. Bariatric surgery: a systematic review and meta-analysis. JAMA. 2004;292:1724–37.

Chapter 5
Obesity Hypoventilation Syndrome

Stephen W. Littleton and Babak Mokhlesi

Abstract Obesity hypoventilation syndrome (OHS) is defined as hypercapnia during wakefulness in an obese patient, without any other known cause, accompanied with some form of sleep-disordered breathing as reported by Mokhlesi et al. (Proc Am Thorac Soc 5:218–25, 2008). Although the effects of OHS are inadequately studied, available data show that morbidity and mortality are high. Among those with obstructive sleep apnea (OSA), risk factors for having OHS include a higher body mass index (BMI), an increased severity of sleep-disordered breathing, and a restrictive defect on pulmonary function testing. While the pathophysiology of the disorder remains unclear, it likely involves the presence of several defects, most notably a blunted central respiratory drive. The most effective treatment option consists of ventilatory support during sleep, in the form of positive airway pressure therapy, with or without supplemental oxygen.

Keywords Obesity hypoventilation syndrome • Pickwickian syndrome • Hypoventilation syndromes • Obstructive sleep apnea • Hypercapnia • Complications of obesity • Effects of obesity on respiratory physiology

S.W. Littleton, M.D. (✉)
Pulmonary, Critical Care, and Sleep Medicine, Cook County Hospital and Rush University Medical Center, 1900 W. Polk St. Room 1416, Chicago, IL 60612, USA
e-mail: slittleton@cookcountyhhs.org

B. Mokhlesi, M.D., M.Sc.
Department of Medicine/Section of Pulmonary and Critical Care, University of Chicago Pritzker School of Medicine, 5841 S. Maryland Ave MC 6076/Room M630, Chicago, IL 60637, USA
e-mail: bmokhles@medicine.bsd.uchicago.edu

A.E. Dixon and E.M. Clerisme-Beaty (eds.), *Obesity and Lung Disease: A Guide to Management*, Respiratory Medicine, DOI 10.1007/978-1-62703-053-3_5,

Objectives

- Review the epidemiology of OHS and its association with obesity
- Discuss the risk factors for OHS
- Review the effect of OHS on morbidity and mortality
- Evaluate treatment options/effectiveness for the management of OHS

Introduction

Historically known as the Pickwickian syndrome, obesity hypoventilation syndrome (OHS) is defined as hypercapnia during wakefulness in an obese patient, without any other known cause accompanied with some form of sleep-disordered breathing [1]. Among those with obstructive sleep apnea (OSA), risk factors for having OHS include a higher body mass index (BMI), an increased severity of sleep-disordered breathing (measured either by the apnea-hypopnea index (AHI) or the % of total sleep time spent with an oxyhemoglobin saturation below 90%), and a restrictive defect on pulmonary function testing [2]. Although the effects of OHS are inadequately studied, available data show that morbidity and mortality are high [3]. The pathophysiology of the disorder is also incompletely understood but likely involves the presence of several defects, most notably a blunted central respiratory drive. The most effective treatment option consists of ventilatory support during sleep, in the form of positive airway pressure therapy, with or without supplemental oxygen. Response to treatment can be full, partial, or minimal, for reasons that are not fully understood [4].

Historical Accounts of Obstructive Sleep Apnea/Obesity Hypoventilation Syndrome

Written accounts of obese, dyspneic, and hypersomnolent patients are almost as old as civilization itself. One of the earliest accounts dates back to Dionysius, a Greek tyrant, born circa 360 BC. It was written of him that "...Dionysius the Heracleote... through daily gluttony and intemperance, increased to an extraordinary degree of corpulency and fatness, by reason whereof he had much adoe to take breath..." because of his obesity, he was afflicted with shortness of breath and fits of choking. His physicians noted that he had difficulty breathing while he slept and devised what could be considered the first treatment for OSA: "So the physicians prescribed that he should get some fine needles, exceedingly long, which they thrust through his ribs and belly whenever he happened to fall into a very deep sleep [5]."

The first person to recognize the similarities between an obese, hypersomnolent patient and Joe, the Fat Boy, in Charles Dickens' *The Posthumous Papers of the Pickwick Club* was a Dr. R Caton of Liverpool, about 60 years after its first publication [6]. Dickens was known for his sharp observations, and the comparison between Joe the Fat Boy and Dr. Caton's patient is apt. Joe's master said of him, "Sleep! He's always asleep. Goes on errands fast asleep, and snores as he waits at the table." He was "red-faced," which could be interpreted as secondary erythrocytosis and also suffered from "young dropsy," the archaic term for congestive heart failure [5]. Mr. Pickwick himself, also obese, was probably not immune to the effects of alcohol on the upper airway. After a few too many glasses of wine, "His head was sunk upon his bosom; and perpetual snoring, with a partial choke occasionally, were the only audible indications of this great man's presence [5]." After arterial blood gas analyzers became widely available in the 1950s, Burwell and colleagues were able to objectively associate hypoventilation with obesity and hypersomnolence [7]. They named the syndrome, Pickwickian syndrome, and the nomenclature was widely adopted [8].

Epidemiology

Although the prevalence of OHS is unknown, a very rough estimate in the USA suggests that between 0.15% and 0.3% of the adult population may suffer from OHS [9]. The prevalence of hypercapnia among obese patients with OSA has been extensively studied in trials from several countries (Italy, the United States, Japan, France, Brazil, and the Netherlands) [10–16] and ranges between 10% and 20%, excluding patients with obstructive airways disease. A recent meta-analysis reported an overall prevalence of 19% among patients with OSA [2]. The prevalence of hypercapnia in hospitalized obese patients appears to be even higher. According to a prospective analysis of 150 obese hospitalized patients, 47 (31%) were found to be hypercapnic, even after excluding other reasons for hypercapnia, such as COPD [17]. This higher prevalence in a hospitalized population probably reflects the higher morbidity these patients experience.

The prevalence of OHS increases in patients with OSA with increasing BMI. Three studies have examined this phenomenon in detail. Although the prevalence among OSA patients with a BMI of 30–34 kg/m^2 is <10%, this increases to 18–25% in those with a BMI≥40 kg/m^2 [1]. Similarly, the prevalence of OHS increases in patients as the severity of OSA increases. Two other studies have reported the prevalence in patients with mild OSA (AHI 5–15 events per hour) to range from 0% to 7.5%, with a sharp increase to 25–28% in those with an AHI of >60 events per hour [9].

Although OSA is slightly more prevalent among men and in older populations, there is no clear association between risk of OHS and increasing age or gender in studies of patients with OSA. In a meta-analysis of 13 studies, the mean age difference between the hypercapnic group and the eucapnic group of patients with OSA was found to be 0.09 years ($p=0.9$), with no gender differences between hypercapnic and eucapnic OSA groups [2].

As the prevalence of obesity and severe obesity in the world increases, the prevalence of OHS is likely to follow suit. In a Swedish study of patients using home mechanical ventilation, the prevalence of OHS increased from 8% to 17% from 1996 to 2001 ($p<0.001$) [18]. Similar results were found in a Swiss study, where the proportion of patients with OHS increased from 14% to 39% ($p<0.001$) from 1992 to 1999 in patients using home noninvasive ventilation [19].

Morbidity and Mortality

The vast majority of patients with OHS are severely obese and have severe OSA [1], both of which are known to negatively affect quality of life, increase health care resource utilization, and increase morbidity and mortality [20–23]. As such, OHS may be associated with significant morbidity and mortality. Further, OHS may exert additional burden on patients independent of the effects of morbid obesity and sleep-disordered breathing.

Quality of Life

When compared to patients with other forms of chronic respiratory failure or OSA, it does not seem that patients with OHS have a significantly worse quality of life. A Japanese study compared patients with untreated OHS to patients with untreated eucapnic OSA matching for age, BMI, and lung function. There was no significant difference in quality of life between the two groups using the short-form 36 (SF-36) quality of life questionnaire, except for the social functioning category, where the OHS group fared worse. Both groups experienced a significant increase in overall quality of life after 3–6 months of treatment, although the authors failed to report whether the OHS group had a significantly greater improvement. The group with OHS was also found to be sleepier than the group with eucapnic OSA (Epworth Sleepiness Scale or ESS 14.6 ± 4.9 vs. 12.5 ± 4.6, $p<0.05$). However, this difference in sleepiness score has not been consistent across studies. A Greek study that examined 175 patients with OSA and 38 patients with OHS found the difference in ESS scores to be insignificant (11.9 ± 6.3 vs.9.5 ± 5.6). Although the OHS group was significantly more obese, the severity of sleep-disordered breathing between the two groups was nearly identical. Therefore, it is unclear whether chronic hypercapnia leads to more daytime sleepiness in these patients independent of obesity and OSA. Furthermore, when compared to other patients receiving home mechanical ventilation for hypercapnic respiratory failure, patients with OHS actually fare better on the severe respiratory insufficiency index (a measure of health-related quality of life in patients with chronic respiratory failure) than those with COPD [24]. This implies that patients with OHS may have a better quality of life than those patients with other forms of chronic respiratory failure.

In summary, OHS does not seem to worsen quality of life when compared to patients with severe OSA. Data on whether they are sleepier than OSA patients is mixed. OHS patients seem to suffer less from their disease when compared to other patients with chronic respiratory failure.

Use of Health Care Resources

Patients with OHS have higher health care costs and are much more likely to be hospitalized than the general population and even equally obese patients. A recent Danish study matched 755 patients with OHS to control subjects by age, sex, socio-economic status, and location. They found that OHS patients were more likely to receive both ambulatory (63% vs. 27%) and inpatient (53% vs. 13%) treatment [25]. A similar Canadian study compared 20 patients with OHS to a group matched for age, sex, and obesity. The OHS group was significantly more likely to be admitted to the hospital (odds ratio 4.9; 95% confidence interval 2.3–10.1, $p=0.001$) or the intensive care unit (mean ICU days per person 3.8 ± 1.49 vs. 0, $p=0.02$) in the 5 years prior to diagnosis than the obese control group. An impressive 70% of OHS patients were hospitalized at least once in the year prior to diagnosis. This rate of hospitalization decreased to 15% 2 years after treatment was initiated ($p<0.01$) [26]. This implies that treatment of OHS may reduce morbidity.

Unsurprisingly, these studies also showed that OHS patients have higher health care costs. In the Danish study, the annual health care costs of the OHS group was significantly higher than that of the control group, with an estimated cost of €13,050 vs. €1730 ($p<0.0001$) (or, \$17617 vs. \$2336 at €1=\$1.35). Annual health care costs for the OHS group was highest immediately after diagnosis at €75,000 but dropped to €40,000–50,000 within 7 years after diagnosis [25]. This implies that effective treatment can reduce health care costs in these patients. However, since these control subjects were not matched by BMI, it is unclear how much of these excess health care costs are secondary to obesity and how much are due to OHS itself. In the Danish study, the annual health costs per year were more than double that of the control group in the 5 years prior to diagnosis, decreasing significantly 2 years after diagnosis (but still remaining above that of the control group)[26].

When performed prospectively, these disparities in health care usage for OHS patients hold up. When hypercapnic obese patients were compared to patients with simple obesity upon hospital admission, the hypercapnic group was more likely to be admitted to the ICU (40% vs. 26%, $p=0.08$), receive invasive mechanical ventilation (6% vs.0%, $p=0.01$), or be discharged to a long-term care facility (9% vs. 2%, $p=0.01$) [17].

Taken together, data from these studies strongly suggest that patients with OHS utilize more health care resources but that treatment can reduce these costs and reduce hospitalizations.

Comorbidity

As OSA and obesity are associated with significant morbidity, it is difficult to determine what additional burden OHS might place on these patients.

Conventional wisdom holds that OHS patients are much more likely to have pulmonary hypertension (because of hypoxemia), but the data are conflicting.

One study found that OHS patients are nine times more likely to have cor pulmonale than matched obese controls (95% CI 1.4–57.1, $p<0.014$) [26]. Another prospective study of 34 OHS patients found 58% had pulmonary hypertension, compared to only 9% of the OSA control group ($p<0.001$) [12]. In contrast, a different prospective study reported only 11% of hospitalized patients with obesity and hypercapnia had pulmonary hypertension compared to 4% of the simple obesity group. However, the difference did not reach statistical significance ($p=0.11$) [17].

Two studies have reported a higher rate of congestive heart failure in patients with OHS [26, 27]. A recent Greek study also found very similar results [27]. 13.2% of the OHS group suffered from congestive heart failure, compared with only 2.9% of the OSA group ($p=0.026$). Interestingly, in two of these studies, there was no difference in the prevalence of hypertension or diabetes mellitus between patients with OHS and obese controls [26], [27]. It is unclear why OHS is associated with CHF, and if the relationship is causal. There are also no studies that have studied the prevalence of other diseases associated with obesity in OHS patients, such as metabolic syndrome or hypertension. From these data, it seems reasonable to consider the diagnosis of OHS in patients with both OSA who also have comorbid congestive heart failure or pulmonary hypertension.

Mortality

Patients with OHS are at higher risk of death than those with obesity and OSA. A prospective study of hospitalized obese, hypercapnic patients found a 23% 18-month mortality rate, compared to 9% in the simple obesity group (hazard ratio 4.0, 95% CI 1.5–10.4), adjusted for age, sex, BMI, and renal function. This is significantly higher than the reported 2-year mortality rate (7–8%) in patients treated for OHS [28, 29] and is likely due to the fact that only 13% of the hypercapnic group were treated for OHS upon discharge.

These findings suggest that treatment can reduce mortality in OHS. However, even when treated, OHS is associated with a higher mortality rate than OSA. The Kaplan-Meier curves are remarkably similar across studies (Fig. 5.1). Given that patients with OHS in these studies tend to be more obese, it is unclear whether the excess mortality is due to obesity or OHS. In addition, compared to other forms of hypercapnic respiratory failure (such as COPD, neuromuscular disorders, and kyphoscoliosis), patients with OHS have a better long-term survival [30].

Prognostic factors for mortality in OHS have been studied, although their utility is unclear. Use of supplemental oxygen is a predictor of poor outcome in OHS, with a 5-year survival rate of <60% compared to >80% in those with and without oxygen, respectively ($p=0.004$) [29]. A multivariate analysis, from a German study, also found daytime hypoxia and leukocyte count to be predicted of poor outcomes, with a daytime $PaO_2<50$ mmHg, a pH$\geq$7.44, and a leukocyte count of$\geq 7.8\times 10^{-3}$ being associated with higher mortality [30]. A reduction of nocturnal $PaCO_2 \geq 23.0\%$ after treatment was initiated and was found to be associated with improved survival. Unlike

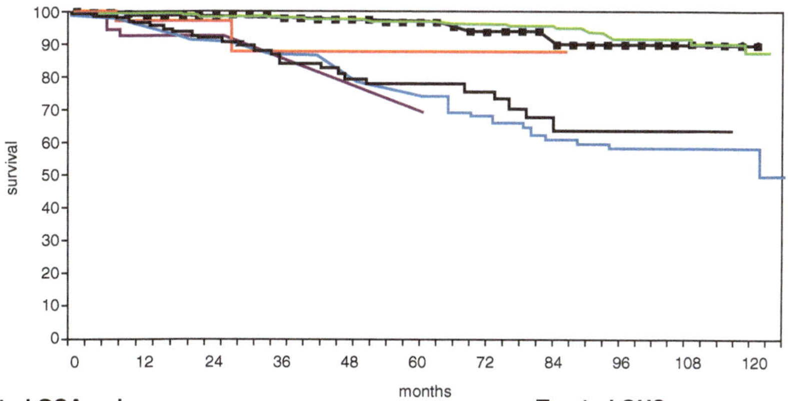

Treated OSA only:
Black squares: Campos-Rodriguez F, *et al.* Mortality in obstructive sleep apnea-hyponea patients treated with positive airway pressure. Chest 2005 Aug; 128(2):624-33.
Green line: Marti S, *et al.* Mortality in severe sleep apnea/hypopnea syndrome patients: impact of treatment. Eur Respir J 2002 Dec; 20(6) 1511-8.

Treated OHS:
Red line: reference 21
Black line: reference 33
Purple line: references 1 and 27
Blue line: reference 20

Fig. 5.1 Kaplan-Meier survival curves comparing various studies on cohorts with treated obstructive sleep apnea and treated obesity hypoventilation syndrome

COPD, where a shorter 6-min walk distance is predictive of mortality, 6-min walk test has not been found to have any prognostic value in patients with OHS [31].

In summary, it appears that OHS is associated with congestive heart failure, although whether it is associated with other conditions is unknown. Mortality also seems to be higher in OHS patients, even when treated and compared to treated OSA patients. It is important to note that the available data is limited by the retrospective study designs, small sample sizes, and use of cohorts from sleep laboratories. As such, larger studies with community cohorts are needed to confirm these findings.

Pathophysiology

Altered Respiratory Mechanics

It is well known that obesity can produce a restrictive defect on pulmonary function testing. However, compared to similarly obese patients, patients with OHS have greater reductions in total lung capacity (TLC) and functional residual capacity (FRC) [32, 33]. One explanation for this disparity in TLC and FRC is the pattern of fat distribution. Patients with OHS have more central obesity (as measured by waist to hip ratio), which may place a greater burden on respiratory mechanics compared to lower body adiposity. Patients with OHS also have lower pulmonary and chest wall compliance than patients that are equally obese [34], likely due to the lower FRC in those with OHS. Furthermore, OHS is also associated with increased lung resistance, three times higher than that of eucapnic obese individuals, again thought to be secondary to the reduced FRC [34]. However, altered respiratory mechanics, although clearly more impaired in patients with OHS, cannot explain the chronic hypercapnia in these patients in the absence of altered respiratory muscle function and/or a defective central respiratory drive.

Increased CO_2 Production

Compared to nonobese controls, CO_2 production is elevated in severely obese subjects individuals [35, 36]. While a portion of the excess CO_2 production may be related to the increased work of breathing, a significant production is due to metabolically active adipose tissue. Most severely obese patients, however, do not develop daytime hypercapnia because of a normal adaptive response to increase ventilation based on the degree of CO_2 production.

Increased Work of Breathing/Respiratory Muscle Function

Early work showed that altered respiratory mechanics lead to an increased work of breathing in obese individuals to approximately 30% above that of normal subjects. The work of breathing in hypercapnic obese patients far exceeds that of even equally obese patients and is almost three times that of normal subjects [34]. This increased work of breathing leads to an increase in the oxygen cost of breathing. Morbidly obese subjects have to commit 15% of their oxygen consumption to the work of breathing, compared to 3% of normal subjects [36]. This may be even higher in patients who are hypercapnic.

More recent research on the work of breathing in patients with OHS confirms earlier findings. Work of breathing in patients with OHS has been shown to be 250% that of nonobese controls while upright and twice that of an equally obese eucapnic group. Evaluations of work of breathing while supine and in stage 2 sleep also show similar results. OHS patients expended almost three times the energy as normal subjects in stage 2 sleep, and 50% more than the eucapnic obese group ($p<0.05$). This increase was equally divided between resistive and elastic work of breathing [37].

The increase in the work of breathing while supine is at least partially explained by the intrinsic positive end-expiratory pressure (PEEPi) seen in obese subjects when supine. In one study, a mean PEEPi of 5.3 ± 3.6 cm H_2O was measured in a group with a mean BMI of 42.8 ± 8.6. This was accompanied by an increase in neural drive when diaphragmatic EMG was measured by an esophageal probe [38]. Therefore, in order for this increased work of breathing to lead to chronic hypercapnia, either the increase in neural drive must be inadequate (implying a central defect) or there must be an insufficient increase in work of the respiratory muscles (implying acute or chronic respiratory muscle fatigue).

Respiratory muscle strength in patients with OHS has not been rigorously studied. However, early studies show it to be 60–70% of normal [39]. Respiratory muscle strength, measured by maximal respiratory pressures, can be normal [40–42] or reduced in eucapnic obese subjects [42, 43]. In contrast, maximum voluntary ventilation is often reduced in severely obese subjects and is correlated with BMI [42, 43]. The fact that many patients with OHS can still voluntarily hyperventilate to eucapnia implies a central rather than peripheral defect [44]. In addition, patients with OHS also show significant improvements in hypercapnia without significant changes in respiratory muscle strength after 2 weeks of positive airway pressure (PAP) therapy [45], thus suggesting that, while it may be present, respiratory muscle weakness or respiratory muscle fatigability may not be necessary for the development of chronic hypercapnia in OHS.

Patients with OHS do not hyperventilate to the same degree as equally obese patients when presented with a hypercapnic challenge [46, 47]. This implies a defect in central respiratory drive. In addition, during a hypercapnic challenge, the work produced by the diaphragm (as measured by transdiaphragmatic pressure, or Pdi) increases at the same rate in patients who previously had OHS as in equally obese subjects. The increase in neural activity of the diaphragm was not as brisk, further implying a neural defect [46]. This blunted neural response improves or corrects after successful treatment with PAP therapy [47–49].

In summary, although OHS patients have a higher work of breathing than equally obese patients and may have weaker respiratory muscles, the available evidence shows the main defect leading to hypercapnia is a blunted respiratory drive.

Sleep-Disordered Breathing

As previously stated, some form of sleep-disordered breathing is central to the pathogenesis of OHS and is a defining characteristic of the syndrome [1]. While most patients have OSA, approximately 10% have persistent nocturnal desaturation as well as sleep hypoventilation without obstructive events. Most, but not all, patients with OHS have an improvement or resolution of hypercapnia with effective treatment of sleep-disordered breathing with either PAP therapy or tracheostomy [47, 50–55]. Duration of usage of PAP therapy is also directly correlated with improvement in hypercapnia [56], with hyperventilatory response to a hypercapnic challenge also improving or normalizing following adequate PAP therapy [47–49], thus suggesting that the hypercapnia and blunted central respiratory drive associated with OHS may develop secondary to severe sleep-disordered breathing.

Norman and colleagues have developed and mathematically tested a model explaining how sleep-disordered breathing leads to daytime hypercapnia [57]. In most patients with OSA, the hyperventilation that follows an obstructive apnea eliminates all the CO_2 accumulated during the apnea [58]. However, if that hyperventilatory response is inadequate, either because of a blunted central response or a short hyperventilatory time before the next obstructive apnea, it may lead to an increased $PaCO_2$ during sleep [59]. As a result, the kidneys retain small amount of

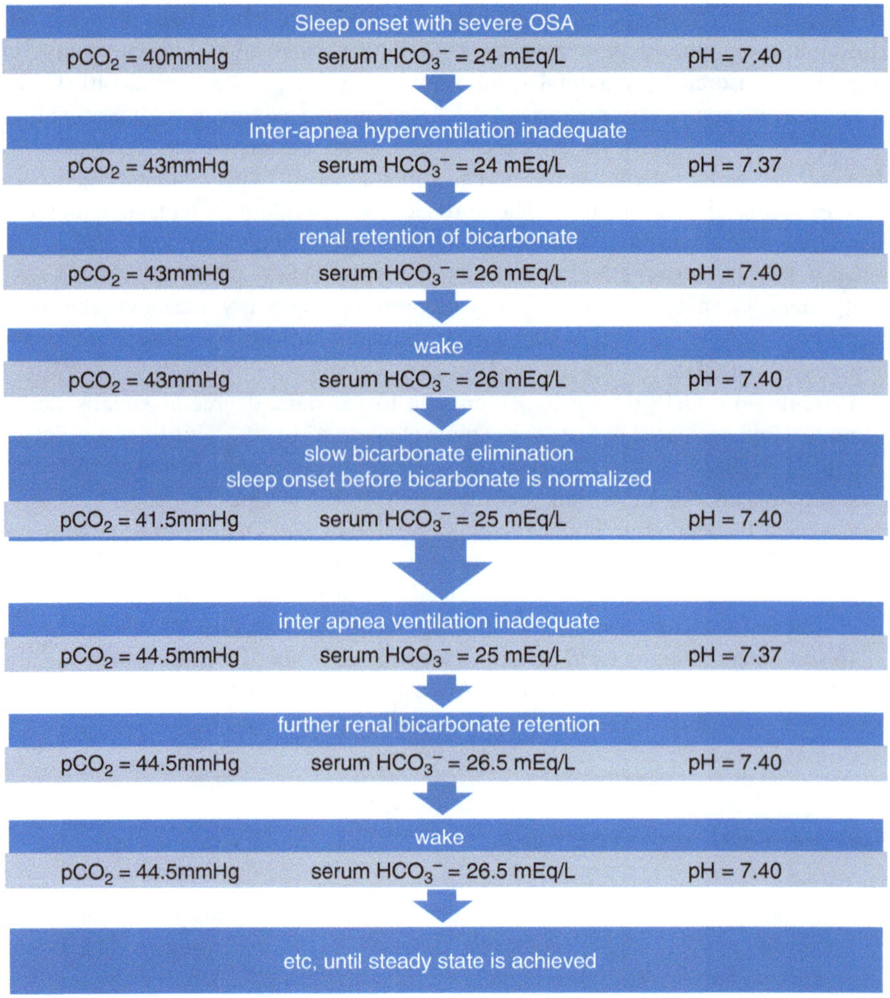
Sleep onset with severe OSA
pCO2 = 40mmHg serum HCO3− = 24 mEq/L pH = 7.40
Inter-apnea hyperventilation inadequate
pCO2 = 43mmHg serum HCO3− = 24 mEq/L pH = 7.37
renal retention of bicarbonate
pCO2 = 43mmHg serum HCO3− = 26 mEq/L pH = 7.40
wake
pCO2 = 43mmHg serum HCO3− = 26 mEq/L pH = 7.40
slow bicarbonate elimination
sleep onset before bicarbonate is normalized
pCO2 = 41.5mmHg serum HCO3− = 25 mEq/L pH = 7.40
inter apnea ventilation inadequate
pCO2 = 44.5mmHg serum HCO3− = 25 mEq/L pH = 7.37
further renal bicarbonate retention
pCO2 = 44.5mmHg serum HCO3− = 26.5 mEq/L pH = 7.40
wake
pCO2 = 44.5mmHg serum HCO3− = 26.5 mEq/L pH = 7.40
etc, until steady state is achieved

Fig. 5.2 Mechanism of daytime hypercapnia in sleep-disordered breathing patient

bicarbonate to buffer the change in pH. However, if the patient does not eliminate the retained bicarbonate during wakefulness before the next sleep period, there will be a net gain in bicarbonate. This can lead to a feedback loop were the patient then retain some CO_2 to buffer the metabolic alkalosis (Fig. 5.2) [57].

Leptin

Leptin is a satiety hormone, produced by adipocytes, that is increased in obesity and stimulates ventilation [60–63]. We have seen that obesity leads to increased O_2 consumption, increased CO_2 production [36], and increased load on the respiratory system. Therefore, the increase in leptin level in obesity helps compensate for the increased CO_2 burden. Patients with OHS and OSA have higher leptin levels than normal subjects and BMI-matched subjects without sleep-disordered breathing. Although it is unclear whether OSA or OHS independently contributes to the increased in leptin levels, the data suggest that increased adiposity is the main contributor [64–67]. Furthermore, patients with OHS have higher levels of leptin than age-, sex-, and BMI-matched subjects with OSA, with leptin levels dropping after PAP therapy [66, 68, 69]. However, this elevation is counterintuitive, since one would expect higher leptin levels to lead to improve ventilation, and therefore protect against the development of hypercapnia. Leptin resistance has been suggested as one possible explanation for this disparity. For leptin to affect the respiratory center and increase minute ventilation, it must penetrate into the cerebrospinal fluid (CSF). The leptin CSF/serum ratio is four times higher in lean individuals compared to obese subjects [70]. It is possible that difference in leptin CSF penetration may explain why some individuals with severe OSA and severe obesity develop OHS and others do not.

Diagnosis

OHS is largely a diagnosis of exclusion. The patient must be obese ($BMI \geq 35\ kg/m^2$), have some form of sleep-disordered breathing (either OSA or sleep hypoventilation) on polysomnography, and have daytime hypercapnia ($PaCO_2 \geq 45$ mmHg). Once these conditions are met, all other causes of hypercapnia should be excluded. The patient should undergo pulmonary function testing to examine for obstructive airways disease. Chest radiography should be obtained to exclude kyphoscoliosis or parenchymal lung diseases. Physical examination should look for muscle weakness or other signs of a neuromuscular disorder. Thyroid function studies should be obtained to rule out severe hypothyroidism, a rare but possible cause of hypoventilation [1]. Elevated serum bicarbonate level due to metabolic compensation of respiratory acidosis is common in OHS, pointing toward the chronic nature of hypercapnia, and may be used as a sensitive test to screen for hypercapnia [16].

Predictors of Hypercapnia in Obese OSA Patients

The probability of OSA increases proportionally with increased obesity and OSA severity. A recent meta-analysis found that the mean AHI of hypercapnic patients to be 64 events per hour (95% CI 52–76), compared to 51 events per hour in the eucapnic group (95% CI 42–60, $p < 0.001$). Likewise, hypercapnic patients had a higher mean BMI than those who were eucapnic, 39 kg/m^2 (95% CI 34–44 kg/m^2) vs. 36 kg/m^2 (95% CI 31–41 kg/m^2), $p < 0.001$ [2]. Although statistically significant, the confidence intervals overlap enough such that it prevents BMI or AHI from being clinically useful predictors. However, it would be reasonable to at least consider OHS in any patient with an AHI >60, as two studies have found the prevalence of OHS in this population to be 25–30% [9, 71].

The percent of total sleep time spent with an oxyhemoglobin saturation <90% (TST<90%) was also identified as a potential predictor of OHS risk in the same meta-analysis. Hypercapnia was associated with a longer duration of low oxygen saturation, with a mean TST<90% of 56.7% in the hypercapnic group versus 21.3% in the eucapnic group ($p<0.000001$). Given the wide differences in TST<90% between the two groups, it may be reasonable to initiate a workup for hypercapnia in a patient who spend≥50% of their total sleep time with an oxyhemoglobin saturation <90% with a polysomnogram, if there are no other known causes for such prolonged hypoxemia.

Treatment

PAP therapy is the most effective treatment for OHS. The use of CPAP for treatment of OHS was first described in 1982 [54], and subsequent studies have confirmed CPAP's efficacy [11, 51, 72]. However, the fact that PAP is not universally effective has led some to question whether bi-level PAP therapy is superior [11, 51, 54, 72, 73]. For example, in a recent prospective study, only 57% of patients were successfully titrated with CPAP using a mean pressure of 13.9 cm H_2O [74]. The other 43% of patients failed CPAP titration because the oxygen saturation remained below 90% for >20% of TST. In addition, these patients had a residual AHI of 25 events per hour, which suggests that a therapeutic pressure was not reached. Unfortunately, since this was a single-night titration study, the question of whether this hypoxemia would have resolved with long-term CPAP therapy was not explored [74].

A recent prospective, randomized study by Piper et al. has compared the long-term efficacy of bi-level PAP with CPAP [75]. After 3 months, there was no significant difference in the degree of improvement in daytime hypercapnia. Moreover, there were no differences in treatment adherence, improvement in daytime sleepiness, or hypoxemia between CPAP and bi-level PAP therapy, thus confirming that the majority of patients with OHS (80%) can be successfully treated with CPAP. Based on the results of this study, bi-level PAP therapy is not superior to CPAP a priori. Rather, treatment should be individualized to each patient.

Bi-level PAP should be used if the patient is intolerant of higher CPAP pressure (>15 cm H_2O), if such a pressure is required to abolish respiratory events or maintain an oxyhemoglobin saturation >90% [77]. During bi-level PAP titration, the inspiratory PAP (IPAP) should be at least 8–10 cm H_2O above the expiratory PAP (EPAP) in order to augment tidal volume and increase minute ventilation [52, 53, 78, 79]. Ideally, tidal volumes should be monitored during bi-level PAP titration in order to achieve the needed level of pressure support (difference between IPAP and EPAP) to improve ventilation. In the minority of patients with OHS who do not have OSA, those with pure sleep hypoventilation, EPAP can be set at 5 cm H_2O and IPAP titrated upward to increase ventilation [78, 79]. Bi-level PAP should also be considered if the $PaCO_2$ does not normalize after 3 months of CPAP therapy.

Impact of Adherence to PAP Therapy on Hypercapnia and Hypoxemia

Average hours of daily use, over a period of 1 month, are directly correlated with improvement in arterial blood gas values. In a retrospective study of 75 outpatients with stable OHS, the $PaCO_2$ decreased by 1.8 mmHg and the PaO_2 increased by 3 mmHg for every mean hour of usage in the last 30 days. In addition, the need for daytime oxygen therapy decreased from 30% of patients prior to PAP therapy to 6% after 30 days of PAP therapy [51]. Therefore, in patients with OHS on daytime oxygen therapy, the need for supplemental oxygen during wakefulness should be reassessed 4–8 weeks after effective PAP therapy is started.

Lack of Improvement in Hypercapnia After PAP Therapy

The most likely cause of a lack of improvement in hypercapnia is nonadherence with PAP therapy. If there is objective evidence of good adherence on the device monitor, other possibilities should be considered, such as inadequate PAP titration, failure of CPAP therapy, or other causes of hypercapnia such as COPD, hypothyroidism, or metabolic alkalosis secondary to diuretic usage [3].

Improvement of daytime hypercapnia in those OHS patients adherent with PAP therapy can be complete, partial, or completely lacking. In two studies, the $PaCO_2$ did not improve in approximately 25% of OHS patients, who had successful PAP titrations and were highly adherent with either CPAP or bi-level PAP therapy (>6 h/night) [56, 76]. In one of these studies, eight patients (34%) who were adherent with PAP therapy for at least 4.5 h daily did not have a significant improvement in $PaCO_2$ (less than 4 mmHg) [56]. These patients tended to have a lower AHI than the group that responded.

Lack of response to PAP therapy, along with case reports of persistent hypoventilation after tracheostomy, suggests that there is a subset of patients with OHS where the driving force behind hypoventilation is something other than OSA. These patients will likely need more aggressive nocturnal ventilation [3].

Average Volume-Assured Pressure-Support Ventilation

Average volume-assured pressure-support ventilation (AVAPS) is a hybrid between pressure-support and volume-controlled ventilation. It delivers a more consistent tidal volume with the comfort of pressure-support ventilation. It ensures a preset tidal volume during bi-level S/T mode. Although significantly more expensive than CPAP or even bi-level PAP devices, it has been shown effective in patients with mild hypercapnia who had failed CPAP therapy, particularly in improving hypoventilation during sleep [80].

Oxygen Therapy

In up to 50% of patients with OHS, oxygen therapy (in addition to PAP therapy) is necessary to maintain oxyhemoglobin saturation >90% [74]. As mentioned previously, the need for oxygen therapy may abate with regular PAP usage, and this need should be reassessed after 4–8 weeks of effective PAP therapy. Oxygen should be used cautiously, especially in patients who present with acute respiratory failure, as 100% oxygen therapy can worsen hypercapnia in some patients with OHS [81, 82].

Weight-Reduction Surgery

Bariatric surgery has variable long-term efficacy in treating obesity and OSA. One study showed that after an average of 11 months after Roux-en-Y gastric bypass, those with severe OSA had a reduction in AHI from 80 to 20 events per hour [83]. It is notable that some of these patients still had moderate OSA and would still benefit from PAP therapy. In another study, approximately half of those who had only mild OSA after maximum weight loss had developed severe OSA 7 years later, without significant weight gain [84]. A recent meta-analysis included 12 studies with 342 patients who underwent polysomnography before surgery and after maximum weight loss. The meta-analysis found there was a 71% reduction in the severity of OSA, the AHI going from a preoperative 55 events per hour to a postoperative 16 events per hour. However, only 38% achieved a cure, defined as an AHI<5 events per hour [86]. Only one study has examined the effects of bariatric surgery on OHS specifically. One year after surgery, 31 patients had significant improvement in both PaO_2 and $PaCO_2$. Five years after surgery, results were available in 12 patients, and their values had slightly worsened without significant weight gain [86]. The worsening of arterial blood gases was probably secondary to the redevelopment of sleep-disordered breathing.

Given that patients experience a 7% weight gain 6–8 years after weight-reduction surgery (relative to their lowest weight after surgery), patients with OSA and OHS should be monitored for recurrence of disease [87]. Bariatric surgery carries some risk, and OSA and OHS may be associated with even higher operative mortality [88, 89]. Patients with OHS should therefore be treated with PAP therapy or, in the case of PAP failure, undergo tracheostomy before having bariatric surgery. PAP therapy should also be applied after extubation to prevent postoperative respiratory failure [90–92], as there is no evidence that postoperative PAP therapy leads to anastomotic disruption or leakage [91, 93].

Tracheostomy

Tracheostomy was the first therapy described for the treatment of OHS [94]. In a retrospective study of 13 patients with OHS, tracheostomy was associated with a significant improvement in OSA, but in seven patients, the AHI remained above

20 events per hour. Despite this, the majority of patients experienced resolution of hypercapnia [95]. Tracheostomy is now reserved for patients who are not adherent with, or intolerant of, PAP therapy, or for patients who present with multiple episodes of acute respiratory failure requiring intubation and invasive mechanical ventilation. Patients with tracheostomies may require nocturnal mechanical ventilation, as central hypoventilation may persist [96]. A polysomnogram with the tracheostomy open is required to determine whether mechanical ventilation is needed [52].

Acetazolamide

Acetazolamide induces metabolic acidosis through carbonic anhydrase inhibition, which increases minute ventilation in normal subjects. It also reduces the AHI in patients with moderate to severe OSA [97, 98]. In patients with OHS and mechanically ventilated for acute respiratory failure, acetazolamide also increases hypercapnic drive and the hypercapnic ventilatory response [99]. As for long-term therapy, there is one case report of a patient who failed to respond to a tracheostomy, but blood gases normalized after acetazolamide therapy [72]. Further study is needed to see if acetazolamide is an effective adjunct therapy for patients who do not respond to PAP therapy.

Medroxyprogesterone

Medroxyprogesterone acts as a hypothalamic respiratory stimulant [100]. Results of treatment of OHS with medroxyprogesterone have been inconsistent, with some patients normalizing blood gases [101] and others (with tracheostomy) remaining unchanged [72]. Administration of a medication that may increase the risk of venous thromboembolism, especially in a population with limited mobility, may be risky [102, 103]. Consideration of medroxyprogesterone therapy in patients who do not respond to PAP therapy should take this risk into account.

Conclusion

OHS is a condition that is frequently under-recognized, despite its relatively high prevalence in patients with severe OSA and severe obesity. Recognition is important, as effective therapy reduces health care costs, reduces hospital admissions, reduces morbidity, and likely reduces mortality. The central pathogenic mechanism seems to be sleep-disordered breathing, but it is unclear why some patients with severe OSA and severe obesity develop OHS and others do not. The cornerstone of treatment is PAP therapy, but further study is needed to determine effective adjunct therapies in the subgroup of patients who either partially respond, or do not respond at all.

References

1. Mokhlesi B, Kryger MH, Grunstein RR. Assessment and management of patients with obesity hypoventilation syndrome. Proc Am Thorac Soc. 2008;5(2):218–25.
2. Kaw R, Hernandez AV, Walker E, Aboussouan L, Mokhlesi B. Determinants of hypercapnia in obese patients with obstructive sleep apnea. Chest. 2009;136(3):787–96.
3. Mokhlesi B. Obesity hypoventilation syndrome: a state-of-the-art review. Respir Care. 2010;55(10):1347–65.
4. Piper AJ. Obesity hypoventilation syndrome – the big and the breathless. Sleep Med Rev. 2011;15(2):79–89.
5. Kryger MH. Sleep apnea. From the needles of Dionysius to continuous positive airway pressure. Arch Intern Med. 1983;143(12):2301–3.
6. Caton R. Reports of societies, "A case of narcolepsy". Br Med J. 1889;357(1):358.
7. Bickelmann AG, Burwell CS, Robin ED, Whaley RD. Extreme obesity associated with alveolar hypoventilation; a Pickwickian syndrome. Am J Med. 1956;21(5):811–8.
8. Auchincloss Jr JH, Cook E, Renzetti AD. Clinical and physiological aspects of a case of obesity, polycythemia and alveolar hypoventilation. J Clin Invest. 1955;34(10):1537.
9. Littleton SW, Mokhlesi B. The pickwickian syndrome-obesity hypoventilation syndrome. Clin Chest Med. 2009;30(3):467–78. vii–viii.
10. Verin E, Tardif C, Pasquis P. Prevalence of daytime hypercapnia or hypoxia in patients with OSAS and normal lung function. Respir Med. 2001;95(8):693–6.
11. Laaban J-P, Chailleux E. Daytime hypercapnia in adult patients with obstructive sleep apnea syndrome in France, before initiating nocturnal nasal continuous positive airway pressure therapy. Chest. 2005;127(3):710–5.
12. Kessler R, Chaouat A, Schinkewitch P, et al. The obesity-hypoventilation syndrome revisited: a prospective study of 34 consecutive cases. Chest. 2001;120(2):369–76.
13. Resta O, Foschino Barbaro MP, Bonfitto P, et al. Hypercapnia in obstructive sleep apnoea syndrome. Neth J Med. 2000;56(6):215–22.
14. Golpe R, Jiménez A, Carpizo R. Diurnal hypercapnia in patients with obstructive sleep apnea syndrome. Chest. 2002;122(3):1100–1. author reply 1101.
15. Akashiba T, Akahoshi T, Kawahara S, et al. Clinical characteristics of obesity-hypoventilation syndrome in Japan: a multi-center study. Intern Med. 2006;45(20):1121–5.
16. Mokhlesi B, Tulaimat A, Faibussowitsch I, Wang Y, Evans AT. Obesity hypoventilation syndrome: prevalence and predictors in patients with obstructive sleep apnea. Sleep Breath. 2007;11(2):117–24.
17. Nowbar S, Burkart KM, Gonzales R, et al. Obesity-Associated hypoventilation in hospitalized patients: prevalence, effects, and outcome* 1. Am J Med. 2004;116(1):1–7.
18. Laub M, Berg S, Midgren B. Home mechanical ventilation in Sweden–inequalities within a homogenous health care system. Respir Med. 2004;98(1):38–42.
19. Janssens J-P. Changing patterns in long-term noninvasive ventilation: a 7-year prospective study in the Geneva lake area. Chest. 2003;123(1):67–79.
20. Flegal KM, Graubard BI, Williamson DF, Gail MH. Excess deaths associated with underweight, overweight, and obesity. JAMA. 2005;293(15):1861–7.
21. Young T, Finn L, Peppard PE, et al. Sleep disordered breathing and mortality: eighteen-year follow-up of the Wisconsin sleep cohort. Sleep. 2008;31(8):1071–8.
22. Punjabi NM, Caffo BS, Goodwin JL, et al. Sleep-disordered breathing and mortality: a prospective cohort study. PLoS Med. 2009;6(8):e1000132.
23. Marin JM, Carrizo SJ, Vicente E, Agusti AGN. Long-term cardiovascular outcomes in men with obstructive sleep apnoea-hypopnoea with or without treatment with continuous positive airway pressure: an observational study. Lancet. 2005;365(9464):1046–53.
24. Budweiser S, Hitzl AP, Jörres RA, et al. Health-related quality of life and long-term prognosis in chronic hypercapnic respiratory failure: a prospective survival analysis. Respir Res. 2007;8:17–92.

25. Jennum P, Kjellberg J. Health, social and economical consequences of sleep-disordered breathing: a controlled national study. Thorax. 2011;66(7):560–6.
26. Berg G, Delaive K, Manfreda J, Walld R, Kryger MH. The use of health-care resources in obesity-hypoventilation syndrome. Chest. 2001;120(2):377–83.
27. Trakada GP, Steiropoulos P, Nena E, Constandinidis TC, Bouros D. Prevalence and clinical characteristics of obesity hypoventilation syndrome among individuals reporting sleep-related breathing symptoms in northern Greece. Sleep Breath. 2010;14(4):381–6.
28. Budweiser S, Riedl SG, Jörres RA, Heinemann F, Pfeifer M. Mortality and prognostic factors in patients with obesity-hypoventilation syndrome undergoing noninvasive ventilation. J Intern Med. 2007;261(4):375–83.
29. Priou P, Hamel J-F, Person C, et al. Long-term outcome of noninvasive positive pressure ventilation for obesity hypoventilation syndrome. Chest. 2010;138(1):84–90.
30. Janssens J-P, Derivaz S, Breitenstein E, et al. Changing patterns in long-term noninvasive ventilation: a 7-year prospective study in the Geneva Lake area. Chest. 2003;123(1):67–79.
31. Budweiser S, Heidtkamp F, Jörres RA, et al. Predictive significance of the six-minute walk distance for long-term survival in chronic hypercapnic respiratory failure. Respiration. 2008;75(4):418–26.
32. Lopata M, Onal E. Mass loading, sleep apnea, and the pathogenesis of obesity hypoventilation. Am Rev Respir Dis. 1982;126(4):640–5.
33. Heinemann F, Budweiser S, Dobroschke J, Pfeifer M. Non-invasive positive pressure ventilation improves lung volumes in the obesity hypoventilation syndrome. Respir Med. 2007;101(6):1229–35.
34. Sharp JT, Henry JP, Sweany SK, Meadows WR, Pietras RJ. The total work of breathing in normal and obese men. J Clin Invest. 1964;43:728–39.
35. Gilbert R, Sipple JH, Auchincloss Jr JH. Respiratory control and work of breathing in obese subjects. J Appl Physiol. 1961;16:21–6.
36. Kress JP, Pohlman AS, Alverdy J, Hall JB. The impact of morbid obesity on oxygen cost of breathing (VO(2RESP)) at rest. Am J Respir Crit Care Med. 1999;160(3):883–6.
37. Lee M-Y, Lin C-C, Shen S-Y, Chiu C-H, Liaw S-F. Work of breathing in eucapnic and hypercapnic sleep apnea syndrome. Respiration. 2009;77(2):146–53.
38. Steier J, Jolley CJ, Seymour J, et al. Neural respiratory drive in obesity. Thorax. 2009;64(8):719–25.
39. Rochester DF, Enson Y. Current concepts in the pathogenesis of the obesity-hypoventilation syndrome. Mechanical and circulatory factors. Am J Med. 1974;57(3):402–20.
40. Collet F, Mallart A, Bervar JF, et al. Physiologic correlates of dyspnea in patients with morbid obesity. Int J Obes (Lond). 2007;31(4):700–6.
41. Kelly TM, Jensen RL, Elliott CG, Crapo RO. Maximum respiratory pressures in morbidly obese subjects. Respiration. 1988;54(2):73–7.
42. Ladosky W, Botelho MA, Albuquerque Jr JP. Chest mechanics in morbidly obese non-hypoventilated patients. Respir Med. 2001;95(4):281–6.
43. Sarikaya S, Cimen O, Gokcay Y, Erdem R. Pulmonary function tests, respiratory muscle strength, and endurance of persons with obesity. Endocrinologist. 2003;13:136–41.
44. Leech J, Onal E, Aronson R, Lopata M. Voluntary hyperventilation in obesity hypoventilation. Chest. 1991;100(5):1334–8.
45. Masa JF, Celli BR, Riesco JA, et al. Noninvasive positive pressure ventilation and not oxygen may prevent overt ventilatory failure in patients with chest wall diseases. Chest. 1997;112(1):207–13.
46. Sampson MG, Grassino K. Neuromechanical properties in obese patients during carbon dioxide rebreathing. Am J Med. 1983;75(1):81–90.
47. Han F, Chen E, Wei H, et al. Treatment effects on carbon dioxide retention in patients with obstructive sleep apnea-hypopnea syndrome. Chest. 2001;119(6):1814–9.
48. Berthon-Jones M, Sullivan CE. Time course of change in ventilatory response to CO_2 with long-term CPAP therapy for obstructive sleep apnea. Am Rev Respir Dis. 1987;135(1):144–7.

49. Lin CC. Effect of nasal CPAP on ventilatory drive in normocapnic and hypercapnic patients with obstructive sleep apnoea syndrome. Eur Respir J. 1994;7(11):2005–10.
50. Masa JF, Celli BR, Riesco JA, et al. The obesity hypoventilation syndrome can be treated with noninvasive mechanical ventilation. Chest. 2001;119(4):1102–7.
51. Mokhlesi B, Tulaimat A, Evans AT, et al. Impact of adherence with positive airway pressure therapy on hypercapnia in obstructive sleep apnea. J Clin Sleep Med. 2006;2(1):57.
52. Berger KI, Ayappa I, Chatr-Amontri B, et al. Obesity hypoventilation syndrome as a spectrum of respiratory disturbances during sleep. Chest. 2001;120(4):1231–8.
53. Pérez de Llano LA, Golpe R, Ortiz Piquer M, et al. Short-term and long-term effects of nasal intermittent positive pressure ventilation in patients with obesity-hypoventilation syndrome. Chest. 2005;128(2):587–94.
54. Rapoport DM, Sorkin B, Garay SM, Goldring RM. Reversal of the "Pickwickian syndrome" by long-term use of nocturnal nasal-airway pressure. N Engl J Med. 1982;307(15):931–3.
55. Leech JA, Onal E, Lopata M. Nasal CPAP continues to improve sleep-disordered breathing and daytime oxygenation over long-term follow-up of occlusive sleep apnea syndrome. Chest. 1992;102(6):1651–5.
56. Mokhlesi B, Tulaimat A, Evans AT, et al. Impact of adherence with positive airway pressure therapy on hypercapnia in obstructive sleep apnea. J Clin Sleep Med. 2006;2(1):57–62.
57. Norman RG, Goldring RM, Clain JM, et al. Transition from acute to chronic hypercapnia in patients with periodic breathing: predictions from a computer model. J Appl Physiol. 2006;100(5):1733–41.
58. Ayappa I, Berger KI, Norman RG, et al. Hypercapnia and ventilatory periodicity in obstructive sleep apnea syndrome. Am J Respir Crit Care Med. 2002;166(8):1112–5.
59. Berger KI, Ayappa I, Sorkin IB, et al. CO(2) homeostasis during periodic breathing in obstructive sleep apnea. J Appl Physiol. 2000;88(1):257–64.
60. Kalra SP. Central leptin insufficiency syndrome: an interactive etiology for obesity, metabolic and neural diseases and for designing new therapeutic interventions. Peptides. 2008;29(1): 127–38.
61. Tankersley C, Kleeberger S, Russ B, Schwartz A, Smith P. Modified control of breathing in genetically obese (ob/ob) mice. J Appl Physiol. 1996;81(2):716–23.
62. Tankersley CG, O'Donnell C, Daood MJ, et al. Leptin attenuates respiratory complications associated with the obese phenotype. J Appl Physiol. 1998;85(6):2261–9.
63. Considine RV, Sinha MK, Heiman ML, et al. Serum immunoreactive-leptin concentrations in normal-weight and obese humans. N Engl J Med. 1996;334(5):292–5.
64. Ip MS, Lam KS, Ho C, Tsang KW, Lam W. Serum leptin and vascular risk factors in obstructive sleep apnea. Chest. 2000;118(3):580–6.
65. Barceló A, Barbé F, Llompart E, et al. Neuropeptide Y and leptin in patients with obstructive sleep apnea syndrome: role of obesity. Am J Respir Crit Care Med. 2005;171(2):183–7.
66. Shimura R, Tatsumi K, Nakamura A, et al. Fat accumulation, leptin, and hypercapnia in obstructive sleep apnea-hypopnea syndrome. Chest. 2005;127(2):543–9.
67. Makinodan K, Yoshikawa M, Fukuoka A, et al. Effect of serum leptin levels on hypercapnic ventilatory response in obstructive sleep apnea. Respiration. 2008;75(3):257–64.
68. Phipps PR, Starritt E, Caterson I, Grunstein RR. Association of serum leptin with hypoventilation in human obesity. Thorax. 2002;57(1):75–6.
69. Yee BJ, Cheung J, Phipps P, et al. Treatment of obesity hypoventilation syndrome and serum leptin. Respiration. 2006;73(2):209–12.
70. Caro JF, Kolaczynski JW, Nyce MR, et al. Decreased cerebrospinal-fluid/serum leptin ratio in obesity: a possible mechanism for leptin resistance. Lancet. 1996;348(9021):159–61.
71. Kawata N, Tatsumi K, Terada J, et al. Daytime hypercapnia in obstructive sleep apnea syndrome. Chest. 2007;132(6):1832–8.
72. Rapoport DM, Garay SM, Epstein H, Goldring RM. Hypercapnia in the obstructive sleep apnea syndrome. A reevaluation of the "Pickwickian syndrome.". Chest. 1986;89(5): 627–35.

73. Schäfer H, Ewig S, Hasper E, Lüderitz B. Failure of CPAP therapy in obstructive sleep apnoea syndrome: predictive factors and treatment with bilevel-positive airway pressure. Respir Med. 1998;92(2):208–15.
74. Banerjee D, Yee BJ, Piper AJ, Zwillich CW, Grunstein RR. Obesity hypoventilation syndrome: hypoxemia during continuous positive airway pressure. Chest. 2007;131(6): 1678–84.
75. Mokhlesi B. Positive airway pressure titration in obesity hypoventilation syndrome: continuous positive airway pressure or bilevel positive airway pressure. Chest. 2007;131(6): 1624–6.
76. Piper AJ, Wang D, Yee BJ, Barnes DJ, Grunstein RR. Randomised trial of CPAP vs bilevel support in the treatment of obesity hypoventilation syndrome without severe nocturnal desaturation. Thorax. 2008;63(5):395–401.
77. Berry RB, Chediak A, Brown LK, et al. Best clinical practices for the sleep center adjustment of noninvasive positive pressure ventilation (NPPV) in stable chronic alveolar hypoventilation syndromes. J Clin Sleep Med. 2010;6(5):491–509.
78. Redolfi S, Corda L, La Piana G, et al. Long-term non-invasive ventilation increases chemosensitivity and leptin in obesity-hypoventilation syndrome. Respir Med. 2007;101(6): 1191–5.
79. de Lucas-Ramos P, de Miguel-Díez J, Santacruz-Siminiani A, et al. Benefits at 1 year of nocturnal intermittent positive pressure ventilation in patients with obesity-hypoventilation syndrome. Respir Med. 2004;98(10):961–7.
80. Storre JH, Seuthe B, Fiechter R, et al. Average volume-assured pressure support in obesity hypoventilation: a randomized crossover trial. Chest. 2006;130(3):815–21.
81. Wijesinghe M, Williams M, Perrin K, Weatherall M, Beasley R. The effect of supplemental oxygen on hypercapnia in subjects with obesity-associated hypoventilation: a randomized, crossover, clinical study. Chest. 2011;139(5):1018–24.
82. Mokhlesi B, Tulaimat A, Parthasarathy S. Oxygen for obesity hypoventilation syndrome: a double-edged sword? Chest. 2011;139(5):975–7.
83. Haines KL, Nelson LG, Gonzalez R, et al. Objective evidence that bariatric surgery improves obesity-related obstructive sleep apnea. Surgery. 2007;141(3):354–8.
84. Pillar G, Peled R, Lavie P. Recurrence of sleep apnea without concomitant weight increase 7.5 years after weight reduction surgery. Chest. 1994;106(6):1702–4.
85. Greenburg DL, Lettieri CJ, Eliasson AH. Effects of surgical weight loss on measures of obstructive sleep apnea: a meta-analysis. Am J Med. 2009;122(6):535–42.
86. Sugerman HJ, Fairman RP, Sood RK, et al. Long-term effects of gastric surgery for treating respiratory insufficiency of obesity. Am J Clin Nutr. 1992;55(2 Suppl):597S–601.
87. Sjöström L, Lindroos A-K, Peltonen M, et al. Lifestyle, diabetes, and cardiovascular risk factors 10 years after bariatric surgery. N Engl J Med. 2004;351(26):2683–93.
88. Fernandez Jr AZ, Demaria EJ, Tichansky DS, et al. Multivariate analysis of risk factors for death following gastric bypass for treatment of morbid obesity. Ann Surg. 2004;239(5):698–702. discussion 702–703.
89. Flum DR, Belle SH, King WC, et al. Perioperative safety in the longitudinal assessment of bariatric surgery. N Engl J Med. 2009;361(5):445–54.
90. Squadrone V, Coha M, Cerutti E, et al. Continuous positive airway pressure for treatment of postoperative hypoxemia: a randomized controlled trial. JAMA. 2005;293(5):589–95.
91. Ebeo CT, Benotti PN, Byrd Jr RP, Elmaghraby Z, Lui J. The effect of bi-level positive airway pressure on postoperative pulmonary function following gastric surgery for obesity. Respir Med. 2002;96(9):672–6.
92. El-Solh AA, Aquilina A, Pineda L, et al. Noninvasive ventilation for prevention of post-extubation respiratory failure in obese patients. Eur Respir J. 2006;28(3):588–95.
93. Huerta S, DeShields S, Shpiner R, et al. Safety and efficacy of postoperative continuous positive airway pressure to prevent pulmonary complications after Roux-en-Y gastric bypass. J Gastrointest Surg. 2002;6(3):354–8.

94. Hensley MJ, Read DJ. Intermittent obstruction of the upper airway during sleep causing profound hypoxaemia. A neglected mechanism exacerbating chronic respiratory failure. Aust N Z J Med. 1976;6(5):481–6.
95. Kim SH, Eisele DW, Smith PL, Schneider H, Schwartz AR. Evaluation of patients with sleep apnea after tracheotomy. Arch Otolaryngol Head Neck Surg. 1998;124(9):996–1000.
96. Mokhlesi B, Tulaimat A. Recent advances in obesity hypoventilation syndrome. Chest. 2007;132(4):1322–36.
97. Tojima H, Kunitomo F, Kimura H, et al. Effects of acetazolamide in patients with the sleep apnoea syndrome. Thorax. 1988;43(2):113–9.
98. Whyte KF, Gould GA, Airlie MA, Shapiro CM, Douglas NJ. Role of protriptyline and acetazolamide in the sleep apnea/hypopnea syndrome. Sleep. 1988;11(5):463–72.
99. Raurich J-M, Rialp G, Ibáñez J, Llompart-Pou JA, Ayestarán I. Hypercapnic respiratory failure in obesity-hypoventilation syndrome: CO(2) response and acetazolamide treatment effects. Respir Care. 2010;55(11):1442–8.
100. Bayliss DA, Millhorn DE. Central neural mechanisms of progesterone action: application to the respiratory system. J Appl Physiol. 1992;73(2):393–404.
101. Sutton FD, Zwillich CW, Creagh CE, Pierson DJ, Weil JV. Progesterone for outpatient treatment of Pickwickian syndrome. Ann Intern Med. 1975;83(4):476–9.
102. Douketis JD, Julian JA, Kearon C, et al. Does the type of hormone replacement therapy influence the risk of deep vein thrombosis? A prospective case-control study. J Thromb Haemost. 2005;3(5):943–8.
103. Poulter NR, Chang CL, Farley TM, Meirik O. Risk of cardiovascular diseases associated with oral progestagen preparations with therapeutic indications. Lancet. 1999;354(9190):1610.

Chapter 6
Effect of Obesity on the Development and Clinical Presentation of Asthma

Akshay Sood and Anne E. Dixon

Abstract Obesity is associated with increased risk for both prevalent and incident asthma in a dose-response relationship. It is still not clear how this association is modified by atopy or sex. It appears that abdominal adiposity rather than global adiposity drives this association, but the role of visceral fat remains unstudied. The association further does not yet fully meet the causality criteria in humans. The mechanistic basis for the association is not fully known, but multiplicity of pathways is suspected including the mechanical and metabolic/inflammatory effects of obesity on the airways. Leptin and adiponectin have been suggested as *mediators* in the obesity-asthma association, but this data is currently better established in mice than in humans. Multiple comorbidities of obesity, such as gastroesophageal reflux disease, sleep apnea, and depression, may partly affect the disease manifestation in the obese subject. Interestingly, the clinical manifestations of asthma are more pronounced in obese than normal-weight asthmatics, but the physiological and inflammatory manifestations do not generally differ. Similarly, weight reduction improves clinical asthma outcomes without improving markers of airway eosinophilic inflammation. Obese patients with asthma also show a reduced beneficial response to asthma medications, particularly to inhaled corticosteroids. Currently, there remain critical gaps in our understanding of this association such as the "uniqueness" of the obesity-associated asthma phenotype.

Keywords Obesity • Asthma • Phenotype • Adipokines • Atopy • Female sex

---

A. Sood, M.D., M.PH. (✉)
Department of Medicine, University of New Mexico Health Sciences Center School of Medicine, 1 University of New Mexico MSC 10 5550, Albuquerque, NM 87131, USA
e-mail: asood@salud.unm

A.E. Dixon, M.A., BM, BCh
Department of Medicine, University of Vermont College of Medicine, 89 Beaumont Avenue Given D209, Burlington, VT 05482, USA
e-mail: anne.dixon@vtmednet.org

A.E. Dixon and E.M. Clerisme-Beaty (eds.), *Obesity and Lung Disease: A Guide to Management*, Respiratory Medicine, DOI 10.1007/978-1-62703-053-3_6,

Objectives

- Review the epidemiology of asthma and obesity and discuss potential mechanism by which the two may be related.
- Discuss the effects of obesity on the clinical presentation and pathophysiology of asthma.
- Assess the effects of obesity on the treatment of asthma.

Introduction

There is an increasing prevalence of obesity (body mass index or BMI $\geq$30 kg/m^2) worldwide, particularly in the United States. Data from the two National Health and Nutrition Examination surveys show that the prevalence of obesity has doubled among adults aged 20–74 years in the United States from 15.0% (in the 1976–1980 survey) to 32.9% (in the 2003–2004 survey) [1]. Similarly, the age-adjusted current asthma prevalence rate of 8.2% based on the 2009 United States National Health Interview Survey data is more than twice the period prevalence of 3.1% reported by the same survey in 1980 [2]. These two epidemics are likely linked.

Epidemiology Linking Obesity and Asthma

Obesity is associated with increased risk for both prevalent and incident asthma. This is supported by a number of cross-sectional, case-control, and longitudinal studies. The presence of a dose-response gradient has in fact been described in various studies whereby the risk of asthma increases with the severity of obesity [3].

Consistency of Association Among Diverse Populations

Although first described in the United States [4], the association between obesity and asthma does not appear to be limited to areas with Western lifestyle or dietary habits. Studies have shown an association between obesity and asthma in most parts of the world, in both developed and developing countries, among urban and rural populations, and across diverse races and ethnicities [5–15]. Despite variations in the strength of the association between obesity and asthma, the relationship is remarkably consistent across diverse patient populations. The association has also been reported among children, adolescents, and adults, including the elderly [7, 8, 10]. However, although described in all socioeconomic strata, the link between obesity and asthma may be stronger among those with low household incomes than with high household incomes [16].

Sex Interaction

The effect of sex on the relationship between obesity and asthma is controversial. Initial studies suggested that obesity was particularly a risk factor for asthma among women [4, 17]. However, other studies have not supported this paradigm [18]; in fact, some studies have even showed the opposite [19, 20]. Despite the findings of a 2007 meta-analysis of seven prospective studies that showed no significant interaction ($p=0.20$) between sex and obesity on incident asthma [3], this issue has not been laid to rest. Several large recent studies have continued to demonstrate that the obesity-asthma association is either significant only among women or stronger among women than men with odds ratio reportedly ranging from 1.3 to 2.1 in obese women compared to normal-weight women [21–25]. A few studies have even reported a statistically significant interaction between female sex and obesity on asthma [22, 24]. Female sex hormones have been implicated, with some studies showing the obesity-asthma association to be stronger among girls with early menarche [26]. However, the greater prevalence of nonatopic asthma in women may be a potential explanation for the stronger obesity-asthma association reported among women compared to men [25].

Atopy Interaction

Atopy, the genetic propensity to develop IgE antibodies in response to usual exposure to allergen, may be a significant modifier of the obesity-asthma association. This is supported by results from a large Canadian cross-sectional study showing that the obesity-asthma association was stronger among nonatopic women than atopic women (interaction $p<0.001$) [25]. Another US-based study on a nationally representative sample found a trend toward a stronger association among nonatopic children and adolescents than their atopic counterparts (interaction $p=0.09$) [27]. While most studies in this field have used self-reports to document atopy [28], an Australian study, using skin-prick test to evaluate atopic status, also confirmed the differential association of nonatopic asthma with obesity (interaction p value not reported) [20]. At present, the potential effect modification by atopy of the obesity-asthma association requires further investigation because of some conflicting findings from studies that do not show such effect modification [22, 29, 30].

Effect of Fat Composition and Distribution on Asthma Risk

Obesity is a heterogeneous disorder, characterized by excess amounts of physiological and ectopic fat. While physiological fat is present within cells of adipose tissue, ectopic fat is present within cells of non-adipose tissue (such as viscera and skeletal muscle) that normally contain minimal amounts of fat. Most studies evaluating the obesity-asthma association have used excess body mass (i.e., high BMI) to define the obesity phenotype. It is now known that high BMI is in fact a collection of various phenotypes with some, but not all, relating to excess fat. Further, BMI might be a less reliable measure of body fat in men than in women, given the large contribution by skeletal muscle toward the BMI value in men. As such, the various phenotypes of obesity may have different effects on asthma risk.

Fat Mass, Lean Mass, and Asthma

Percent body fat, measured using bioelectrical impedance, is significantly associated with asthma in women ($p=0.04$) but not in men ($p=0.75$) [23]. Sood et al. studied the relative contribution of fat mass and lean mass (primarily skeletal muscle and viscera) using dual-energy X-ray absorptiometry (DEXA) toward the odds of asthma [24]. While DEXA accurately identifies relatively large physiological fat depots as fat mass, it may inaccurately classify some smaller and highly metabolically active ectopic fat within the skeletal muscle and viscera as lean mass. This study found that increased total "lean" mass was associated with *higher* odds for asthma among women and possibly lower odds among men [24]. This study further suggested that "lean" mass may be a *better* predictor of asthma risk than fat mass among women. A plausible explanation for these surprising findings is that ectopic fat depots, though small (and therefore inaccurately assessed by DEXA as components of lean mass), may be more important from an inflammatory standpoint than larger, physiological fat depots for the development of asthma in women. Interestingly, "lipidization" of skeletal muscle (described in lay terms as "marbling of muscle") is more pronounced in women than men, independent of overall obesity [31–33]. "Lipidization" of viscera, although less in amount in women than men, is associated with greater metabolic effects in women and may thus contribute to the higher asthma risk in women [34–36].

Android Body Shape and Asthma

An android body shape is characterized by fat localization around the waist (Fig. 6.1). Like BMI, increased waist circumference is associated with asthma [20, 36]. In a prospective study, Romieu et al. showed that the transition from a self-perceived leaner body silhouette to one that was progressively more android (i.e., predominantly abdominal fat distribution) after menarche was associated with a substantial increase in asthma risk among French women [37]. In another study of women teachers from California [36], a large waist circumference (>88 cm) was associated with 37% greater odds of asthma prevalence, even among those with a normal BMI. Further, the odds of asthma among BMI-defined obese women were greater in those with concomitant abdominal obesity. These findings suggest that android pattern of obesity in women may be associated with asthma.

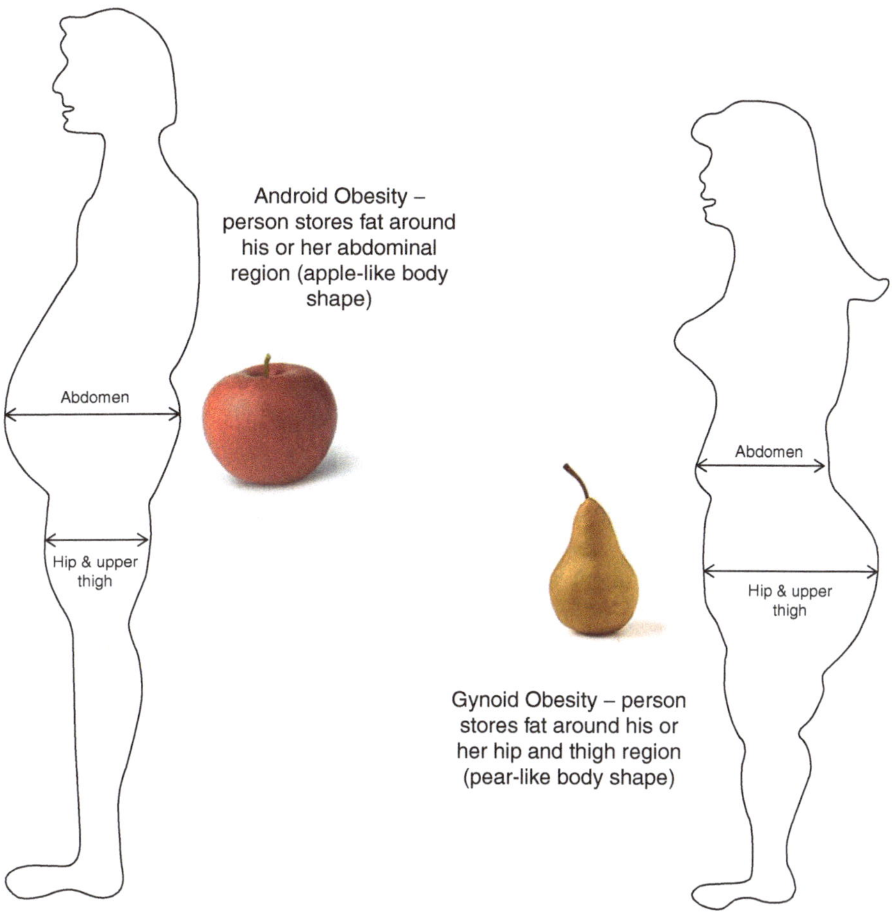

Fig. 6.1 Android and gynoid patterns of obesity. Typically, women manifest the gynoid pattern and men the android pattern. Interestingly, asthma risk appears to be strongly associated with the development of android pattern of obesity *in women*. On the other hand, the gynoid pattern of obesity is not so strongly associated with asthma

Aside from its potential association with asthma, abdominal adiposity is also related to the development of the metabolic syndrome, additionally characterized by hypertension, hypertriglyceridemia, hyperglycemia, and low serum HDL cholesterol. It is not known whether the metabolic syndrome overall or its components are better predictors for asthma than BMI [38–40]. However, data suggest that systemic inflammation or systemic oxidative stress, often seen with the metabolic syndrome, does not predict asthma independent of abdominal adiposity [41, 42]. While abdominal adiposity is used by some as a surrogate marker for visceral fat, there are currently no studies in the literature that have evaluated the independent association between visceral fat, measured by computed tomography or magnetic resonance spectroscopy, and asthma risk.

Gynoid Body Shape and Asthma

Women have relatively larger gluteofemoral fat deposits than men, giving rise to the "pear-shaped" or gynoid pattern (Fig. 6.1). Findings by Sood et al. suggest that. gluteofemoral fat is the weakest predictor among the various physiological fat deposits for asthma among women [24]. Gynoid obesity is characterized by adipocyte hyperplasia as opposed to adipocyte hypertrophy. There is evidence to suggest that adipocyte hyperplasia in the gluteofemoral region may be associated with a more favorable adipokine milieu as well as higher sex-specific levels of lipoprotein lipase (a key enzyme involved in lipogenesis) than fat in other regions [43]. Relative to other fat compartments, gluteofemoral fat is "metabolically benign" [44] and does not exert any mechanical effects on the respiratory system. Thus, the gynoid pattern of obesity in women is an unlikely explanation for the obesity-asthma association.

In summary, studies using BMI do not adequately capture the complexity of the association between the varied phenotypes of obesity and asthma. Abdominal obesity, particularly abdominal ectopic fat deposits, may play a significant role in asthma risk, particularly among women. The independent association between visceral fat, measured by computed tomography or magnetic resonance spectroscopy, and asthma risk has however not been studied.

Is the Obesity-Asthma Association Causal?

Despite the epidemiologic evidence and convincing experimental data in mice [45], the association between obesity and asthma has not yet fully met the Bradford-Hill causality criteria in humans [46, 47]. This is in part due to a lack of consistency among studies evaluating the physiological and inflammatory phenotypes of asthma and the conflicting data on the association between obesity and atopy (usually considered an intermediate asthma phenotype) [13, 48–52]. In addition, there are still questions regarding the underlying pathophysiological mechanisms by which obesity may lead to the development of asthma in humans. Moreover, the strength of the association between the two diseases, which can be described as weak based on generally reported odds ratios of less than 2.0, has raised concerns that the association may result from bias or confounding.

On the other hand, there are several factors that support a possible causal link between obesity and asthma. These include data showing that obesity antedates the development of asthma [17] and that there may be a dose-response gradient between obesity and increased risk of asthma [3]. Furthermore, there have been several reports demonstrating clinical improvement in asthma following weight reduction [23, 53, 54].

Further, although the mechanistic basis for the obesity-asthma association is not yet known, several plausible hypotheses have been proposed and investigated. These include misclassification error, the mechanical effects of obesity on airway hyperresponsiveness, as well as the metabolic/inflammatory effects of adipose tissue on the airways. In addition, obesity may be associated with genetic, epigenetic, hormonal, environmental, and developmental factors as well as comorbidities that may also be causally associated with asthma.

Misclassification Bias

It was initially thought that the association between obesity and self-reported asthma in epidemiologic studies was primarily the result of a misclassification bias due to obese subjects differentially reporting asthma-like symptoms without manifesting bronchial hyperreactivity [55]. Recent studies using objective tests have shown that this misclassification is in fact non-differential between obese and nonobese subjects [20, 56–58]. The resulting bias is typically in a predictable direction (i.e., toward lack of association) and unlikely to produce a spurious effect. However, although obesity is not an independent predictor of the misdiagnosis of asthma overall, Pakhale et al. showed that obesity may predict misdiagnosis of asthma only in the subgroup of patients who had urgent medical visits for respiratory symptoms in the preceding year [58]. Thus, obese subjects who require urgent visits for respiratory symptoms are more likely to be mislabeled as having asthma than their counterparts of normal weight (interaction p value not reported) [58].

Mechanical Effects of Obesity on Airway Hyperresponsiveness

Obesity is associated with reduced functional residual capacity due to changes in the elastic properties of the chest wall. [59] Since the retractive forces of the lung parenchyma on the airway are reduced at low functional residual capacity, airway smooth muscle shortens in the obese subjects which in turn causes airway narrowing and increases airway hyperreactivity [60]. Similarly, the lack of deep tidal breathing and associated lack of tidal stretch on the airway in the obese may also contribute toward shortening of the airway smooth muscle [61]. These issues are discussed in greater detail in the chapters titled "Effects of Obesity on Lung Function" and "Effects of Obesity on Airway Hyperreactivity and Airway Inflammation."

Adipokines and Asthma

Adipose tissue is a metabolically active organ involved in the regulation of systemic inflammation via a variety of secreted proteins called adipokines. Although adipokines include a number of cytokines, chemokines, and cytokine receptors, recent studies have focused on the inflammatory and metabolic role of two energy-regulating hormones – adiponectin and leptin.

Adiponectin

Adiponectin is a predominantly anti-inflammatory adipokine. Adiponectin and all of its known receptors are expressed in the lung [62–64]. Adiponectin is also transported from blood into the alveolar lining fluid via the T-cadherin molecule on the endothelium [65]. Although visceral adipocytes are the most important source of adiponectin [66], serum adiponectin concentrations are lower among obese subjects [67], likely secondary to hypoxia-related necrosis of adipocytes in obese subjects leading to activation of macrophages [68]. These activated macrophages produce tumor necrosis factor-alpha (TNF-α) and interleukin-6 which in turn directly inhibit the local production of adiponectin in a paracrine fashion [69].

There are three forms of circulating adiponectin – low-molecular weight (trimers), medium-molecular weight (hexamers), and high-molecular weight or HMW (higher-order multimers). HMW adiponectin is disproportionately reduced in obesity. In addition, testosterone has been shown to lower serum concentrations of total and HMW adiponectin [70]. This effect of testosterone explains the higher concentration of total adiponectin and higher proportion of HMW to total adiponectin in women compared to men, despite greater levels of overall adiposity in women [70]. Metabolic studies suggest that the HMW isoform is the most biologically active form of adiponectin in regulating insulin resistance. Whether the same is true for asthma is not known, but the airway preponderance of the HMW isoform noted in mice suggests that may be the case [71].

The potential role for adiponectin in asthma is further supported by murine studies where exogenous adiponectin administration has been shown to prevent the development of allergen-induced airway hyperreactivity [72]. However, human data on the independent association between serum adiponectin concentrations and asthma are currently inconclusive [73–77]. Two studies involving German children and American adults, respectively, showed a protective association between serum adiponectin concentrations and odds of prevalent asthma, among nonatopic peripubertal girls and premenopausal women independent of BMI [75, 77]. A longitudinal study examining this association showed that low serum adiponectin predicted significantly higher risk of *incident* asthma in women and in premenopausal women and particularly among current smokers [78]. In that study, low serum adiponectin was also found to be more important than BMI in predicting the risk of *incident* asthma among women [78]. These findings are in conflict with those of two other large studies, based in Finland and New Zealand, which failed to find an association between serum adiponectin and clinical diagnosis of asthma [74, 76].

Systemic adiponectin is also associated with good clinical control of asthma in adolescent boys [79], though recent data by Dominic et al. suggests that the opposite may be true in middle-aged men [78]. While it is possible that these conflicting findings are due to significant methodological differences between the two studies, testosterone-related changes in adiponectin isoform distribution (toward a lower proportion of HMW isoform) in men compared to boys [70, 80] may also play a role.

Further, systemic and bronchoalveolar lavage concentrations of total adiponectin were not associated with any airway biomarker of oxidation or inflammation [81]. Thus, the current role of adiponectin with respect to asthma control remains unclear.

Leptin

Leptin is a primarily proinflammatory adipokine. Serum concentrations of leptin are greater in obese subjects compared to normal-weight. Leptin and leptin receptors are expressed by the lung [82]. A causal role for leptin in asthma is supported by murine studies, where administration of exogenous leptin in normal-weight mice augments airway hyperreactivity following allergen challenge as well as lung inflammation following ozone exposure [83, 84]. Similar to adiponectin, human data is currently inconclusive regarding the independent association between serum leptin concentrations and asthma prevalence or asthma control [73, 77, 79, 85, 86]. A large cross-sectional population-based study in the United States showed a positive association between the highest quartile of serum leptin concentration and the risk for asthma in women (OR of 3.2, 95% CI 1.3–7.7), independent of triceps skinfold thickness [86]. However, the findings were not replicated in two large studies, based in Finland and New Zealand [74, 76]. Studies in children and adolescents similarly showed variable results [73, 77, 79, 85]. Among the positive studies, the association appears to be stronger among prepubertal boys, peripubertal girls, and premenopausal women [75, 77, 85, 86]. In a small study, systemic and bronchoalveolar lavage concentrations of leptin were not associated with airway biomarkers of oxidation and inflammation [81]. Thus, the current role of leptin with respect to asthma is conflicting and unclear in humans.

In summary, although the mouse data suggests that leptin and adiponectin may be *mediators* in the obesity-asthma association, the role of these adipokines in human asthma is less clear. The fact that the obesity-asthma association is not entirely explained by systemic adipokines implies multiplicity of mechanistic pathways. Further, even among the studies that do show an adipokine-asthma association, this association is not entirely explained by obesity, suggesting that adipokine regulation by factors other than obesity may also be important in asthma. Such factors could include physical activity, insulin resistance, sex hormones, race, and menopausal status. This makes untangling the independent contributions of obesity and adipokines to asthma difficult because of the complex relationships between these interrelated variables.

Obesity-Related Comorbidities and Asthma Risk

Obesity is associated with multiple comorbidities, such as gastroesophageal reflux disease (GERD), sleep apnea, and depression, that could potentially affect asthma symptoms and airway disease among individuals who are obese.

Gastroesophageal Reflux Disease (GERD)

GERD has been linked with asthma, even in the absence of obesity. Studies show that the prevalence of GERD is not only increased in asthma but that GERD often precedes and is perhaps involved in the pathogenesis of asthma even in normal-weight individuals [87]. While the reasons for this are complex, studies in animals suggest at least two possible mechanisms through which GERD could lead to bronchospasm and asthma. First, reflux may cause bronchospasm by direct spill of acid contents into the airway. In addition, it is possible that acid in the lower esophagus may lead to reflex bronchospasm without entering the airway [88–90]. As there are numerous reports of increased GERD in obesity [91], there has been much speculation about the potential role that GERD could be playing in asthma in obese individuals [92]. However, a recent study showed that although asthmatics had a high prevalence of GERD overall, the prevalence of acid reflux did not further increase in proportion to obesity. Moreover, acid reflux was not associated with asthma severity in either obese or lean patients [91]. It may be that asthma increases the tendency toward acid reflux, and so obesity does not much further increase the risk of acid reflux beyond that of having asthma. As such, GERD is unlikely to be a significant risk factor for asthma in obese individuals.

Obstructive Sleep Apnea

Obstructive sleep apnea is another comorbidity that is dramatically increased in obesity. There is strong evidence supporting an association between increasing BMI and increased prevalence of sleep apnea [93]. Sleep apnea has been shown to be associated with increased asthma symptoms and worse asthma control in obese patients [94]. In fact, studies suggest that the association between sleep apnea and worse asthma control may be independent of obesity [95]. Given that sleep apnea is associated with worse asthma control, several small studies have investigated whether treatment of sleep apnea could improve asthma control. Their findings suggest that treatment of sleep apnea may improve not only asthma symptoms but also airway hyperreactivity [96–98]. However, these findings have not yet been replicated using larger studies. Given that sleep apnea itself is a serious comorbidity, and may potentially contribute to poor asthma control, it makes sense to consider sleep apnea in assessment of poor asthma control in obese patients with plans to treat it if present.

Depression

Obesity is also associated with depression, and depression is associated with the presence of asthma, particularly in females [99]. Depression and anxiety have also been shown to be associated with poor asthma control [99–101]. The reasons for this are not known but could include multiple factors including adherence to treatment.

However, it remains unknown whether treatment of depression and anxiety would lead to improved asthma control. As in the case of sleep apnea, it is reasonable to consider depression and anxiety as factors that could be contributing to poor asthma control in obese patients. However, depression and anxiety are serious comorbidities that warrant treatment regardless of their effect on asthma.

As stated previously, obesity is a complex disease associated with serious comorbidities and complications that may contribute to the pathogenesis and control of asthma. Although we lack studies of the effect of treating these comorbidities on asthma-specific outcomes, these are serious health problems which warrant treatment in their own right. It is important to consider the potential role of these comorbidities in the clinical evaluation of obese patients with poorly controlled asthma.

Clinical Presentation of Asthma in the Obese

The clinical definition of asthma includes recurrent episodes of respiratory symptoms such as wheezing, breathlessness, chest tightness, and cough. There is greater prevalence of asthma-related symptom [17, 55, 102], doctor diagnosis of asthma, as well as asthma-related medication use [102], health care utilization [103], and absenteeism [104] among the obese, as compared to normal-weight population.

Obesity is less strongly associated with physiological and inflammatory manifestations of asthma. These issues are discussed in greater detail in the chapters titled "Effects of Obesity on Lung Function" and "Effects of Obesity on Airway Hyperreactivity and Airway Inflammation."

Data from several clinical studies suggest that the clinical manifestations of asthma may be more pronounced in obese asthmatics, including more severe, poorly controlled disease and increased exacerbations [7, 21, 36, 79, 105, 106]. These effects may be further more pronounced among women than men [79]. Evaluation in the emergency room of acute asthma exacerbations, however, shows that obese adult asthmatics have similar symptom severity as nonobese asthmatics, despite having slightly higher peak expiratory flow rates [103]. It is worth noting that the peak expiratory flow rates of obese adults with asthma exacerbation respond equally well to intensive treatment in the emergency room as nonobese adults [103]. Yet, obese subjects are more likely to be admitted to the hospital and have a greater hospital length of stay than nonobese subjects, suggesting a slower symptomatic recovery from acute asthma exacerbation in obese subjects [107, 108]. While it is possible that obese subjects have a greater perception of dyspnea in response to bronchoconstriction, the data in this regard are conflicting [109, 110]. The basis for the seemingly greater clinical severity of asthma in the obese subject is thus not well understood.

Interestingly, while the clinical severity of disease may be greater in the obese asthmatic than in the nonobese asthmatic, it has not been established that the physiological and inflammatory manifestations of asthma differ between obese and nonobese asthmatics. This is an important area of ongoing research that is discussed in greater detail in the chapters titled "Effects of Obesity on Lung Function" and "Effects of Obesity on Airway Hyperreactivity and Airway Inflammation."

Effect of Weight Reduction

Asthma prevalence and severity, including asthma-related symptoms and exacerbations, use of rescue medications, need for hospitalizations, and low quality of life, improve following even modest weight reduction among obese subjects [23, 53, 54]. In addition, weight reduction studies among obese subjects show an improvement in lung function [53, 54, 111, 112]. There has also been report of striking reduction in levels of serum markers of oxidative stress among subjects with asthma following dietary restriction and associated weight loss [54]. One recent study showed significantly improved airway hyperreactivity particularly in nonatopic asthmatics with bariatric surgery, though markers of airway eosinophilic inflammation did not change, and markers of lymphocytic inflammation increased [112]. This suggests that weight loss has complex effects on airway inflammation and physiology, and the net result of weight loss likely depends on the underlying phenotype of asthma.

Is the Obesity-Associated Asthma a Unique Phenotype of Asthma?

There is a growing recognition that the term "asthma" does not describe a single pathological disease process. In fact, "asthma" is an umbrella term which covers many distinct phenotypes of airway disease commonly encountered in clinical practice.

By way of background, it is helpful to consider what is known about the pathophysiology of early-onset allergic asthma. This type of asthma is characterized by childhood-onset disease with atopy and Th2 lymphocyte-driven allergic inflammation. Th2 inflammation is associated with the production of cytokines such as interleukins 4 and 5 which promote airway eosinophilia. Asthma in obese asthmatics does not readily conform to this stereotypical pattern. Obesity does not increase airway eosinophilia. Indeed, some cross-sectional studies have found an inverse relationship between BMI and airway eosinophilia [113–115]. Studies have also reported that exhaled nitric oxide, a noninvasive measure of airway eosinophilic inflammation, decreases with increasing BMI [116]. This also supports the emerging concept that allergic airway inflammation is inversely related to BMI. Obesity does not lead to asthma through increased allergic inflammation.

A number of studies published in the last few years have described the different phenotypes of asthma [117, 118] and provided important insight into our understanding of the relationship between obesity and asthma. Although these studies varied somewhat in their particulars, one study by Moore et al. has been quite influential [119] and divided patients into five main phenotypes (shown in Table 6.1). Cluster groups 3 and 5 consist of predominantly obese female with relatively low prevalence of atopy and late-onset asthma. The other three groups (cluster groups 1, 2, and 4) consist of atopic asthmatics with early-onset disease and varying disease

Table 6.1 Five main phenotypes of patients with asthma

Cluster group	1	2	4	3	5
Prevalence of obesity	Normal	Normal	Normal	High	High
Age of asthma onset	Early	Early	Early	Late	Late
Prevalence of atopy	High	High	High	Low	Low
Gender predominance	Female	Female	Equal	Female	Female
Symptoms	Low	Intermediate	High	High	High
Lung function	Normal	Normal	Decreased	Normal	Decreased
		Atopic		Nonatopic	

severity [108]. This study suggests that there may be a "unique" type of asthma that occurs primarily among obese women, characterized by late-onset and nonatopic disease.

Although obesity does not cause increased allergic airway inflammation, there are likely to be people with allergic asthma who happen to be obese simply given the very high prevalence of obesity in the developed world. However, there also appears to be a unique phenotype of asthma, characterized by the older female non-atopic asthmatic, with asthma that develops in the setting of obesity [112, 118]. To summarize, there are at least two distinct phenotypes of asthma in obesity: atopic asthmatics with early-onset disease (who happen to be obese) and nonatopic asthmatics with later-onset disease (developing consequent to obesity). The implications for treatment of these two different phenotypes are not known.

Response to Asthma Therapy in Obese Patients

Unfortunately, the current guidelines do not specifically address the management of obese patients with asthma. Obese patients with asthma show a reduced beneficial response to asthma medications, particularly to inhaled corticosteroids [105, 120]. Weight loss, even when modest, is associated with clinical improvement in asthma control [53, 107, 121] and therefore should be recommended. Habitual exercise is presumably beneficial due to its associated deep breathing and beneficial changes in adipokines but has not been specifically studied. Additional details on this subject are available in the accompanying chapter titled "Treatment of the Obese Patient with Asthma."

Conclusion

Obesity plays an important role in the development and clinical presentation of asthma. Despite the extensive number of studies published on this topic in the last decade, there remain critical gaps in our understanding of the association between obesity and asthma. In order to move the field forward, it is important to (1) unravel

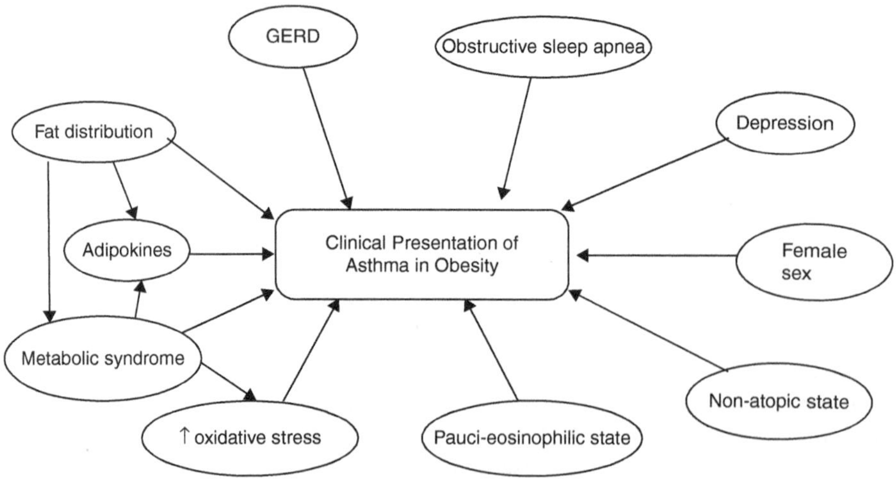

Fig. 6.2 Factors contributing to presentation of asthma in obesity

the biological basis for the potential sex- and atopy-related interactions with obesity on asthma; (2) clarify the role of ectopic vs. physiological fat deposits as well as the associated role of adipokines, such as high-molecular weight adiponectin; and (3) understand the clinical and therapeutic implications of obesity-associated asthma phenotype (Fig. 6.2).

References

1. National Center for Health Care Statistics. Chart Book on trends in the health of Americans, health, United States, 2006. Hyattsville: Public Health Service; 2006.
2. Akinbami LJ, Moorman JE, Liu X. Asthma prevalence, health care use, and mortality: United States, 2005–2009. Hyattsville: National Center for Health Care Statistics; 2011.
3. Beuther DA, Sutherland ER. Overweight, obesity, and incident asthma: a meta-analysis of prospective epidemiologic studies. Am J Respir Crit Care Med. 2007;175:661–6.
4. Camargo Jr CA, Weiss ST, Zhang S, Willett WC, Speizer FE. Prospective study of body mass index, weight change, and risk of adult-onset asthma in women. Arch Intern Med. 1999;159: 2582–8.
5. Asfaw A. The effects of obesity on doctor-diagnosed chronic diseases in Africa: empirical results from Senegal and South Africa. J Public Health Policy. 2006;27:250–64.
6. Barros LL, Souza-Machado A, Correa LB, Santos JS, Cruz C, Leite M, et al. Obesity and poor asthma control in patients with severe asthma. J Asthma. 2011;48:171–6.
7. Belamarich PF, Luder E, Kattan M, Mitchell H, Islam S, Lynn H, et al. Do obese inner-city children with asthma have more symptoms than nonobese children with asthma? Pediatrics. 2000;106:1436–41.
8. Brunner WM, Lindgren PG, Langner DM, Williams AN, Yawn BP. Asthma among rural Minnesota adolescents. J Asthma. 2005;42:787–92.
9. Bustos P, Amigo H, Oyarzun M, Rona RJ. Is there a causal relation between obesity and asthma? Evidence from Chile. Int J Obes (Lond). 2005;29:804–9.

10. Cassol VE, Rizzato TM, Teche SP, Basso DF, Centenaro DF, Maldonado M, et al. Obesity and its relationship with asthma prevalence and severity in adolescents from southern Brazil. J Asthma. 2006;43:57–60.
11. Celedon JC, Palmer LJ, Litonjua AA, Weiss ST, Wang B, Fang Z, et al. Body mass index and asthma in adults in families of subjects with asthma in Anqing, China. Am J Respir Crit Care Med. 2001;164:1835–40.
12. Coogan PF, Palmer JR, O'Connor GT, Rosenberg L. Body mass index and asthma incidence in the Black Women's Health Study. J Allergy Clin Immunol. 2009;123:89–95.
13. Jang AS, Son MH, Choi IS, Koh YI. High body mass index is associated with wheezing among older adults living in high-altitude area in Korea. J Korean Med Sci. 2002;17: 479–82.
14. Mishra V. Effect of obesity on asthma among adult Indian women. Int J Obes Relat Metab Disord. 2004;28:1048–58.
15. Noonan CW, Brown BD, Bentley B, Conway K, Corcoran M, FourStar K, et al. Variability in childhood asthma and body mass index across northern plains American Indian communities. J Asthma. 2010;47:496–500.
16. Chen Y, Bishop M, Liepold H. Increased effect of obesity on asthma in adults with low household income. J Asthma. 2010;47:263–8.
17. Beckett WS, Jacobs Jr DR, Yu X, Iribarren C, Williams OD. Asthma is associated with weight gain in females but not males, independent of physical activity. Am J Respir Crit Care Med. 2001;164:2045–50.
18. Nystad W, Meyer HE, Nafstad P, Tverdal A, Engeland A. Body mass index in relation to adult asthma among 135,000 Norwegian men and women. Am J Epidemiol. 2004;160:969–76.
19. Huovinen E, Kaprio J, Koskenvuo M. Factors associated to lifestyle and risk of adult onset asthma. Respir Med. 2003;97:273–80.
20. Appleton SL, Adams RJ, Wilson DH, Taylor AW, Ruffin RE. Central obesity is associated with nonatopic but not atopic asthma in a representative population sample. J Allergy Clin Immunol. 2006;118:1284–91.
21. Boulet LP, Des Cormiers A. The link between obesity and asthma: a Canadian perspective. Can Respir J. 2007;14:217–20.
22. Loerbroks A, Apfelbacher CJ, Amelang M, Sturmer T. Obesity and adult asthma: potential effect modification by gender, but not by hay fever. Ann Epidemiol. 2008;18:283–9.
23. McLachlan CR, Poulton R, Car G, Cowan J, Filsell S, Greene JM, et al. Adiposity, asthma, and airway inflammation. J Allergy Clin Immunol. 2007;119:634–9.
24. Sood A, Qualls C, Li R, Schuyler M, Beckett WS, Smith LJ, et al. Lean mass predicts asthma better than fat mass among females. Eur Respir J. 2010;37:65–71.
25. Chen Y, Dales R, Jiang Y. The association between obesity and asthma is stronger in nonallergic than allergic adults. Chest. 2006;130:890–5.
26. Herrera-Trujillo M, Barraza-Villarreal A, Lazcano-Ponce E, Hernandez B, Sanin LH, Romieu I. Current wheezing, puberty, and obesity among mexican adolescent females and young women. J Asthma. 2005;42:705–9.
27. Visness CM, London SJ, Daniels JL, Kaufman JS, Yeatts KB, Siega-Riz AM, et al. Association of childhood obesity with atopic and nonatopic asthma: results from the National Health and Nutrition Examination Survey 1999–2006. J Asthma. 2010;47:822–9.
28. Garcia-Marcos L, Arnedo Pena A, Busquets-Monge R, Morales Suarez-Varela M, Garcia de Andoin N, Batlles-Garrido J, et al. How the presence of rhinoconjunctivitis and the severity of asthma modify the relationship between obesity and asthma in children 6–7 years old. Clin Exp Allergy. 2008;38:1174–8.
29. Braback L, Hjern A, Rasmussen F. Body mass index, asthma and allergic rhinoconjunctivitis in Swedish conscripts-a national cohort study over three decades. Respir Med. 2005;99: 1010–4.
30. Ronmark E, Andersson C, Nystrom L, Forsberg B, Jarvholm B, Lundback B. Obesity increases the risk of incident asthma among adults. Eur Respir J. 2005;25:282–8.

31. Miljkovic-Gacic I, Wang X, Kammerer CM, Gordon CL, Bunker CH, Kuller LH, et al. Fat infiltration in muscle: new evidence for familial clustering and associations with diabetes. Obesity (Silver Spring). 2008;16:1854–60.
32. Forsberg AM, Nilsson E, Werneman J, Bergstrom J, Hultman E. Muscle composition in relation to age and sex. Clin Sci (Lond). 1991;81:249–56.
33. Perseghin G, Scifo P, Pagliato E, Battezzati A, Benedini S, Soldini L, et al. Gender factors affect fatty acids-induced insulin resistance in nonobese humans: effects of oral steroidal contraception. J Clin Endocrinol Metab. 2001;86:3188–96.
34. Rattarasarn C, Leelawattana R, Soonthornpun S, Setasuban W, Thamprasit A. Gender differences of regional abdominal fat distribution and their relationships with insulin sensitivity in healthy and glucose-intolerant Thais. J Clin Endocrinol Metab. 2004;89:6266–70.
35. Leenen R, van der Kooy K, Seidell JC, Deurenberg P. Visceral fat accumulation measured by magnetic resonance imaging in relation to serum lipids in obese men and women. Atherosclerosis. 1992;94:171–81.
36. Von Behren J, Lipsett M, Horn-Ross PL, Delfino RJ, Gilliland F, McConnell R, et al. Obesity, waist size and prevalence of current asthma in the California Teachers Study cohort. Thorax. 2009;64:889–93.
37. Romieu I, Avenel V, Leynaert B, Kauffmann F, Clavel-Chapelon F. Body mass index, change in body silhouette, and risk of asthma in the E3N cohort study. Am J Epidemiol. 2003; 158:165–74.
38. Agrawal A, Mabalirajan U, Ahmad T, Ghosh B. Emerging interface between metabolic syndrome and asthma. Am J Respir Cell Mol Biol. 2011;44:270–5.
39. Al-Shawwa B, Al-Huniti N, Titus G, Abu-Hasan M. Hypercholesterolemia is a potential risk factor for asthma. J Asthma. 2006;43:231–3.
40. Cottrell L, Neal WA, Ice C, Perez MK, Piedimonte G. Metabolic abnormalities in children with asthma. Am J Respir Crit Care Med. 2011;183:441–8.
41. Ford ES. Asthma, body mass index, and C-reactive protein among US adults. J Asthma. 2003;40:733–9.
42. Sood A, Qualls C, Arynchyn A, Beckett WS, Gross MD, Steffes MW, et al. Obesity-asthma association: is it explained by systemic oxidant stress? Chest. 2009;136:1055–62.
43. Arner P, Lithell H, Wahrenberg H, Bronnegard M. Expression of lipoprotein lipase in different human subcutaneous adipose tissue regions. J Lipid Res. 1991;32:423–9.
44. Weinberg EG, Shore SC. Sodium cromoglycate in asthma therapy. A retrospective survey. S Afr Med J. 1983;64:896–9.
45. Shore SA. Obesity and asthma: lessons from animal models. J Appl Physiol. 2007;102:516–28.
46. Camilo DF, Ribeiro JD, Toro AD, Baracat EC, Barros Filho AA. Obesity and asthma: association or coincidence? J Pediatr (Rio J). 2010;86:6–14.
47. Sood A. Does obesity weigh heavily on the health of the human airway? J Allergy Clin Immunol. 2005;115:921–4.
48. Huang SL, Shiao G, Chou P. Association between body mass index and allergy in teenage girls in Taiwan. Clin Exp Allergy. 1999;29:323–9.
49. Husemoen LL, Glumer C, Lau C, Pisinger C, Morch LS, Linneberg A. Association of obesity and insulin resistance with asthma and aeroallergen sensitization. Allergy. 2008;63:575–82.
50. Irei AV, Takahashi K, Le DS, Ha PT, Hung NT, Kunii D, et al. Obesity is associated with increased risk of allergy in Vietnamese adolescents. Eur J Clin Nutr. 2005;59:571–7.
51. Jarvis D, Chinn S, Potts J, Burney P. Association of body mass index with respiratory symptoms and atopy: results from the European Community Respiratory Health Survey. Clin Exp Allergy. 2002;32:831–7.
52. von Mutius E, Schwartz J, Neas LM, Dockery D, Weiss ST. Relation of body mass index to asthma and atopy in children: the National Health and Nutrition Examination Study III. Thorax. 2001;56:835–8.
53. Stenius-Aarniala B, Poussa T, Kvarnstrom J, Gronlund EL, Ylikahri M, Mustajoki P. Immediate and long term effects of weight reduction in obese people with asthma: randomised controlled study. BMJ. 2000;320:827–32.

54. Johnson JB, Summer W, Cutler RG, Martin B, Hyun DH, Dixit VD, et al. Alternate day calorie restriction improves clinical findings and reduces markers of oxidative stress and inflammation in overweight adults with moderate asthma. Free Radic Biol Med. 2007;42:665–74.
55. Schachter LM, Salome CM, Peat JK, Woolcock AJ. Obesity is a risk for asthma and wheeze but not airway hyperresponsiveness. Thorax. 2001;56:4–8.
56. Aaron SD, Vandemheen KL, Boulet LP, McIvor RA, Fitzgerald JM, Hernandez P, et al. Overdiagnosis of asthma in obese and nonobese adults. CMAJ. 2008;179:1121–31.
57. Lang JE, Feng H, Lima JJ. Body mass index-percentile and diagnostic accuracy of childhood asthma. J Asthma. 2009;46:291–9.
58. Pakhale S, Doucette S, Vandemheen K, Boulet LP, McIvor RA, Fitzgerald JM, et al. A comparison of obese and nonobese people with asthma: exploring an asthma-obesity interaction. Chest. 2010;37:1316–23.
59. Naimark A, Cherniack RM. Compliance of the respiratory system and its components in health and obesity. J Appl Physiol. 1960;15:377–82.
60. Ding DJ, Martin JG, Macklem PT. Effects of lung volume on maximal methacholine-induced bronchoconstriction in normal humans. J Appl Physiol. 1987;62:1324–30.
61. Gump A, Haughney L, Fredberg J. Relaxation of activated airway smooth muscle: relative potency of isoproterenol vs. tidal stretch. J Appl Physiol. 2001;90:2306–10.
62. Miller M, Cho JY, Pham A, Ramsdell J, Broide DH. Adiponectin and functional adiponectin receptor 1 are expressed by airway epithelial cells in chronic obstructive pulmonary disease. J Immunol. 2009;182:684–91.
63. Dent G, Hadjicharalambous C, Yoshikawa T, Handy RL, Powell J, Anderson IK, et al. Contribution of eotaxin-1 to eosinophil chemotactic activity of moderate and severe asthmatic sputum. Am J Respir Crit Care Med. 2004;169:1110–7.
64. Delvaux M, Henket M, Lau L, Kange P, Bartsch P, Djukanovic R, et al. Nebulised salbutamol administered during sputum induction improves bronchoprotection in patients with asthma. Thorax. 2004;59:111–5.
65. Hug C, Wang J, Ahmad NS, Bogan JS, Tsao TS, Lodish HF. T-cadherin is a receptor for hexameric and high-molecular-weight forms of Acrp30/adiponectin. Proc Natl Acad Sci USA. 2004;101:10308–13.
66. Steffes MW, Gross MD, Schreiner PJ, Yu X, Hilner JE, Gingerich R, et al. Serum adiponectin in young adults–interactions with central adiposity, circulating levels of glucose, and insulin resistance: the CARDIA study. Ann Epidemiol. 2004;14:492–8.
67. Arita Y, Kihara S, Ouchi N, Takahashi M, Maeda K, Miyagawa J, et al. Paradoxical decrease of an adipose-specific protein, adiponectin, in obesity. Biochem Biophys Res Commun. 1999;257:79–83.
68. Cinti S, Mitchell G, Barbatelli G, Murano I, Ceresi E, Faloia E, et al. Adipocyte death defines macrophage localization and function in adipose tissue of obese mice and humans. J Lipid Res. 2005;46:2347–55.
69. Bruun JM, Lihn AS, Verdich C, Pedersen SB, Toubro S, Astrup A, et al. Regulation of adiponectin by adipose tissue-derived cytokines: in vivo and in vitro investigations in humans. Am J Physiol Endocrinol Metab. 2003;285:E527–33.
70. Andersen KK, Frystyk J, Wolthers OD, Heuck C, Flyvbjerg A. Gender differences of oligomers and total adiponectin during puberty: a cross-sectional study of 859 Danish school children. J Clin Endocrinol Metab. 2007;92:1857–62.
71. Zhu M, Hug C, Kasahara DI, Johnston RA, Williams AS, Verbout NG, et al. Impact of adiponectin deficiency on pulmonary responses to acute ozone exposure in mice. Am J Respir Cell Mol Biol. 2009;43:487–97.
72. Shore SA, Terry RD, Flynt L, Xu A, Hug C. Adiponectin attenuates allergen-induced airway inflammation and hyperresponsiveness in mice. J Allergy Clin Immunol. 2006;118:389–95.
73. Kim KW, Shin YH, Lee KE, Kim ES, Sohn MH, Kim KE. Relationship between adipokines and manifestations of childhood asthma. Pediatr Allergy Immunol. 2008;19:535–40.
74. Jartti T, Saarikoski L, Jartti L, Lisinen I, Jula A, Huupponen R, et al. Obesity, adipokines and asthma. Allergy. 2009;64:770–7.

75. Sood A, Cui X, Qualls C, Beckett WS, Gross MD, Steffes MW, et al. Association between asthma and serum adiponectin concentration in women. Thorax. 2008;63:877–82.
76. Sutherland TJ, Sears MR, McLachlan CR, Poulton R, Hancox RJ. Leptin, adiponectin, and asthma: findings from a population-based cohort study. Ann Allergy Asthma Immunol. 2009;103:101–7.
77. Nagel G, Koenig W, Rapp K, Wabitsch M, Zoellner I, Weiland SK. Associations of adipokines with asthma, rhinoconjunctivitis, and eczema in German schoolchildren. Pediatr Allergy Immunol. 2009;20:81–8.
78. Sood A, Qualls B, Thyagarajan M, Steffes M, Smith LJ, Jacobs DR. Low Serum adiponectin predicts future risk of asthma in women. Am J Resp Crit Care Med. 2012 Apr 6. [Epub ahead of print]. PMID:22492987.
79. Kattan M, Kumar R, Bloomberg GR, Mitchell HE, Calatroni A, Gergen PJ, et al. Asthma control, adiposity, and adipokines among inner-city adolescents. J Allergy Clin Immunol. 2010;125:584–92.
80. Page ST, Herbst KL, Amory JK, Coviello AD, Anawalt BD, Matsumoto AM, et al. Testosterone administration suppresses adiponectin levels in men. J Androl. 2005;26:85–92.
81. Holguin F, Rojas M, Brown LA, Fitzpatrick AM. Airway and plasma leptin and adiponectin in lean and obese asthmatics and controls. J Asthma. 2011;48:217–23.
82. Bergen HT, Cherlet TC, Manuel P, Scott JE. Identification of leptin receptors in lung and isolated fetal type II cells. Am J Respir Cell Mol Biol. 2002;27:71–7.
83. Shore SA, Schwartzman IN, Mellema MS, Flynt L, Imrich A, Johnston RA. Effect of leptin on allergic airway responses in mice. J Allergy Clin Immunol. 2005;115:103–9.
84. Shore SA, Rivera-Sanchez YM, Schwartzman IN, Johnston RA. Responses to ozone are increased in obese mice. J Appl Physiol. 2003;95:938–45.
85. Guler N, Kirerleri E, Ones U, Tamay Z, Salmayenli N, Darendeliler F. Leptin: does it have any role in childhood asthma? J Allergy Clin Immunol. 2004;114:254–9.
86. Sood A, Ford ES, Camargo Jr CA. Association between leptin and asthma in adults. Thorax. 2006;61:300–5.
87. Gunnbjornsdottir MI, Omenaas E, Gislason T, Norrman E, Olin AC, Jogi R, et al. Obesity and nocturnal gastro-oesophageal reflux are related to onset of asthma and respiratory symptoms. Eur Respir J. 2004;24:116–21.
88. Herve P, Denjean A, Jian R, Simonneau G, Duroux P. Intraesophageal perfusion of acid increases the bronchomotor response to methacholine and to isocapnic hyperventilation in asthmatic subjects. Am Rev Respir Dis. 1986;134:986–9.
89. Lopes FD, Alvarenga GS, Quiles R, Dorna MB, Vieira JE, Dolhnikoff M, et al. Pulmonary responses to tracheal or esophageal acidification in guinea pigs with airway inflammation. J Appl Physiol. 2002;93:842–7.
90. Tuchman DN, Boyle JT, Pack AI, Scwartz J, Kokonos M, Spitzer AR, et al. Comparison of airway responses following tracheal or esophageal acidification in the cat. Gastroenterology. 1984;87:872–81.
91. El-Serag HB, Ergun GA, Pandolfino J, Fitzgerald S, Tran T, Kramer JR. Obesity increases oesophageal acid exposure. Gut. 2007;56:749–55.
92. Shore SA, Johnston RA. Obesity and asthma. Pharmacol Ther. 2006;110:83–102.
93. Belle SH, Chapman W, Courcoulas AP, Flum DR, Gagner M, Inabnet WB, et al. Relationship of body mass index with demographic and clinical characteristics in the Longitudinal Assessment of Bariatric Surgery (LABS). Surg Obes Relat Dis. 2008;4:474–80.
94. Dixon AE, Clerisme-Beaty EM, Sugar EA, Cohen RI, Lang JE, Brown ED, et al. Effects of obstructive sleep apnea and gastroesophageal reflux disease on asthma control in obesity. J Asthma. 2011;48:707–13.
95. Teodorescu M, Consens FB, Bria WF, Coffey MJ, McMorris MS, Weatherwax KJ, et al. Predictors of habitual snoring and obstructive sleep apnea risk in patients with asthma. Chest. 2009;135:1125–32.
96. Alkhalil M, Schulman ES, Getsy J. Obstructive sleep apnea syndrome and asthma: the role of continuous positive airway pressure treatment. Ann Allergy Asthma Immunol. 2008;101:350–7.

97. Ciftci TU, Ciftci B, Guven SF, Kokturk O, Turktas H. Effect of nasal continuous positive airway pressure in uncontrolled nocturnal asthmatic patients with obstructive sleep apnea syndrome. Respir Med. 2005;99:529–34.
98. Chan CS, Woolcock AJ, Sullivan CE. Nocturnal asthma: role of snoring and obstructive sleep apnea. Am Rev Respir Dis. 1988;137:1502–4.
99. de Miguel Diez J, Hernandez Barrera V, Puente Maestu L, Carrasco Garrido P, Gomez Garcia T, Jimenez Garcia R. Psychiatric comorbidity in asthma patients. Associated factors. J Asthma. 2011;48:253–8.
100. Lavoie KL, Cartier A, Labrecque M, Bacon SL, Lemiere C, Malo JL, et al. Are psychiatric disorders associated with worse asthma control and quality of life in asthma patients? Respir Med. 2005;99:1249–57.
101. ten Brinke A, Sterk PJ, Masclee AA, Spinhoven P, Schmidt JT, Zwinderman AH, et al. Risk factors of frequent exacerbations in difficult-to-treat asthma. Eur Respir J. 2005;26: 812–8.
102. Sin DD, Jones RL, Man SF. Obesity is a risk factor for dyspnea but not for airflow obstruction. Arch Intern Med. 2002;162:1477–81.
103. Thomson CC, Clark S, Camargo Jr CA. Body mass index and asthma severity among adults presenting to the emergency department. Chest. 2003;124:795–802.
104. Nathell L, Jensen I, Larsson K. High prevalence of obesity in asthmatic patients on sick leave. Respir Med. 2002;96:642–50.
105. Camargo Jr CA, Sutherland ER, Bailey W, Castro M, Yancey SW, Emmett AH, et al. Effect of increased body mass index on asthma risk, impairment and response to asthma controller therapy in African Americans. Curr Med Res Opin. 2010;26:1629–35.
106. Grammer LC, Weiss KB, Pedicano JB, Kimmel LG, Curtis LS, Catrambone CD, et al. Obesity and asthma morbidity in a community-based adult cohort in a large urban area: the Chicago Initiative to Raise Asthma Health Equity (CHIRAH). J Asthma. 2010;47:491–5.
107. Carroll CL, Bhandari A, Zucker AR, Schramm CM. Childhood obesity increases duration of therapy during severe asthma exacerbations. Pediatr Crit Care Med. 2006;7:527–31.
108. Rodrigo GJ, Plaza V. Body mass index and response to emergency department treatment in adults with severe asthma exacerbations: a prospective cohort study. Chest. 2007;132: 1513–9.
109. Deesomchok A, Fisher T, Webb KA, Ora J, Lam YM, Lougheed MD, et al. Effects of obesity on perceptual and mechanical responses to bronchoconstriction in asthma. Am J Respir Crit Care Med. 2010;181:125–33.
110. Salome CM, Munoz PA, Berend N, Thorpe CW, Schachter LM, King GG. Effect of obesity on breathlessness and airway responsiveness to methacholine in non-asthmatic subjects. Int J Obes (Lond). 2008;32:502–9.
111. Maniscalco M, Zedda A, Faraone S, Cerbone MR, Cristiano S, Giardiello C, et al. Weight loss and asthma control in severely obese asthmatic females. Respir Med. 2008;102:102–8.
112. Dixon AE, Pratley RE, Forgione PM, Kaminsky DA, Whittaker-Leclair LA, Griffes LA, et al. Effects of obesity and bariatric surgery on airway hyperresponsiveness, asthma control, and inflammation. J Allergy Clin Immunol. 2011;128:508–15 e1-2.
113. Lessard A, Turcotte H, Cormier Y, Boulet LP. Obesity and asthma: a specific phenotype? Chest. 2008;134:317–23.
114. Todd DC, Armstrong S, D'Silva L, Allen CJ, Hargreave FE, Parameswaran K. Effect of obesity on airway inflammation: a cross-sectional analysis of body mass index and sputum cell counts. Clin Exp Allergy. 2007;37:1049–54.
115. van Veen IH, Ten Brinke A, Sterk PJ, Rabe KF, Bel EH. Airway inflammation in obese and nonobese patients with difficult-to-treat asthma. Allergy. 2008;63:570–4.
116. Berg CM, Thelle DS, Rosengren A, Lissner L, Toren K, Olin AC. Decreased fraction of exhaled nitric oxide in obese subjects with asthma symptoms: data from the population study INTERGENE/ADONIX. Chest. 2011;139:1109–16.
117. Haldar P, Pavord ID, Shaw DE, Berry MA, Thomas M, Brightling CE, et al. Cluster analysis and clinical asthma phenotypes. Am J Respir Crit Care Med. 2008;178:218–24.

118. Holguin F, Bleecker ER, Busse WW, Calhoun WJ, Castro M, Erzurum SC, et al. Obesity and asthma: an association modified by age of asthma onset. J Allergy Clin Immunol. 2011;127:1486–93. e2.
119. Moore WC, Meyers DA, Wenzel SE, Teague WG, Li H, Li X, et al. Identification of asthma phenotypes using cluster analysis in the Severe Asthma Research Program. Am J Respir Crit Care Med. 2010;181:315–23.
120. Peters-Golden M, Swern A, Bird SS, Hustad CM, Grant E, Edelman JM. Influence of body mass index on the response to asthma controller agents. Eur Respir J. 2006;27:495–503.
121. Eneli IU, Skybo T, Camargo Jr CA. Weight loss and asthma: a systematic review. Thorax. 2008;63:671–6.

Chapter 7
Treatment of the Obese Patient with Asthma

E. Rand Sutherland

Abstract Asthma in obese adults is more severe than in lean individuals, and emerging data from clinical and translational studies suggest that obese patients are also less likely to respond to controller therapies, particularly inhaled corticosteroids. As a result, obese asthmatics receive complicated treatment regimens to which they are less likely to respond favorably. Given the high prevalence of both asthma and obesity, this interaction has significant potential to adversely impact both individual and population asthma burden. Despite this, no specific guidance currently exists in NIH or international guidelines as to the optimal therapeutic approach to the obese asthmatic. This chapter will review clinical data regarding mechanisms by which obesity modifies asthma phenotype, focusing on clinical and translational studies of response to controller therapies such as glucocorticoids and agents targeting leukotriene pathways.

Keywords Obesity • Inflammation • Asthma • Steroid • Epidemiology

Objectives

- Review epidemiological data suggesting glucocorticoid resistance in obesity
- Discuss possible mechanisms of glucocorticoid resistance in asthma
- Review efficacy of weight loss in the treatment of asthma in obesity

---

E.R. Sutherland, M.D., M.P.H. (✉)
Department of Medicine, National Jewish Health,
1400 Jackson Street, J-201, Denver, CO 80206, USA
e-mail: sutherlande@njhealth.org

A.E. Dixon and E.M. Clerisme-Beaty (eds.), *Obesity and Lung Disease: A Guide to Management*, Respiratory Medicine, DOI 10.1007/978-1-62703-053-3_7,

Introduction

Asthma in obese adults is more severe than in lean individuals [1, 2], and a number of studies have demonstrated that asthma in obese adults is less responsive to inhaled corticosteroids (ICS) [3–5], the first-line controller treatment for asthma [6]. Given that over 50% of adult asthmatics are overweight or obese [5], the attenuated response to glucocorticoids observed in obese asthmatics substantially increases asthma burden and is a major public health issue. Despite this, no specific guidance currently exists in NIH or international guidelines as to the optimal therapeutic approach to the obese asthmatic [6, 7], and many obese asthmatics receive complicated asthma treatment regimens to which they do not respond [2].

Only recently has work in earnest attempted to elucidate mechanisms relevant to the obesity-asthma interaction, with the goal of facilitating the development of more effective therapeutic approaches in obese asthmatics. It is important to recognize that obesity is a well-documented cause of clinically relevant systemic inflammation [8], particularly in the context of the metabolic syndrome and insulin resistance [9, 10]. Given that clinical and epidemiologic studies suggest a link between obesity and the worsening/development of asthma, it has been hypothesized that systemic inflammation and other metabolic abnormalities in obesity could increase airway inflammation in asthma [11, 12], while also modulating steroid responsiveness. This chapter will review selected aspects of our current understanding of the contributions of obesity-related airway and systemic inflammation to asthma, with a focus on the impact of inflammation as a modifier of therapeutic response, principally to ICS, but also to other controller agents.

Glucocorticoid Response in Asthma

Inhaled corticosteroids are glucocorticoid (GC) preparations widely used as the principal controller therapy for patients with persistent asthma [6]. Although the majority of patients with asthma can be successfully treated with ICS-containing treatment regimens, studies have suggested that there is variability in response to ICS, with a substantial minority of patients achieving less-than-optimal asthma control, despite high doses of ICS [13–15]. This is an important clinical issue in that recognizing suboptimal therapeutic response to ICS, understanding the mechanisms thereof, and developing strategies to address this are likely to translate directly to improved treatment algorithms for patients with asthma. In brief, GCs exert their effects by diffusing across the plasma membrane and binding to a cytoplasmic receptor protein, GC receptor-alpha (GCRα), a ligand-dependent transcription factor [16]. Under GC-responsive conditions, the GC-GCR complex translocates to the nucleus where it binds to specific GC response elements (GRE) within the promoter regions of GC-responsive genes to enhance transcription after induction of histone acetylation [16, 17].

The mechanisms of GC insensitivity are complex, reflecting the multiple steps involved in GC action. For example, recent reports have suggested that the majority of peripheral blood mononuclear cells (PBMC) from GC-insensitive and steroid-dependent asthmatics have impaired nuclear localization of GCRα despite treatment with GCs [18]. Glucocorticoids have also been reported to increase expression of a key regulator of MAP kinase (MAPK) inactivation, MAP kinase phosphatase-1 (MKP-1) [19–21]. As reviewed recently [22], interactions between activation of p38 MAPK and corticosteroid activation pathways have been postulated to lead to corticosteroid insensitivity in chronic airway disease. Augmented proinflammatory response of cells from GC-insensitive asthmatics could be due to a lack of ability of steroids to induce phosphatase expression that may allow persistent MAPK activation and cell activation, and the importance of this pathway to GC response in obese asthmatics is discussed below. Finally, in humans, alternative splicing of the ninth exon of the GCR pre-mRNA gives rise to two homologous GCR protein isoforms, termed GCRα and GCRβ [23, 24]. In contrast to GCRα, GCRβ does not bind GCs, is transcriptionally inactive [25–27], and competes with GCRα in the nucleus for coactivators such as histone acetyltransferases. GCRβ expression is enhanced by proinflammatory cytokines, such as TNFα and IL-1 [28], combination IL-2/IL-4 [29], and IL-13 [16]. Furthermore, RNA silencing of GCRβ in monocytes/macrophages enhances GCR function, suggesting that GCRβ has a physiologic role in steroid resistance [30]. These data suggest that under conditions of immune activation and inflammation, the GCRβ isoform accumulates preferentially, causing GC insensitivity.

Potential Mechanisms of Glucocorticoid Insensitivity in Obese Asthmatics

Emerging data suggest that elevated BMI might be associated with suboptimal response to GC, the most effective controller therapy for patients with persistent asthma. Inflammation in obesity is characterized by abnormal cytokine production [31], and research over the last decade has demonstrated that TNFα is overexpressed in the adipose tissue and muscle of obese humans [9, 32–34]. In addition, some obese patients manifest elevated plasma concentrations of hsCRP, accompanied by elevated IL-6 concentrations and reduced adiponectin concentrations [35, 36]. There is potential for an interrelationship between inflammation in obesity and GC insensitivity in that production of proinflammatory cytokines seen in obesity (TNFα, IL-6) is upregulated in lung macrophages from GC-insensitive asthmatics [37]. This suggests that the cytokine environment described in obesity may modify response to GCs, perhaps via alterations in MKP-1 induction by GCs.

Alterations in mechanisms of GC signaling and response may underlie reports suggesting that health status is impaired in obese individuals with asthma [38], with more severe, less well-controlled, and less treatment-responsive disease being observed in obese patients. Recent cluster analyses of patient data from clinical populations have been elucidating in this regard. Haldar and colleagues reported that obese asthmatics appeared to aggregate from other patients with asthma with regard to important factors such as symptom expression (increased), eosinophilic airway inflammation (reduced), age of onset (adult), and sex (female predominant) [1]. Additionally, this population appeared to be less responsive to inhaled glucocorticoids. A separate analysis of data from the NHLBI-sponsored Severe Asthma Research Program also indicated that elevated BMI was important in severe asthma, with the identification of a cluster of patients in whom elevated BMI was associated with female sex, adult-onset asthma, a greater likelihood of complicated asthma treatment regimens, and more frequent health care utilization and need for systemic corticosteroids [2].

Although it is intuitive to conclude that this increase in asthma severity must be associated with increased airway inflammation, studies have failed to demonstrate a robust relationship between obesity and traditional biomarkers of airway inflammation in adult asthmatics. For example, Todd and colleagues utilized induced sputum cell counts as an alternative means of assessing airway inflammation in 727 obese subjects with and without asthma. While sputum eosinophil counts were higher overall in subjects with asthma, there was not a significant correlation between BMI and sputum eosinophils either in asthmatic participants or in the study population as a whole [39]. McLachlan and colleagues reported similar findings in a population-based cohort of approximately 1,000 individuals, demonstrating that while adiposity (reflected in percentage of body fat) was associated with asthma and airflow limitation in a subset of subjects, there was not a meaningful association between exhaled nitric oxide (F_ENO) or adiposity [40]. Thus, traditionally monitored biomarkers of airway inflammation (e.g., induced sputum eosinophil percentage, F_ENO) do not necessarily increase as body mass increases in subjects with asthma, suggesting that novel biologically relevant biomarkers of airway inflammation in obese asthmatics need to be identified. Strategies which take advantage of research bronchoscopy to directly sample the airway are likely to be of high yield in this regard. As discussed elsewhere in this volume, one challenge in assessing treatment response in obese asthmatics relates to the assessment of physiologic variables in this population.

Although more work is needed to refine the basic mechanisms by which obesity modifies response to GC in asthma, it is possible that mechanism associated with systemic inflammation also impacts the airway. Recent studies have shown that monokines secreted by adipose tissue activate blood monocytes and recruit activated macrophages to adipose tissue, significantly amplifying proinflammatory cytokine generation [41–45]. The phenotype of blood monocytes and adipose tissue macrophages in obesity is consistent with "classical" or "M1" activation, [45–48] in which there is expression of inflammatory mediators (e.g., α, IL-1β, IL-6) that are crucial to innate immune responses against pathogens. Classical activation is inhibited by Th2 cytokines which "alternatively" program macrophages [49–52], and allergen-driven "asthma" in murine models and mild atopic human asthma is associated with a Th2 milieu and alternative macrophage programming [53]. However, inflammation in refractory asthma has also been associated with Th1 cytokines [54–56], and M1 skewing of blood monocytes and alveolar macrophages has been documented in glucocorticoid-insensitive asthma [57, 58]. These data suggest that in asthma, obesity may alter certain aspects of airway inflammation and response to effective controller therapies, possibly increasing asthma severity and making the disease more difficult to treat.

Finally, the elevations in TNFα observed in obesity may be relevant to the treatment of obese asthmatics. A recent clinical trial demonstrated that increased expression of membrane-bound TNFα, TNFα receptor 1, and TNFα-converting enzyme in peripheral blood mononuclear cells from patients with severe asthma was associated with GC insensitivity. This study also suggested a beneficial effect of soluble TNFα receptor, etanercept, in these patients, as shown by improvements in AHR, FEV_1, and asthma-related quality of life [56], raising the possibility that controller agents other than corticosteroids may be effective in obese asthmatics in whom systemic inflammation and GC insensitivity are shown to be important factors.

Evidence from Clinical Studies

In one of the first reports to assess the relationship between body mass index and response to controller therapies in adult asthmatics, Peters-Golden and colleagues used data obtained during clinical trials of montelukast and inhaled beclomethasone to perform a retrospective analysis of the effect of obesity (as reflected by increased BMI) on asthma control, using asthma control days as the primary clinical variable of interest [59]. The study population consisted of 1,603 patients who had a normal BMI, 971 patients with BMI in the overweight range, and 499 who were obese. Obese patients were older, with a median age of 40 years, compared with 36 years in overweight patients and 28 years in lean patients. With regard to lung function, median FEV_1 was 68.1% of predicted for lean participants, 66.6% for overweight participants, and 65.2% for obese participants. In lean patients, beclomethasone resulted in a higher percentage of asthma control data than did montelukast, at 18.6% versus 9.5% ($p<0.001$). However, the beneficial effect of the inhaled corticosteroid versus the leukotriene modifier became less as BMI increased, with a comparative effect of 18.8% versus 15.7% in overweight ($p=0.25$) and 13.9% versus 13.4% ($p=0.90$) in obese adults. In overweight and obese participants, the authors also reported a significant statistical interaction ($p=0.04$) of BMI and treatment response, with an inverse correlation between increasing body mass index category and the reduction in asthma control days, a finding that was significant with beclomethasone and placebo but not with montelukast. On the basis on these findings, the authors concluded that increasing BMI is associated with a decrease in the overall level of asthma control in response to controller therapy and suggested that there may be a differential effect of BMI on response to inhaled corticosteroids when compared with montelukast, with the negative impact of BMI being greater in those patients treated with inhaled corticosteroids [59].

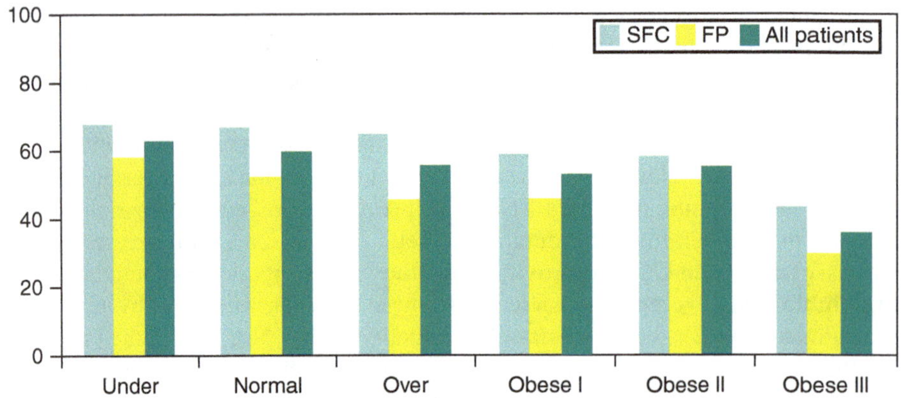

Fig. 7.1 Percentage of patients in various BMI categories achieving asthma control after 12 weeks of treatment with either fluticasone propionate (FP) or salmeterol/fluticasone propionate (SFP) (Reprinted from [62] with permission)

A subsequent article by Boulet and Franssen evaluated the relationship between increasing BMI and response to an inhaled corticosteroid (fluticasone) with and without an added long-acting beta agonist (salmeterol). The authors utilized data from five clinical trials, including the GOAL study [60], ultimately including 1,242 steroid-naïve nonsmoking adults with asthma. Mean FEV_1 in the analysis population was 83% of predicted, with 31.7% and 25.5% being overweight and obese, respectively. All patients demonstrated bronchodilator response with a mean improvement of 20%. Overall, obese subjects were less likely than nonobese individuals to achieve asthma control in response to treatment with either agent. When the odds of achieving asthma control were compared between patients with WHO class 3 obesity (BMI ≥ 40 kg/m^2)[61] and other weight categories, the odds ratio for achieving asthma control were 3.23 (95% confidence interval 1.50–6.97) for patients with BMI < 20, 2.66 (1.45–4.87) for patients with BMI 20–24.9, 2.11 (1.15–3.87) for patients with BMI 25–29.9, 1.91 (1.01–3.61) for BMI 30–34.9, and 2.46 (1.17–5.18) for patients with BMI of 35–39.9 (Fig. 7.1). For patients treated with fluticasone alone, 39.7% of patients with a normal BMI were able to achieve asthma control; this proportion dropped to 28.8% in those who were overweight, 13.9% in those with WHO class 1 obesity (BMI 30–34.9), 6.0% in those with class 2 obesity, and 3.3% in those with class 3 obesity. Similar trends were seen with patients treated with the combination of fluticasone and salmeterol, with 38.2% of treated lean patients achieving asthma control compared to 2.8% of those with class 3 obesity (Fig. 7.1). The authors concluded that obesity is associated with a reduced likelihood of achieving asthma control in response to both inhaled steroid monotherapy and inhaled steroid/long-acting beta agonist combination therapy, a finding most pronounced in those with the most severe form of obesity [62]. These findings validated the observations of Peters-Golden and colleagues and extended the observation not just to inhaled steroid or leukotriene modifier monotherapy but also to the combination of an inhaled steroid and a long-acting beta agonist. Additional post hoc analyses of data from multiple clinical trial populations have further validated these observations [5, 63–65]. In one of these, we analyzed data from studies conducted by the NIH-funded Asthma Clinical Research Network in a similar post hoc approach to those described above and reported an approximately 55% reduction in the effectiveness of ICS monotherapy in lowering exhaled nitric oxide in overweight/obese subjects, as well as a reduction of the beneficial effect of ICS/LABA combinations on FEV_1 and FEV_1/FVC ratio in overweight and obese subjects [5].

Less is known about the effect of overweight and obesity on response to theophylline, with much of the insight coming from a secondary analysis of the LODO study [66], which studied the effectiveness of low-dose theophylline as add-on therapy in poorly controlled asthma. In this analysis, published by Dixon and colleagues, 73% of the 488 included subjects were overweight or obese, and although there were no baseline differences between the groups with regard to cough, dyspnea, or wheeze, obese participants utilized rescue bronchodilators 30% more frequently than other subjects. Overweight and obese participants achieved serum theophylline concentrations similar to those in lean participants, but despite this, there was a significant increase in asthma exacerbations in obese participants compared to those who were lean or overweight, with a relative risk of exacerbation of 3.7 [95% confidence interval 2.2–6.3, $p<0.001$]. Differences in exacerbation rates were not seen in the placebo or montelukast add-on arms of the study [66].

Although many of the reports cited above have identified a reduction in clinical response to GC-containing therapeutic regimens in overweight and obese asthmatics, the mechanisms by which this insensitivity to GCs occurs have been less rigorously investigated. One potential mechanism by which this could be hypothesized to occur is altered molecular response to GCs due to systemic inflammation. As noted above, glucocorticoids inhibit proinflammatory gene expression, in part through negative regulation of MAP kinase signaling pathways by molecules such as MAP kinase phosphatase-1 (MKP-1). Given that proinflammatory cytokines such as IL-1, IL-6, and TNFα are increased in many obese individuals and given that these same cytokines are regulated by potential regulators of p38 MAP kinase [19], it is possible that this proinflammatory environment might modify GC function in obese asthmatics. In order to evaluate this possibility, we hypothesized that overweight and obese asthmatics would demonstrate evidence of reduced molecular responsiveness to GCs in immune cells derived from both the peripheral blood and lung, a process potentially mediated by enhanced expression of or sensitivity to TNFα. They enrolled 45 nonsmoking adults, 33 with asthma (mean (SD) FEV_1% of 70.7 (9.8)%) and 12 without, in a study in which sensitivity to glucocorticoids was assessed in vitro in both peripheral blood mononuclear cells (PBMC) and bronchoalveolar lavage (BAL) cells. Dexamethasone-induced PBMC MKP-1 expression was reduced in overweight/obese versus lean asthmatics, with mean (±SEM) fold induction of 3.11 ± 0.46 versus 5.27 ± 0.66, respectively ($p=0.01$, Fig. 7.2). In asthmatics, regression analysis revealed a -0.16 ± 0.08-fold decrease in DEX-induced MKP-1 per unit BMI increase ($p=0.04$). PBMC TNFα expression increased as BMI increased in subjects with asthma, with a 0.27 unit increase in log [TNFα (ng/mL)] per unit BMI increase ($p=0.01$). The ratio of PBMC [log [TNFα]:DEX-induced MKP-1]

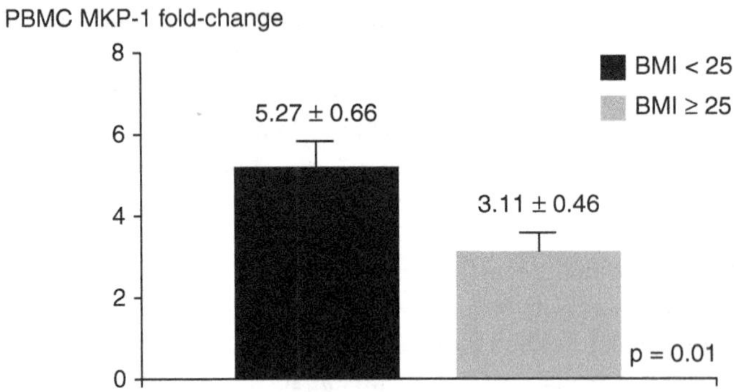

Fig. 7.2 Reduced DEX-induced MKP-1 expression in peripheral blood mononuclear cells from overweight and obese versus lean adults with asthma (Reprinted from [4] with permission)

also increased as BMI increased in asthmatics (+0.09 ± 0.02, $p = 0.004$). In AL cells, DEX-induced MKP-1 expression was also reduced in overweight/obese versus lean asthmatics (1.36 ± 0.09 vs. 1.76 ± 0.15-fold induction, $p = 0.05$). Similar findings were not observed in nonasthmatic controls. On the basis of these findings, the authors concluded that GC sensitivity decreased in both the lung and the periphery as body mass increases in individuals with asthma. This effect was found to occur via a reduced induction of MKP-1 expression in response to dexamethasone in both PBMC and BAL cells and was related to enhanced expression of TNFα in both peripheral and lung immune cells as body mass increases, suggesting a scenario in which one or more molecular pathways governing GC responses are modified in both the airway and peripheral blood in overweight and obese asthmatics [4].

Obesity and Treatment Response in Children and Adolescents with Asthma

Fewer studies have reported on the association between increased body weight and treatment response in children and adolescents. Using data from the Childhood Asthma Management Program (CAMP), Forno and colleagues conducted a retrospective analysis of the impact of increased body mass index on response to inhaled corticosteroids in children with asthma [67]. The CAMP dataset consists of longitudinal data on 1,041 children obtained during a randomized, controlled trial in which participants were treated either with inhaled budesonide, nedocromil, or placebo. On average, this cohort had a normal prebronchodilator FEV_1 at 93.7% of predicted and a slightly reduced FEV_1/FVC ratio of 79.6%. The cohort also demonstrated evidence of bronchodilator responsiveness, with a 10.8% improvement in FEV_1 after administration of albuterol. Approximately one-third (31.4%) of participants were overweight or obese, with overweight/obese participants more likely to be African American ($p = 0.002$), older ($p = 0.002$), and have lower vitamin D levels. The investigators reported there was a significant interaction between body mass index and response to budesonide with regard both to the FEV_1/FVC ratio ($p=0.0007$) and bronchodilator responsiveness ($p=0.049$) for bronchodilator response. Additionally, a nonstatistically significant trend for an interaction with regard to FEV_1 improvement was noted as well ($p=0.15$). The authors calculated that for every 1% increase in body mass index, children treated with budesonide would experience a reduction in inhaled steroid response of approximately 0.04% in FEV_1/FVC and 0.025% in the degree of bronchodilator response. Given the retrospective nature of the analysis and limited availability of biological specimens, the investigators were unable to identify specific mechanisms of reduced inhaled steroid responsiveness in this population but speculated that many of the same mechanisms present in adults could impact steroid responsiveness in overweight and obese children [67].

In a study that sheds some light on the association in adolescents, Kattan and colleagues investigated the relationship between adiposity, adipokines, and asthma control in a population of adolescents in the Asthma Adiposity Study [68]. This group of 368 adolescents between 12 and 20 years of age demonstrated increases in BMI, with females demonstrating a BMI percentile of 82 ± 22.3% and males demonstrating a BMI percentile of 75.6 ± 25.9%. Female participants had, on average, 35.4 ± 89% body fat, while males demonstrated a body fat percentage of 21.9 ± 10.2% ($p<0.001$ for comparison). In association with this relatively increased BMI and percent body fat, female participants also demonstrated higher concentrations of adiponectin, leptin, CRP, and IL-6 when compared with male participants. In female participants, but not in males, there was a significant relationship between increases in percent body fat and increases in both asthma symptoms and asthma exacerbations. These findings suggest that measurements of adiposity other than body mass index are associated with asthma morbidity, underscoring a relationship between obesity and a decreased level of asthma control [68].

Weight Loss as a Therapeutic Adjunct in Obese Asthmatics

Studies of the effect of weight loss on response to asthma therapy are in their infancy. In controlled trials, nonsurgical weight loss protocols [69] can induce an approximately 10% reduction in body weight, and this degree of weight loss has been shown to improve lung function in asthma and to improve adipokines and other markers of systemic inflammation in obesity [70]. This amount of weight loss has also been shown to be enough to permit improvement in waist circumference, blood pressure, circulating cytokines, and fasting levels of glucose, triglycerides, and HDL cholesterol [70] and therefore could be predicted to result improvement in asthma, although this remains speculative. A 2008 systematic review on weight loss in asthma cited only four prior reports of medical weight loss, all of which evaluated primarily spirometric outcomes and which enrolled 120 subjects in toto. Thus, additional studies are needed.

Surgical weight loss approaches induce an even greater degree of weight loss (>20% of body weight in some cases), which may alter pulmonary physiology in ways that make linking weight loss and clinical response more challenging. However, a recent report by Dixon and colleagues [71] has improved our understanding of the impact of weight loss surgery in asthma. In their cohort of 23 asthmatics, 21 of whom followed for up to 12 months after surgery, significant clinical and physiologic improvements were observed after surgery. Asthma control questionnaire score improved from 1.55 to 0.74 ($p < .0001$), a 50% improvement, and patients also reported reduced need for rescue beta agonists and improved asthma-related quality of life. Methacholine PC_{20} improved almost one doubling dose, from 3.90 ± 3.59 to 7.28 ± 6.50 mg/mL ($p = 0.03$), a response observed only in patients with normal serum IgE concentrations (p for interaction $= 0.01$). These findings add asthma control and airway hyperresponsiveness to the list of clinical variables (principally symptoms heretofore) that improve with surgical weight loss.

Conclusion

Ample evidence from both clinical and translational studies suggests that response to asthma controller therapies decreases as body mass increases. The strongest evidence relates to the impact of obesity on response to inhaled corticosteroids, although similar findings have been observed when long-acting beta agonists, montelukast, and theophylline are all added to inhaled corticosteroids. Despite this, no specific guidance currently exists in NIH or international guidelines as to the optimal therapeutic approach to the obese asthmatic, and many obese asthmatics receive complicated asthma treatment regimens to which they do not respond. Until clinical trials specifically evaluating treatment regimens in obese asthmatics are conducted, clinicians must carefully apply guideline-based care to obese patients with asthma, frequently assessing asthma control and treatment response and modifying treatment algorithms as necessary.

References

1. Haldar P, Pavord ID, Shaw DE, Berry MA, Thomas M, Brightling CE, et al. Cluster analysis and clinical asthma phenotypes. Am J Respir Crit Care Med. 2008;178:218–24.
2. Moore WC, Meyers DA, Wenzel SE, Teague WG, Li H, Li X, et al. Identification of asthma phenotypes using cluster analysis in the severe asthma research program. Am J Respir Crit Care Med. 2009;181:315–23.
3. Sutherland ER, Goleva E, Jackson LP, Stevens AD, Leung DY. Vitamin D levels, lung function, and steroid response in adult asthma. Am J Respir Crit Care Med. 2010;181:699–704.
4. Sutherland ER, Goleva E, Strand M, Beuther DA, Leung DY. Body mass and glucocorticoid response in asthma. Am J Respir Crit Care Med. 2008;178:682–7.
5. Sutherland ER, Lehman EB, Teodorescu M, Wechsler ME. Body mass index and phenotype in subjects with mild-to-moderate persistent asthma. J Allergy Clin Immunol. 2009; 123:1328–34. e1.
6. Expert panel report 3: guidelines for the diagnosis and management of asthma. U.S. Department of Health and Human Services 2007. NIH Publication Number 07–4051.

7. Global strategy for asthma management and prevention 2008 update. http://www.ginasthma.org. Accessed 1 Nov 2011.
8. Hotamisligil GS. Inflammation and metabolic disorders. Nature. 2006;444:860–7.
9. Hotamisligil GS, Arner P, Caro JF, Atkinson RL, Spiegelman BM. Increased adipose tissue expression of tumor necrosis factor-alpha in human obesity and insulin resistance. J Clin Invest. 1995;95:2409–15.
10. Hotamisligil GS, Shargill NS, Spiegelman BM. Adipose expression of tumor necrosis factor-alpha: direct role in obesity-linked insulin resistance. Science. 1993;259:87–91.
11. Beuther DA, Weiss ST, Sutherland ER. Obesity and asthma. Am J Respir Crit Care Med. 2006;174:112–9.
12. Cottrell L, Neal WA, Ice C, Perez MK, Piedimonte G. Metabolic abnormalities in children with asthma. Am J Respir Crit Care Med. 2011;183:441–8.
13. Adcock IM, Barnes PJ. Molecular mechanisms of corticosteroid resistance. Chest. 2008; 134:394–401.
14. Bateman ED, Boushey HA, Bousquet J, Busse WW, Clark TJ, Pauwels RA, et al. Can guideline-defined asthma control be achieved? The gaining optimal asthma control study. Am J Respir Crit Care Med. 2004;170:836–44.
15. Szefler SJ, Martin RJ, King TS, Boushey HA, Cherniack RM, Chinchilli VM, et al. Significant variability in response to inhaled corticosteroids for persistent asthma. J Allergy Clin Immunol. 2002;109:410–8.
16. Leung DY, Bloom JW. Update on glucocorticoid action and resistance. J Allergy Clin Immunol. 2003;111:3–22.
17. Ito K, Barnes PJ, Adcock IM. Glucocorticoid receptor recruitment of histone deacetylase 2 inhibits interleukin-1beta-induced histone H4 acetylation on lysines 8 and 12. Mol Cell Biol. 2000;20:6891–903.
18. Matthews JG, Ito K, Barnes PJ, Adcock IM. Defective glucocorticoid receptor nuclear translocation and altered histone acetylation patterns in glucocorticoid-resistant patients. J Allergy Clin Immunol. 2004;113:1100–8.
19. Clark AR. MAP kinase phosphatase 1: a novel mediator of biological effects of glucocorticoids? J Endocrinol. 2003;178:5–12.
20. Kassel O, Sancono A, Kratzschmar J, Kreft B, Stassen M, Cato AC. Glucocorticoids inhibit MAP kinase via increased expression and decreased degradation of MKP-1. EMBO J. 2001;20:7108–16.
21. Zhao Q, Shepherd EG, Manson ME, Nelin LD, Sorokin A, Liu Y. The role of mitogen-activated protein kinase phosphatase-1 in the response of alveolar macrophages to lipopolysaccharide: attenuation of proinflammatory cytokine biosynthesis via feedback control of p38. J Biol Chem. 2005;280:8101–8.
22. Chung KF. p38 Mitogen-Activated protein kinase pathways in asthma and COPD. Chest. 2011;139:1470–9.
23. Bamberger CM, Bamberger AM, de Castro M, Chrousos GP. Glucocorticoid receptor beta, a potential endogenous inhibitor of glucocorticoid action in humans. J Clin Invest. 1995;95:2435–41.
24. Oakley RH, Webster JC, Sar M, Parker Jr CR, Cidlowski JA. Expression and subcellular distribution of the beta-isoform of the human glucocorticoid receptor. Endocrinology. 1997;138:5028–38.
25. Oakley RH, Jewell CM, Yudt MR, Bofetiado DM, Cidlowski JA. The dominant negative activity of the human glucocorticoid receptor beta isoform. Specificity and mechanisms of action. J Biol Chem. 1999;274:27857–66.
26. Oakley RH, Sar M, Cidlowski JA. The human glucocorticoid receptor beta isoform. Expression, biochemical properties, and putative function. J Biol Chem. 1996;271:9550–9.
27. Yudt MR, Jewell CM, Bienstock RJ, Cidlowski JA. Molecular origins for the dominant negative function of human glucocorticoid receptor beta. Mol Cell Biol. 2003;23:4319–30.
28. Webster JC, Oakley RH, Jewell CM, Cidlowski JA. Proinflammatory cytokines regulate human glucocorticoid receptor gene expression and lead to the accumulation of the dominant negative beta isoform: a mechanism for the generation of glucocorticoid resistance. Proc Natl Acad Sci USA. 2001;98:6865–70.

29. Leung DY, Hamid Q, Vottero A, Szefler SJ, Surs W, Minshall E, et al. Association of glucocorticoid insensitivity with increased expression of glucocorticoid receptor beta. J Exp Med. 1997;186: 1567–74.
30. Goleva E, Li LB, Eves PT, Strand MJ, Martin RJ, Leung DY. Increased glucocorticoid receptor beta alters steroid response in glucocorticoid-insensitive asthma. Am J Respir Crit Care Med. 2006;173:607–16.
31. Wellen KE, Hotamisligil GS. Inflammation, stress, and diabetes. J Clin Invest. 2005;115: 1111–9.
32. Kern PA, Saghizadeh M, Ong JM, Bosch RJ, Deem R, Simsolo RB. The expression of tumor necrosis factor in human adipose tissue. Regulation by obesity, weight loss, and relationship to lipoprotein lipase. J Clin Invest. 1995;95:2111–9.
33. Krogh-Madsen R, Plomgaard P, Moller K, Mittendorfer B, Pedersen BK. Influence of TNF-alpha and IL-6 infusions on insulin sensitivity and expression of IL-18 in humans. Am J Physiol Endocrinol Metab. 2006;291:E108–14.
34. Saghizadeh M, Ong JM, Garvey WT, Henry RR, Kern PA. The expression of TNF alpha by human muscle. Relationship to insulin resistance. J Clin Invest. 1996;97:1111–6.
35. Cote M, Mauriege P, Bergeron J, Almeras N, Tremblay A, Lemieux I, et al. Adiponectinemia in visceral obesity: impact on glucose tolerance and plasma lipoprotein and lipid levels in men. J Clin Endocrinol Metab. 2005;90:1434–9.
36. Lemieux I, et al. Contribution of interleukin-6 and tumor necrosis factor-alpha to the elevated C-reactive protein levels found in abdominally obese men. Obes Res. 2001;9:66S.
37. Hauk PJ, Goleva E, Liu AH, et al. Corticosteroid resistant asthma is associated with classical activation of airway macrophages and exposure to lipopolysaccharide. J Allergy Clin Immunol. 2006;117:S194.
38. Vortmann M, Eisner MD. BMI and health status among adults with asthma. Obesity (Silver Spring). 2008;16:146–52.
39. Todd DC, Armstrong S, D'Silva L, Allen CJ, Hargreave FE, Parameswaran K. Effect of obesity on airway inflammation: a cross-sectional analysis of body mass index and sputum cell counts. Clin Exp Allergy. 2007;37:1049–54.
40. McLachlan CR, Poulton R, Car G, Cowan J, Filsell S, Greene JM, et al. Adiposity, asthma, and airway inflammation. J Allergy Clin Immunol. 2007;119:634–9.
41. Lee YH, Nair S, Rousseau E, Allison DB, Page GP, Tataranni PA, et al. Microarray profiling of isolated abdominal subcutaneous adipocytes from obese vs non-obese Pima Indians: increased expression of inflammation-related genes. Diabetologia. 2005;48:1776–83.
42. Kanda H, Tateya S, Tamori Y, Kotani K, Hiasa K, Kitazawa R, et al. MCP-1 contributes to macrophage infiltration into adipose tissue, insulin resistance, and hepatic steatosis in obesity. J Clin Invest. 2006;116:1494–505.
43. Dahlman I, Kaaman M, Olsson T, Tan GD, Bickerton AS, Wahlen K, et al. A unique role of monocyte chemoattractant protein 1 among chemokines in adipose tissue of obese subjects. J Clin Endocrinol Metab. 2005;90:5834–40.
44. Gordon S. Macrophage heterogeneity and tissue lipids. J Clin Invest. 2007;117:89–93.
45. Lumeng CN, Bodzin JL, Saltiel AR. Obesity induces a phenotypic switch in adipose tissue macrophage polarization. J Clin Invest. 2007;117:175–84.
46. Ghanim H, Aljada A, Hofmeyer D, Syed T, Mohanty P, Dandona P. Circulating mononuclear cells in the obese are in a proinflammatory state. Circulation. 2004;110:1564–71.
47. Gustafson B, Smith U. Cytokines promote Wnt signaling and inflammation and impair the normal differentiation and lipid accumulation in 3 T3-L1 preadipocytes. J Biol Chem. 2006;281:9507–16.
48. Powell K. Obesity: the two faces of fat. Nature. 2007;447:525–7.
49. Mantovani A, Sozzani S, Locati M, Allavena P, Sica A. Macrophage polarization: tumor-associated macrophages as a paradigm for polarized M2 mononuclear phagocytes. Trends Immunol. 2002;23:549–55.

50. Duffield JS. The inflammatory macrophage: a story of Jekyll and Hyde. Clin Sci (Lond). 2003;104:27–38.
51. Van Ginderachter JA, Movahedi K, Hassanzadeh Ghassabeh G, Meerschaut S, Beschin A, Raes G, et al. Classical and alternative activation of mononuclear phagocytes: picking the best of both worlds for tumor promotion. Immunobiology. 2006;211:487–501.
52. Martinez FO, Gordon S, Locati M, Mantovani A. Transcriptional profiling of the human monocyte-to-macrophage differentiation and polarization: new molecules and patterns of gene expression. J Immunol. 2006;177:7303–11.
53. Zimmermann N, King NE, Laporte J, Yang M, Mishra A, Pope SM, et al. Dissection of experimental asthma with DNA microarray analysis identifies arginase in asthma pathogenesis. J Clin Invest. 2003;111:1863–74.
54. Truyen E, Coteur L, Dilissen E, Overbergh L, Dupont LJ, Ceuppens JL, et al. Evaluation of airway inflammation by quantitative Th1/Th2 cytokine mRNA measurement in sputum of asthma patients. Thorax. 2006;61:202–8.
55. Arshad SH, Kurukulaaratchy RJ, Fenn M, Matthews S. Early life risk factors for current wheeze, asthma, and bronchial hyperresponsiveness at 10 years of age. Chest. 2005; 127:502–8.
56. Berry MA, Hargadon B, Shelley M, Parker D, Shaw DE, Green RH, et al. Evidence of a role of tumor necrosis factor alpha in refractory asthma. N Engl J Med. 2006;354:697–708.
57. Hauk PJ, Goleva E, Liu AH, Hall CF, Riches DWH, Martin RJ, et al. Corticosteroid resistant (CR) asthma is associated with classical activation of airway macrophages and exposure to lipopolysaccharide (LPS). J Allergy Clin Immunol. 2006;117:S194.
58. Hakonarson H, Bjornsdottir US, Halapi E, Bradfield J, Zink F, Mouy M, et al. Profiling of genes expressed in peripheral blood mononuclear cells predicts glucocorticoid sensitivity in asthma patients. Proc Natl Acad Sci USA. 2005;102:14789–94.
59. Peters-Golden M, Swern A, Bird SS, Hustad CM, Grant E, Edelman JM. Influence of body mass index on the response to asthma controller agents. Eur Respir J. 2006;27:495–503.
60. Bateman ED. Can guideline-defined asthma control be achieved?: the gaining optimal asthma control study. Am J Respir Crit Care Med. 2004;170:836–44.
61. Obesity: preventing and managing the global epidemic. Report of a WHO consultation. World Health Organ Tech Rep Ser. 2000;894:i–xii, 1–253.
62. Boulet L, Franssen E. Influence of obesity on response to fluticasone with or without salmeterol in moderate asthma. Respir Med. 2007;101:2240–7.
63. Camargo CA, Boulet L-P, Sutherland ER, Busse WW, Yancey SW, Emmett AH, et al. Body mass index and response to asthma therapy: fluticasone propionate/salmeterol versus montelukast. J Asthma. 2010;47:76–82.
64. Camargo Jr CA, Sutherland ER, Bailey W, Castro M, Yancey SW, Emmett AH, et al. Effect of increased body mass index on asthma risk, impairment and response to asthma controller therapy in African Americans. Curr Med Res Opin. 2010;26:1629–35.
65. Sutherland ER, Camargo CA, Busse WW, Meltzer EO, Ortega HG, Yancey SW, et al. Comparative effect of body mass index on response to asthma controller therapy. Allergy Asthma Proc. 2010;31:20–5.
66. Dixon AE, Shade DM, Cohen RI, Skloot GS, Holbrook JT, Smith LJ, et al. Effect of obesity on clinical presentation and response to treatment in asthma. J Asthma. 2006;43:553–8.
67. Forno E, Lescher R, Strunk R, Weiss S, Fuhlbrigge A, Celedon JC. Decreased response to inhaled steroids in overweight and obese asthmatic children. J Allergy Clin Immunol. 2011;127:741–9.
68. Kattan M, Kumar R, Bloomberg GR, Mitchell HE, Calatroni A, Gergen PJ, et al. Asthma control, adiposity, and adipokines among inner-city adolescents. J Allergy Clin Immunol. 2010;125:584–92.
69. Eckel RH. Clinical practice. Nonsurgical management of obesity in adults. N Engl J Med. 2008;358:1941–50.

70. Poirier P, Giles T, Bray G, Hong Y, Stern J, Pi-Sunyer F, et al. Obesity and cardiovascular disease: pathophysiology, evaluation, and effect of weight loss: an update of the 1997 American Heart Association Scientific statement on obesity and heart disease from the obesity committee of the council on nutrition, physical activity, and metabolism. Circulation. 2006;113:898.
71. Dixon AE, Pratley RE, Forgione PM, Kaminsky DA, Whittaker-Leclair LA, Griffes LA, et al. Effects of obesity and bariatric surgery on airway hyperresponsiveness, asthma control, and inflammation. J Allergy Clin Immunol. 2011;128:508–15.

Chapter 8
Obesity and Chronic Obstructive Pulmonary Disease

Frits M.E. Franssen and Emiel F.M. Wouters

Abstract COPD and obesity are two heterogeneous chronic conditions with increasing prevalences all over the world. For accurate clinical assessment and disease management, it is important to understand the effects of excessive fat accumulation in patients with concomitant COPD and obesity. In COPD, obesity results in reductions in static lung hyperinflation, irrespective of the severity of airflow limitation. The impact of obesity on exercise capacity in COPD is likely dependent on the type of exercise, with obesity being associated with decreased tolerance to weight-bearing exercise while having beneficial effects on dynamic ventilatory mechanics during weight-supported exercise. Although obese COPD patients have higher levels of systemic inflammation and increased risk of metabolic syndrome, it is currently unknown whether and to what extent adipose tissue dysfunction and insulin resistance contribute to increased cardiovascular risk and extrapulmonary manifestations in COPD. In contrast to early stage COPD, obesity seems to protect against mortality in patients with severe disease. Even though additional studies on the interaction between obesity and COPD are warranted, the current findings suggest that the presence of obesity has implications for interpretation of diagnostic measurements and management of patients with COPD. Future studies need to show the overall effects of nutritional interventions in obese COPD patients and determine the optimal BMI for an obese patient with COPD.

F.M.E. Franssen, M.D., Ph.D. (✉)
Program Development Center, Ciro+, Center of Expertise for Chronic Organ Failure, Hornerheide 1, 6085 NM Horn, Limburg, The Netherlands
e-mail: fritsfranssen@ciro-horn.nl

E.F.M. Wouters, M.D., Ph.D.
Department of Respiratory Medicine, Maastricht University Medical Center, P. Debyelaan 25, 6229 HX Maastricht, Limburg, The Netherlands
e-mail: e.wouters@mumc.nl

A.E. Dixon and E.M. Clerisme-Beaty (eds.), *Obesity and Lung Disease: A Guide to Management*, Respiratory Medicine, DOI 10.1007/978-1-62703-053-3_8,

Keywords Chronic obstructive pulmonary disease • Obesity • Epidemiology • Metabolic syndrome • Adipose tissue • Lung function • Exercise tolerance • Hyperinflation • Systemic inflammation

Objectives

- Describe the epidemiological relationship between obesity and COPD
- Discuss the effects of obesity on lung function and exercise tolerance in COPD
- Describe the impact of obesity on mortality in COPD
- Discuss the relationship between the metabolic syndrome and comorbidities in COPD
- Consider the potential pathophysiologic role of adipose tissue dysfunction in COPD

Introduction

Chronic obstructive pulmonary disease (COPD) is characterized by progressive airflow limitation, caused by inhalation of noxious particles or gases, particularly smoke from tobacco and from burning of biomass [1]. Millions of people worldwide suffer from COPD. According to the "Burden of Obstructive Lung Disease" (BOLD) Initiative, the global prevalence of spirometrically confirmed COPD in adults ranges from 11% to 25% [2]. It is predicted that COPD will become the third leading cause of mortality and the fifth most important contributor to disability-adjusted life years by 2020 [3]. Typical presenting symptoms of patients with COPD are dyspnea on exertion, cough, and sputum production [1]. In addition, progressive exercise limitation is frequently observed in patients with COPD [4] and is multifactorially determined [5]. Traditionally, COPD was considered a respiratory disease, based on the presence of chronic airflow limitation. Nowadays, it is recognized that COPD is a heterogeneous disease with both pulmonary as well as extrapulmonary manifestations that are insufficiently captured by the degree of airflow limitation [6]. Anthropometric differences between patients with COPD probably contribute to the observed heterogeneity in this disabling disease.

The prevalence of obesity, defined as body mass index (BMI) ≥ 30 kg/m^2, has more than doubled worldwide since 1980. According to WHO estimates, it is projected that the number of obese adults will exceed 700 million by the year 2015 [7]. Aside from its effect on chronic diseases such as diabetes, heart disease, sleep-disordered breathing, and stroke, obesity is associated with both mechanical and systemic changes that may contribute to COPD heterogeneity and the development of comorbidities such as cardiovascular disease. Furthermore, COPD-specific factors, such as systemic hypoxemia and reduced skeletal muscle oxidative capacity, may aggravate obesity-related metabolic and inflammatory derangements in patients with COPD [8].

This chapter focuses on the epidemiology of obesity in COPD and examines the impact of excessive fat mass on pulmonary function, exercise tolerance, and prognosis. In addition, the potential role of metabolic syndrome and adipose tissue dysfunction in COPD pathophysiology will be evaluated.

Epidemiology

COPD patients are at increased risk of developing obesity compared with healthy elderly, as a result of a reduced level of daily physical activities [9]. An increased prevalence of obesity in COPD could therefore be anticipated. Only a few studies concerning the prevalence of obesity in patients with COPD have been performed, and results are inconclusive. In the multicenter population-based epidemiologic "Proyecto Latinoamericano de Investigacion en Obstruccio´n Pulmonar" (PLATINO) study, the overall prevalence of COPD in adults aged 40 or older was 14% [10]. The prevalence of obesity among those meeting spirometric criteria for COPD (FEV_1/FVC<0.7) was 23%, compared to 32% in subjects without COPD [10]. In another study from the Netherlands based on a large primary care population of COPD patients, the prevalence of obesity was 18% [11]. In that cohort, obesity was found to be more prevalent (16–24%) in patients with milder disease severity (GOLD 1 and 2) and was lowest (6%) in those with severe disease (GOLD 4) [11]. This is compared to the national prevalence of obesity in the general adult population in the Netherlands at that time of approximately 11% [12]. A much higher prevalence of obesity was reported in an adult multiethnic cohort of early stage COPD patients from Northern California, USA [13]. In this study, 54% of subjects met criteria for obesity compared to the 20–24% reported prevalence for the general adult population of that region.

As such, available data indicate that the prevalence of obesity in COPD is variable and may be related to differences in general risk factors for obesity among populations, such as dietary factors and physical activity. In addition, factors related to COPD disease severity, such as the severity of airflow limitation, frequency of hospitalizations, comorbidities, use of systemic glucocorticosteroids, and smoking status, may also contribute to the observed differences in prevalence of obesity between studies.

Effect of Obesity on Lung Function in COPD

The respective changes in pulmonary function at rest related to obesity and COPD are well understood. As described in Chap. 2, reduction in functional residual capacity (FRC) [14] as a result of a reduction in lung compliance [15] is the most prominent effect of obesity on respiratory physiology. The effects of obesity on airway function are limited with forced expiratory volume in 1 s (FEV_1) and forced vital capacity (FVC) being usually preserved [16] and FEV_1/FVC ratio remaining normal. However, obese subjects are at increased risk of expiratory flow limitation as a result of their breathing at lower lung volume [14], and small airways disease may be present. Diffusing lung capacity of carbon monoxide (DLCO) is also in the normal range or increased in obesity [17]. In contrast, COPD is characterized by chronic expiratory airflow limitation and lung hyperinflation at rest [1]. Lung hyperinflation is defined as an abnormal increase in resting FRC, which is the result of increased lung compliance and airflow limitation [18].

The pathophysiologic interactions between obesity and COPD are complex and have not yet been extensively investigated. However, it is important to understand these interactions to correctly interpret lung function measurements in patients with COPD and coexisting obesity, an increasingly growing population. In a study of moderate-to-severe COPD patients, there was no difference in diffusion capacity or maximum inspiratory mouth occlusion pressure between normal-weight and obese patients with a comparable degree of airflow limitation [19]. Although resting hyperinflation was present in both groups, FRC and ERV were significantly lower in obese patients compared to normal-weight patients [19] likely due to the effects of obesity on static lung volumes in COPD causing less hyperinflation. Similarly, TLC (%predicted) was smaller, and IC/TLC ratio was significantly increased in obese compared to normal-weight COPD patients. In line with isolated obesity, increasing BMI was associated with decreasing static lung volumes in COPD [19], resulting in less hyperinflation. The association between BMI and plethysmographically measured lung volumes was shown to be independent of the severity of COPD [20]. However, increasing BMI was found to be associated with increasing FEV_1/FVC ratio, especially in patients with severe to very severe disease [20].

Whether these observed effects of obesity on lung function in COPD patients differ based on distribution of fat mass (i.e., central vs. peripheral obesity) has not yet been studied.

Effect of Obesity on Exercise Performance in COPD

Obesity is associated with increased absolute oxygen uptake, and carbon dioxide production is higher at rest and during exercise, as a consequence of a larger metabolically active muscle mass. Also, obese subjects have increased work of breathing [21] and more rapid and shallow breathing pattern as a result of mechanical restriction, leading to increased dyspnea and difficulties performing daily physical activities [22]. Despite the anticipated negative consequences of obesity on exercise tolerance, peak exercise capacity has been shown to be normal in healthy obese subjects [23]. Although oxygen consumption and minute ventilation at any given work rate were found consistently increased during incremental cycle exercise, there was no difference in breathlessness ratings or ventilatory equivalent for carbon dioxide production response between obese and normal-weight women [24]. Aside from its effect on increased metabolic needs, obesity also affects operating lung volumes during exercise with progressive increase in end-expiratory lung volume (EELV) and recruitment of resting IC during cycle exercise [24]. This likely attenuates the progressive expiratory flow limitation by breathing at lower lung volumes close to the maximal flow volume loop and increased respiratory rate [24].

In COPD, exercise is associated with insufficient expiratory time due to increased respiration rate that leads to increased EELV and worsening hyperinflation. This phenomenon, known as dynamic hyperinflation [25], is associated with decreased tidal volume and increased inspiratory effort that leads to increased dyspnea and exercise intolerance. Neuromechanical dissociation due to dynamic hyperinflation further contributes to the development of breathlessness and decreased exercise tolerance in COPD [18].

Given the effects of obesity on resting FRC and ERV, one would expect a beneficial effect of obesity on dynamic hyperinflation and exercise tolerance in COPD patients. Indeed, peak oxygen uptake and peak work rate during symptom-limited cycle exercise were higher in obese COPD patients compared to normal-weight patients matched for FEV_1 [19]. Although both patient groups had a ventilatory exercise limitation, minute ventilation and ventilatory efficiency at any given work rate were greater in the obese patients. Dyspnea intensity at any given level of ventilation was also lower in obese COPD patients compared to normal-weight patients [19], despite higher respiratory rate in the obese patients. The lower dyspnea intensity in the obese COPD subjects is probably the result of improved ventilatory mechanics. Although the magnitude of dynamic hyperinflation was comparable to the normal-weight COPD patients, the relative dynamic EELV was lower during exercise in the obese patients [19], resulting in a higher maximal minute ventilation.

Despite decrease in dyspnea perception and lower operating lung volumes, obese COPD patients show impairments in weight-bearing exercises. Specifically, obese COPD patients have a shorter 6-min walking distance, reduced self-reported functional activities, and greater fatigue than nonobese patients [26]. This is likely due to increased metabolic and ventilatory requirements associated with weight-bearing exercise, given comparable physiologic responses, i.e., dyspnea and leg fatigue during 6-min walking test between obese and nonobese COPD patients [27]. Thus, the potential beneficial influence of obesity on exercise tolerance related to decreased resting hyperinflation may be offset by the increased metabolic load associated with weight-bearing exercise in obesity. Future studies need to clarify the influence of obesity on activities of daily life in COPD.

Effect of Obesity on Prognosis in COPD

In the general population, obesity is associated with a large decrease in life expectancy [28]. In the Prospective Studies Collaboration, the association between BMI and mortality was assessed by long-term prospective follow-up of almost 900,000 participants [29]. For each 5 kg/m^2 increase in BMI above the normal range, overall mortality was about 30% higher, mainly due to cardiovascular disease [29].

Few studies have investigated the impact of obesity on prognosis in patients with COPD. In the epidemiological Copenhagen City Heart Study, obesity was associated with a 20–34% increase in the relative risk of all-cause mortality in patients with mild-to-moderate COPD compared to normal BMI patients with comparable disease severity [30]. However, the relative risk of all-cause mortality and COPD-related mortality was 0.62 and 0.31, respectively, in patients with severe COPD compared to normal-weight patients with severe disease [30]. A possibly protective role for obesity in patients with severe COPD was also observed in early studies on the association between body weight and mortality [31, 32]. In the "Association Nationale pour le Traitement a Domicile de l'Insuffisance Respiratoire Chronique" (ANTADIR) network, the prognostic value of obesity in hypoxemic patients with COPD treated with long-term oxygen therapy was clearly demonstrated [33]. During the 7.5-year follow-up, the highest survival and lowest hospitalization rates were observed in obese COPD patients. The 5-year survival rates were 24%, 34%, 44%, and 59%, respectively, for patients with BMIs < 20, 20 to 24, 25 to 29, and > 30 kg/m^2.

This possible association between obesity and improved survival in COPD thus contrasts with epidemiological data from the general population. Although not completely understood, this phenomenon known as the "obesity paradox" is not unique for COPD [34]. One explanation, for the prognostic advantage of obesity, concerns the relative reduction in static lung volumes in obese COPD patients. During a 3-year follow-up study, the inspiratory capacity to total lung capacity ratio (IC/TLC), an index of static lung hyperinflation, was found to be an independent predictor of increased respiratory and all-cause mortality in patients with COPD [35]. Although the mechanism underlying the association between hyperinflation and prognosis remains unclear, it can be speculated that increased IC/TLC in obese patients with COPD [19] may contribute to a benefit in survival.

In addition, obesity is associated with significantly lower annual decline in FEV_1 in men and not in women [36]. Thus, there may be gender-specific differences in the effect of obesity on the progression of chronic airflow limitation. Furthermore, it is not yet clear whether excessive fat mass or muscle mass contributes to the survival advantage in chronic diseases [34].

Based on the evidence outlined above, it can be hypothesized that obesity exerts divergent effects on COPD prognosis based on patient characteristics and disease severity. Obesity may protect against mortality in advanced COPD patients, in which loss of fat-free mass is a particularly important short-term risk factor for death [37]. By contrast, in earlier stage COPD, the harmful long-term effects of obesity-related conditions such as low-grade systemic inflammation and metabolic syndrome may result in increased cardiovascular and all-cause mortality.

Metabolic Syndrome in COPD

Patients with COPD are at high risk of hospitalization and death from cardiovascular disease [38] and at increased risk of diabetes [39]. Although the mechanisms responsible for this association remain largely unknown, obesity is associated with abnormal metabolic and inflammatory responses that may contribute to increased cardiovascular morbidity in COPD.

Metabolic syndrome is a cluster of risk factors (i.e., hypertension, dyslipidemia, diabetes) for cardiovascular disease [40]. Central obesity is one of the key factors in the pathogenesis of this syndrome, in addition to physical inactivity, nutrition, aging, genetics, and proinflammatory state, and hormonal changes play a role [41]. Metabolic syndrome is associated with restrictive lung function impairment, independent of waist circumference and BMI [42]. In a large population-based study, the risk of metabolic syndrome was 40% higher in subjects with restrictive lung function impairment compared to subjects with normal lung function [43]. Abdominal obesity, not BMI, was the strongest predictor of lung function impairment in that study.

Several studies have investigated the prevalence of metabolic syndrome in patients with COPD. In a small study of patients with severe COPD referred for pulmonary rehabilitation, 47% of patients fulfilled the diagnostic criteria for metabolic syndrome. This percentage was significantly higher compared to the age- and gender-matched control subjects, in whom the prevalence of metabolic syndrome was only 21% [44]. Similar results were reported in a larger study including patients with chronic bronchitis and COPD [45]. Although the prevalence of metabolic syndrome does not appear to vary based on the severity of lung disease, it is associated with increased circulatory levels of high-sensitivity C-reactive protein (hs-CRP) and interleukin-6 (IL-6) and with physical inactivity. These associations were independent of lung function impairment [45]. Future studies should focus on whether patients with COPD and the metabolic syndrome indeed have an increased risk of developing comorbidities including cardiovascular diseases and diabetes and whether this contributes to increased cardiovascular and all-cause mortality in these patients.

Adipose Tissue Dysfunction in COPD?

In recent years, it has become known that adipose tissue is not an inert organ simply for the storage of energy. Instead, adipose tissue is now recognized as a highly active metabolic and endocrine organ [46]. Adipocytes secrete a variety of proteins, called adipokines, that exert effects at the local and systemic level [47]. Normal function of adipose tissue is disturbed in obesity with growing evidence suggesting that this plays an important role in the metabolic and hemodynamic disturbances observed in obesity and metabolic syndrome. In short, adipocytes in obesity are characterized by hypertrophy, decreased blood flow, hypoxia, infiltration of macrophages, and disturbed adipokines secretion [47]. In morbidly obese subjects undergoing open gastric bypass surgery, IL-6 concentrations in the portal vein, which drains the visceral fat, were significantly increased compared to IL-6 levels in peripheral arterial blood, demonstrating that visceral fat is an important source of IL-6 in obesity [48]. Furthermore, portal vein IL-6 levels were related to arterial CRP concentrations, suggesting a mechanistic link between visceral fat mass and systemic inflammation.

In addition to pulmonary inflammation, low-grade systemic inflammation is considered a hallmark of COPD [49, 50] and may explain the increase cardiovascular morbidity and metabolic syndrome noted in patients with COPD. Increased levels of proinflammatory cells and mediators have been reported in the circulation of COPD patients, including increased plasma concentrations of fibrinogen, CRP, TNF-α, and circulating leukocytes [49]. Increased levels of IL-6 [51, 52], IL-8 [53], IL-10 [52], and IL-18 [54] have also been reported. Although it is often hypothesized that inflammation in the systemic compartment is the result of spillover of the inflammatory process in the airways, lung parenchyma, and pulmonary vasculature, evidence from cross-sectional studies indicates no correlation between pulmonary and circulatory inflammatory markers in stable COPD [53, 55].

However, adipose tissue may be a potential source of systemic inflammation in COPD. Increased levels of systemic inflammation have been reported in relation with excessive fat mass in COPD patients. Specifically, TNF-α, IL-6, and leptin plasma levels have been shown to be significantly increased in overweight/obese patients compared with normal-weight patients, while plasma adiponectin concentrations were reduced [50]. The likelihood of having elevated CRP is three times higher in obese patients compared to normal-weight patients, after adjusting for relevant confounders [56], with abdominal fat mass being positively associated with plasma CRP levels in patients with COPD [57]. To date, no studies have investigated differences in adipokine expression and secretion by adipose tissue and their relationship with systemic inflammation in obese and normal-weight patients with COPD. Two studies have examined adipose tissue inflammation in COPD and found significant differences in subcutaneous adipose tissue mRNA expression of proinflammatory IL-6, TNF-α, and CD68 (macrophage cell surface receptor) among cachectic, normal-weight, overweight, and obese patients with moderate-to-severe COPD [58]. However, there was no difference in serum levels of IL-6, TNF-α, and high-sensitivity CRP (hs-CRP) [58]. In another study, gene expression of proinflammatory CD40, mitogen-activated protein kinase 4 (MKK4), and c-Jun NH_2-terminal kinases (JNK) was increased in subcutaneous adipose tissue in underweight and muscle-wasted COPD patients with resting hypoxia, compared to less severe patients with overweight and preserved muscle mass [59]. Upregulation of CD40, MKK4, and JNK was inversely related to arterial oxygen tension (P_aO_2), BMI, and adipocyte diameter. However, since no healthy control groups matched for body composition were included, a COPD-specific effect on adipose tissue inflammation could not be assessed. Further, given comparable levels of circulating hs-CRP and IL-6 levels in the underweight hypoxemic patients and the overweight normoxemic patients, a link between white adipose tissue inflammation and systemic inflammation has not been proven. To conclude, evidence suggests higher levels of systemic inflammation in obese COPD patients, but the potential contribution of excessive fat mass remains unknown.

The current findings suggest that the presence of obesity has implications for interpretation of diagnostic measurements and management of patients with COPD. Future studies need to show the overall effects of nutritional interventions in obese COPD patients and determine the optimal BMI for an obese patient with COPD.

References

1. Rabe KF, Hurd S, Anzueto A, Barnes PJ, Buist SA, Calverley P, et al. Global strategy for the diagnosis, management, and prevention of chronic obstructive pulmonary disease: GOLD executive summary. Am J Respir Crit Care Med. 2007;176(6):532–55.
2. Buist AS, McBurnie MA, Vollmer WM, Gillespie S, Burney P, Mannino DM, et al. International variation in the prevalence of COPD (the BOLD Study): a population-based prevalence study. Lancet. 2007;370(9589):741–50.
3. Murray CJ, Lopez AD. Alternative projections of mortality and disability by cause 1990–2020: global burden of disease study. Lancet. 1997;349(9064):1498–504.
4. Loke J, Mahler DA, Man SF, Wiedemann HP, Matthay RA. Exercise impairment in chronic obstructive pulmonary disease. Clin Chest Med. 1984;5(1):121–43.
5. American Thoracic Society/European Respiratory Society Statement. Skeletal muscle dysfunction in chronic obstructive pulmonary disease. Am J Respir Crit Care Med. 1999;159 (4 Pt 2):S1–40.
6. Agusti A, Calverley PM, Celli B, Coxson HO, Edwards LD, Lomas DA, et al. Characterisation of COPD heterogeneity in the ECLIPSE cohort. Respir Res. 2010;11:122.
7. WHO. Obesity: preventing and managing the global epidemic. Report of a WHO Consultation. WHO Technical Report Series 894. 2000.
8. Franssen FM, O'Donnell DE, Goossens GH, Blaak EE, Schols AM. Obesity and the lung: 5. Obesity and COPD. Thorax. 2008;63(12):1110–7.
9. Pitta F, Troosters T, Spruit MA, Probst VS, Decramer M, Gosselink R. Characteristics of physical activities in daily life in chronic obstructive pulmonary disease. Am J Respir Crit Care Med. 2005;171(9):972–7.
10. Montes de Oca M, Talamo C, Perez-Padilla R, Jardim JR, Muino A, Lopez MV, et al. Chronic obstructive pulmonary disease and body mass index in five Latin America cities: the PLATINO study. Respir Med. 2008;102(5):642–50.
11. Steuten LM, Creutzberg EC, Vrijhoef HJ, Wouters EF. COPD as a multicomponent disease: inventory of dyspnoea, underweight, obesity and fat free mass depletion in primary care. Prim Care Respir J. 2006;15(2):84–91.
12. Schokker DF, Visscher TL, Nooyens AC, van Baak MA, Seidell JC. Prevalence of overweight and obesity in the Netherlands. Obes Rev. 2007;8(2):101–8.
13. Eisner MD, Blanc PD, Sidney S, Yelin EH, Lathon PV, Katz PP, et al. Body composition and functional limitation in COPD. Respir Res. 2007;8:7.
14. Salome CM, King GG, Berend N. Physiology of obesity and effects on lung function. J Appl Physiol. 2010;108(1):206–11.
15. Pelosi P, Croci M, Ravagnan I, Vicardi P, Gattinoni L. Total respiratory system, lung, and chest wall mechanics in sedated-paralyzed postoperative morbidly obese patients. Chest. 1996;109(1):144–51.
16. Sin DD, Jones RL, Man SF. Obesity is a risk factor for dyspnea but not for airflow obstruction. Arch Intern Med. 2002;162(13):1477–81.

17. Collard P, Wilputte JY, Aubert G, Rodenstein DO, Frans A. The single-breath diffusing capacity for carbon monoxide in obstructive sleep apnea and obesity. Chest. 1996;110(5): 1189–93.
18. O'Donnell DE. Hyperinflation, dyspnea, and exercise intolerance in chronic obstructive pulmonary disease. Proc Am Thorac Soc. 2006;3(2):180–4.
19. Ora J, Laveneziana P, Ofir D, Deesomchok A, Webb KA, O'Donnell DE. Combined effects of obesity and COPD on dyspnea and exercise tolerance. Am J Respir Crit Care Med. 2009;180:964–71.
20. O'Donnell DE, Deesomchok A, Lam YM, Guenette JA, Amornputtisathaporn N, Forkert L, et al. Effects of body mass index on static lung volumes in patients with airway obstruction. Chest. 2011;140(2):461–8.
21. Naimark A, Cherniack RM. Compliance of the respiratory system and its components in health and obesity. J Appl Physiol. 1960;15:377–82.
22. Lean ME, Han TS, Seidell JC. Impairment of health and quality of life using new US federal guidelines for the identification of obesity. Arch Intern Med. 1999;159(8):837–43.
23. Babb TG, Ranasinghe KG, Comeau LA, Semon TL, Schwartz B. Dyspnea on obese women: association with an increased oxygen cost of breathing. Am J Respir Crit Care Med. 2008;178(2):116–23.
24. Ofir D, Laveneziana P, Webb KA, O'Donnell DE. Ventilatory and perceptual responses to cycle exercise in obese women. J Appl Physiol. 2007;102(6):2217–26.
25. Hughes RL, Katz H, Sahgal V, Campbell JA, Hartz R, Shields TW. Fiber size and energy metabolites in five separate muscles from patients with chronic obstructive lung diseases. Respiration. 1983;44(5):321–8.
26. Ramachandran K, McCusker C, Connors M, Zuwallack R, Lahiri B. The influence of obesity on pulmonary rehabilitation outcomes in patients with COPD. Chron Respir Dis. 2008;5(4):205–9.
27. Bautista J, Ehsan M, Normandin E, Zuwallack R, Lahiri B. Physiologic responses during the six minute walk test in obese and non-obese COPD patients. Respir Med. 2011;105(8):1189–94.
28. Peeters A, Barendregt JJ, Willekens F, Mackenbach JP, Al Mamun A, Bonneux L. Obesity in adulthood and its consequences for life expectancy: a life-table analysis. Ann Intern Med. 2003;138(1):24–32.
29. Whitlock G, Lewington S, Sherliker P, Clarke R, Emberson J, Halsey J, et al. Body-mass index and cause-specific mortality in 900,000 adults: collaborative analyses of 57 prospective studies. Lancet. 2009;373(9669):1083–96.
30. Landbo C, Prescott E, Lange P, Vestbo J, Almdal TP. Prognostic value of nutritional status in chronic obstructive pulmonary disease. Am J Respir Crit Care Med. 1999;160(6):1856–61.
31. Wilson DO, Rogers RM, Wright EC, Anthonisen NR. Body weight in chronic obstructive pulmonary disease. The National Institutes of Health Intermittent Positive-Pressure Breathing Trial. Am Rev Respir Dis. 1989;139(6):1435–8.
32. Schols AM, Slangen J, Volovics L, Wouters EF. Weight loss is a reversible factor in the prognosis of chronic obstructive pulmonary disease. Am J Respir Crit Care Med. 1998;157(6 Pt 1): 1791–7.
33. Chailleux E, Laaban JP, Veale D. Prognostic value of nutritional depletion in patients with COPD treated by long-term oxygen therapy: data from the ANTADIR observatory. Chest. 2003;123(5):1460–6.
34. Kalantar-Zadeh K, Horwich TB, Oreopoulos A, Kovesdy CP, Younessi H, Anker SD, et al. Risk factor paradox in wasting diseases. Curr Opin Clin Nutr Metab Care. 2007;10(4): 433–42.
35. Casanova C, Cote C, de Torres JP, Aguirre-Jaime A, Marin JM, Pinto-Plata V, et al. Inspiratory-to-total lung capacity ratio predicts mortality in patients with chronic obstructive pulmonary disease. Am J Respir Crit Care Med. 2005;171(6):591–7.
36. Watson L, Vonk JM, Lofdahl CG, Pride NB, Pauwels RA, Laitinen LA, et al. Predictors of lung function and its decline in mild to moderate COPD in association with gender: results from the Euroscop study. Respir Med. 2006;100(4):746–53.

37. Schols AM, Broekhuizen R, Weling-Scheepers CA, Wouters EF. Body composition and mortality in chronic obstructive pulmonary disease. Am J Clin Nutr. 2005;82(1):53–9.
38. Mannino DM, Thorn D, Swensen A, Holguin F. Prevalence and outcomes of diabetes, hypertension and cardiovascular disease in COPD. Eur Respir J. 2008;32(4):962–9.
39. Feary JR, Rodrigues LC, Smith CJ, Hubbard RB, Gibson JE. Prevalence of major comorbidities in subjects with COPD and incidence of myocardial infarction and stroke: a comprehensive analysis using data from primary care. Thorax. 2010;65(11):956–62.
40. Alberti KG, Eckel RH, Grundy SM, Zimmet PZ, Cleeman JI, Donato KA, et al. Harmonizing the metabolic syndrome: a joint interim statement of the International Diabetes Federation Task Force on Epidemiology and Prevention; National Heart, Lung, and Blood Institute; American Heart Association; World Heart Federation; International Atherosclerosis Society; and International Association for the Study of Obesity. Circulation. 2009;120(16):1640–5.
41. Huang TT, Ball GD, Franks PW. Metabolic syndrome in youth: current issues and challenges. Appl Physiol Nutr Metab. 2007;32(1):13–22.
42. Fimognari FL, Pasqualetti P, Moro L, Franco A, Piccirillo G, Pastorelli R, et al. The association between metabolic syndrome and restrictive ventilatory dysfunction in older persons. J Gerontol A Biol Sci Med Sci. 2007;62(7):760–5.
43. Leone N, Courbon D, Thomas F, Bean K, Jego B, Leynaert B, et al. Lung function impairment and metabolic syndrome: the critical role of abdominal obesity. Am J Respir Crit Care Med. 2009;179(6):509–16.
44. Marquis K, Maltais F, Duguay V, Bezeau AM, LeBlanc P, Jobin J, et al. The metabolic syndrome in patients with chronic obstructive pulmonary disease. J Cardiopulm Rehabil. 2005;25(4):226–32. discussion 33–4.
45. Watz H, Waschki B, Kirsten A, Muller KC, Kretschmar G, Meyer T, et al. The metabolic syndrome in patients with chronic bronchitis and COPD: frequency and associated consequences for systemic inflammation and physical inactivity. Chest. 2009;136(4):1039–46.
46. Kershaw EE, Flier JS. Adipose tissue as an endocrine organ. J Clin Endocrinol Metab. 2004;89(6):2548–56.
47. Goossens GH. The role of adipose tissue dysfunction in the pathogenesis of obesity-related insulin resistance. Physiol Behav. 2007;94:206–18.
48. Fontana L, Eagon JC, Trujillo ME, Scherer PE, Klein S. Visceral fat adipokine secretion is associated with systemic inflammation in obese humans. Diabetes. 2007;56(4):1010–3.
49. Gan WQ, Man SF, Senthilselvan A, Sin DD. Association between chronic obstructive pulmonary disease and systemic inflammation: a systematic review and a meta-analysis. Thorax. 2004;59(7):574–80.
50. Poulain M, Doucet M, Drapeau V, Fournier G, Tremblay A, Poirier P, et al. Metabolic and inflammatory profile in obese patients with chronic obstructive pulmonary disease. Chron Respir Dis. 2008;5(1):35–41.
51. Yasuda N, Gotoh K, Minatoguchi S, Asano K, Nishigaki K, Nomura M, et al. An increase of soluble Fas, an inhibitor of apoptosis, associated with progression of COPD. Respir Med. 1998;92(8):993–9.
52. Koehler F, Doehner W, Hoernig S, Witt C, Anker SD, John M. Anorexia in chronic obstructive pulmonary disease–association to cachexia and hormonal derangement. Int J Cardiol. 2007;119(1):83–9.
53. Vernooy JH, Kucukaycan M, Jacobs JA, Chavannes NH, Buurman WA, Dentener MA, et al. Local and systemic inflammation in patients with chronic obstructive pulmonary disease: soluble tumor necrosis factor receptors are increased in sputum. Am J Respir Crit Care Med. 2002;166(9):1218–24.
54. Petersen AM, Penkowa M, Iversen M, Frydelund-Larsen L, Andersen JL, Mortensen J, et al. Elevated levels of IL-18 in plasma and skeletal muscle in chronic obstructive pulmonary disease. Lung. 2007;185(3):161–71.
55. Donaldson GC, Seemungal TA, Patel IS, Bhowmik A, Wilkinson TM, Hurst JR, et al. Airway and systemic inflammation and decline in lung function in patients with COPD. Chest. 2005;128(4):1995–2004.

56. Breyer MK, Spruit MA, Celis AP, Rutten EP, Janssen PP, Wouters EF. Highly elevated C-reactive protein levels in obese patients with COPD: a fat chance? Clin Nutr. 2009; 28(6):642–7.
57. Rutten EP, Breyer MK, Spruit MA, Hofstra T, van Melick PP, Schols AM, et al. Abdominal fat mass contributes to the systemic inflammation in chronic obstructive pulmonary disease. Clin Nutr. 2010;29(6):756–60.
58. Skyba P, Ukropec J, Pobeha P, Ukropcova B, Joppa P, Kurdiova T, et al. Metabolic phenotype and adipose tissue inflammation in patients with chronic obstructive pulmonary disease. Mediators Inflamm. 2010;2010:173498.
59. Tkacova R, Ukropec J, Skyba P, Ukropcova B, Pobeha P, Kurdiova T, et al. Increased adipose tissue expression of proinflammatory CD40, MKK4 and JNK in patients with very severe chronic obstructive pulmonary disease. Respiration. 2010;81(5):386–93.

Chapter 9
Obesity, the Metabolic Syndrome, and Pulmonary Hypertension

Anna Ryan Hemnes and Ivan M. Robbins

Abstract Pulmonary hypertension may be caused by many different conditions, classified broadly into five categories by the World Health Organization. The primary determinants of pulmonary vascular pressure are left atrial pressure, pulmonary vascular resistance, and flow through the pulmonary circulation. In this chapter, the effects of obesity on each of these components are considered. Currently, there is ample evidence that obesity and its attendant systemic diseases play a role in increasing left atrial pressure and may affect flow through the pulmonary vasculature. Hypoxia is a potent pulmonary vasoconstrictor, and increased pulmonary vascular resistance is well described in patients with hypoxemia associated with sleep-disordered breathing or obesity hypoventilation. There is also a growing body of literature that fat cytokines such as adiponectin and insulin resistance associated with obesity may contribute to the development of primary pulmonary vascular disease such as pulmonary arterial hypertension. In addition to examining the role obesity may play in pulmonary hypertension etiology, this chapter will review the difficulty obesity poses to accurately diagnosing pulmonary vascular disease and the role of obesity in pulmonary hypertension therapy.

Keywords Pulmonary hypertension • Pulmonary arterial hypertension • Right ventricular dysfunction • Metabolic syndrome • Obesity • Sleep-disordered breathing • Hypoxemia • Obesity hypoventilation • Adipokines • Insulin resistance

A.R. Hemnes, M.D. (✉) • I.M. Robbins, M.D.
Department of Medicine, Vanderbilt University Medical Center,
1161 21st Avenue South MCN, Room T-1218,
Nashville, TN 37232, USA
e-mail: anna.r.hemnes@vanderbilt.edu; Ivan.Robbins@vanderbilt.edu

A.E. Dixon and E.M. Clerisme-Beaty (eds.), *Obesity and Lung Disease: A Guide to Management*, Respiratory Medicine, DOI 10.1007/978-1-62703-053-3_9,

Abbreviations

BMI	Body mass index
BMPR2	Bone morphogenic protein receptor type 2
COPD	Chronic obstructive pulmonary disease
HFPEF	Heart failure with preserved ejection fraction
NHANES	National health and nutrition examination survey
OHS	Obesity hypoventilation syndrome
OSA	Obstructive sleep apnea
PPARγ	Peroxisome proliferator-activated receptor γ
PAH	Pulmonary arterial hypertension
PH	Pulmonary hypertension
PVH	Pulmonary venous hypertension
RHC	Right heart catheterization
WHO	World health organization

Objectives

- Review WHO classification of pulmonary hypertension
- Discuss causes of pulmonary hypertension in obesity
- Review pathophysiology of pulmonary hypertension in obesity
- Discuss evaluation of pulmonary hypertension in obesity
- Discuss treatment of pulmonary hypertension in obesity

Introduction

Pulmonary hypertension is a consequence of a diverse group of conditions affecting the cardiopulmonary system. The main determinants of pulmonary artery pressure are left atrial pressure, flow through the pulmonary vasculature, and resistance of the vascular bed (Fig. 9.1). Alterations in each of these components may result in pulmonary hypertension (PH). For instance, elevation of left atrial pressure with mitral stenosis will result in PH as will high pulmonary vascular flow associated with hyperthyroidism. Careful assessment through detailed evaluation is mandatory for the proper diagnosis and treatment of PH [1, 2].

Pulmonary Hypertension Classification

The World Health Organization (WHO) has broadly categorized conditions that cause PH based on pathology and disease etiology into five groups (Table 9.1). These groups are patients with intrinsic pulmonary arterial disorders in the absence of parenchymal

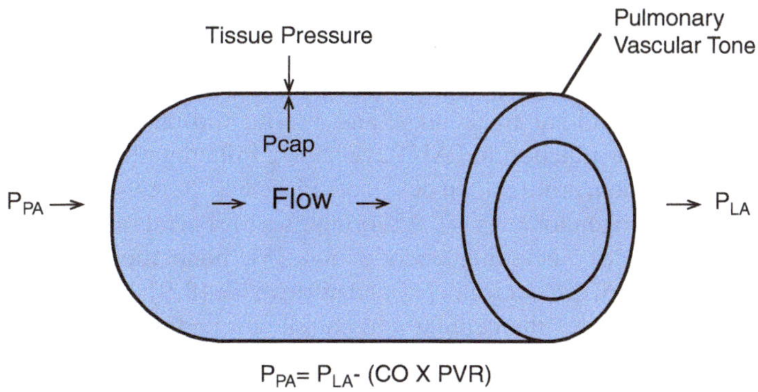

Fig. 9.1 Determinants of pulmonary arterial pressure. P_{PA} = pulmonary arterial pressure, P_{LA} = left atrial pressure, P_{CAP} = hydrostatic pressure in pulmonary capillaries, PVR = pulmonary vascular resistance

Table 9.1 Pulmonary hypertension classification

Group 1 Pulmonary arterial hypertension
Idiopathic
Heritable
Associated with other conditions (e.g., scleroderma, HIV, portopulmonary hypertension)
Congenital left-to-right shunt
Drug- and toxin-induced
Group 1' Pulmonary veno-occlusive disease and/or pulmonary capillary hemangiomatosis
Group 2 Pulmonary hypertension owing to left heart disease
Aortic or mitral valvular disease
Left ventricular systolic failure
Heart failure with preserved ejection fraction
Group 3 Pulmonary hypertension owing to lung disease and/or hypoxia
Advanced parenchymal lung disease
Sleep-disordered breathing
Obesity hypoventilation syndrome
Group 4 Chronic thromboembolic pulmonary hypertension
Group 5 Pulmonary hypertension with unclear or multifactorial mechanisms
Sarcoidosis
Pulmonary Langerhans cell histiocytosis
Hematologic disorders

Adapted from WHO 2008 Dana Point Classification

disease (WHO group 1, pulmonary arterial hypertension (PAH)), left-sided heart disease leading to elevated post-capillary pressure and the subsequent development of PH due passive congestion (WHO group 2, pulmonary venous hypertension (PVH)), hypoxemia or parenchymal lung disease causing destruction and/or vasoconstriction of the vascular bed (WHO group 3), chronic thromboembolic disease (WHO group 3), and PH with unclear or multifactorial mechanisms (WHO group 5).

The bulk of basic science research has focused on PAH, with a great expansion of our understanding of the basic underlying pathogenesis of PAH in the last several decades. Pathologically, PAH is characterized by vascular remodeling including medial hypertrophy, intimal thickening, and in situ thrombosis [3]. Studies of molecular and cellular function in PAH have shown inflammation, endothelial cell damage and dysfunction, proliferation of smooth muscle cells, resistance to apoptosis, and recruitment of progenitor cells [4]. Abnormalities of several important mediators and signaling cascades, including endothelin-1 [5], bone morphogenic protein receptor-2 (BMPR2) [6], prostacyclin [7], and nitric oxide [8, 9], have been identified as contributing to many of the cellular and pathologic findings. Current therapies include prostacyclin derivatives, endothelin receptor antagonists, and phosphodiesterase type 5 inhibitors [10], which have had a small, but significant impact on survival [11]. Detailed description of PAH diagnosis and therapy is outside the scope of this chapter, but can be found elsewhere [1, 12, 13].

The underlying mechanisms for non-WHO group 1 PH are varied and in some cases overlapping. In group 2 patients, left ventricular systolic and increasingly diastolic failure (more recently termed heart failure with preserved ejection fraction (HFPEF)) are frequently associated with passive PH. The elevation in PAP is generally mild. Chronic hypoxia with pulmonary arterial remodeling as well as vascular obliteration contributes to PH associated with parenchymal lung disease in group 3 patients [14, 15]. Aside from surgical endarterectomy for patients with chronic thromboembolic PH (group 4), the treatment of WHO groups 2–5 is, for the most part, aimed at the underlying conditions with the assumption that PH will improve with treatment of the primary disorder.

Patients with obesity and PH do not fall into one WHO group; rather, they have risk factors for PH that are found in groups 2, 3, and 4 and perhaps, group 1, as will be discussed in detail later in this chapter. Alveolar hypoventilation, a subcategory of group 3, is most often associated with obesity but can occur in nonobese patients as well. Likewise, other risk factors for PH such as HFPEF and hypoxia, while seen frequently in patients with obesity, are not uniquely associated with an elevated body mass index (BMI).

Clinically, PH and obesity have been closely linked for decades, if not centuries. One of the central characters in Charles Dickens' "The Pickwick Papers" was Joe, an obese boy described as consuming great quantities of food and constantly sleeping and snoring [16]. In 1956, Burwell and Robin described a poker player who gained weight, snored, and became sleepy during the day. They coined the term "Pickwickian syndrome," now referred to as obesity hypoventilation syndrome (OHS), to describe this constellation of findings associated with obesity and subsequently shown to result from alveolar hypoventilation with hypoxia and CO_2 retention, the latter leading to daytime hypersomnolence. Interestingly, the original patient description included evidence of PH with right heart failure or cor pulmonale. Whether other factors such as HFPEF contributed to this patient's PH is unknown. More recently, there is mounting evidence that obesity-associated metabolic derangements, and the metabolic syndrome more broadly (central obesity, systemic hypertension, insulin resistance, and dyslipidemia [17]), have direct effects on the pulmonary vasculature and may play a role in development of true PAH, WHO group 1 disease [18–21].

In this chapter, we will review the basic science evidence for pulmonary vascular effects of obesity, discuss PH phenotypes associated with obesity, and consider the role of obesity in diagnosis and management of patients with PH.

Mechanisms of Obesity-Related Pulmonary Vascular Disease

An increase in any of the determinants of pulmonary arterial pressure – left atrial pressure, pulmonary blood flow, or pulmonary vascular resistance – will raise pulmonary artery pressure (Fig. 9.1). Obesity, often with concomitant type 2 diabetes mellitus, systemic hypertension, and sleep apnea, is closely associated with PVH (WHO group 2) due to heart failure with reduced ejection fraction as a result of coronary artery disease [22] and, increasingly, due to HFPEF [23–25]. Similarly, obesity can be associated with increased pulmonary blood flow [26] that, in turn, may increase pulmonary arterial pressure. Hypoxia associated with obstructive sleep apnea and obesity hypoventilation is one of the strongest stimuli for pulmonary vasoconstriction and undoubtedly plays a role in the pathophysiology of PH in this syndrome. Finally, there is also growing evidence that the effects of obesity including increased production of fat cytokines, dyslipidemia, insulin resistance, and related oxidative stress have direct effects on the pulmonary vasculature that raise pulmonary vascular resistance, unrelated to the effects of obesity on left atrial pressure or pulmonary blood flow.

Pulmonary Arterial Hypertension

Links Between BMPR2 and Obesity

As mentioned above, the BMPR2 receptor, a member of TGFβ receptor family, is frequently altered in several forms of PAH [27–29], and numerous mutations have been identified in heritable, and to a lesser extent, idiopathic PAH [28, 30]. Interestingly, a downstream target of this signaling pathway is the transcription factor peroxisome proliferator-activator receptor γ (PPARγ), which is closely associated with glucose metabolism and adipogenesis. PPARγ is highly expressed in the lungs and also has been shown to regulate other pathways known to be important in PAH including MCP-1, endothelin-1, and eNOS [31, 32]. Lung tissue from patients with PAH has shown decreased expression of PPARγ and also its downstream effector ApoE [33, 34], which plays an important role in reduction of circulating oxidized lipids. When mice with ApoE deficiency are given a high-fat diet to promote insulin resistance, PH develops and can be reversed when rosiglitazone, a PPARγ agonist, is coadministered to upregulate PPARγ signaling [35]. Additional support for this observation is provided by the demonstration in human smooth muscle cell lines derived from PAH patients [36] that PPARγ stimulation can decrease abnormally

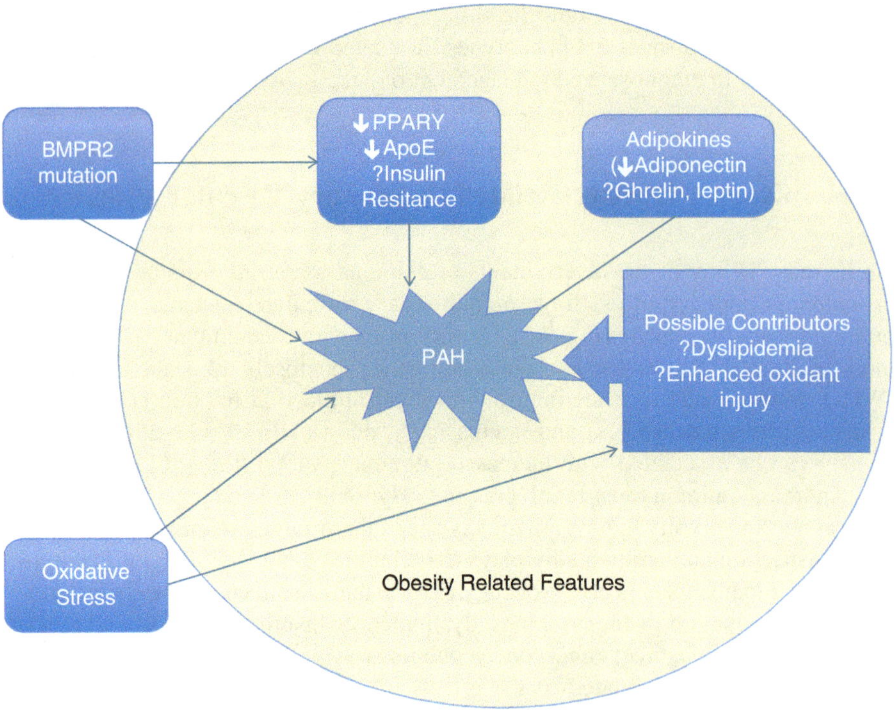

Fig. 9.2 Schematic diagram of interaction of non-obesity-related factors shown to promote PAH (BMPR2 mutation and enhanced oxidant stress) with obesity-related factors that may contribute to or promote PAH. The role of enhanced reactive oxygen species signaling in obesity and dyslipidemia in promotion of pulmonary vascular disease is less well defined

high proliferation rates. Additionally, mice with targeted smooth muscle cell deletion of PPARγ spontaneously develop PH [36]. A schematic of these relationships is demonstrated in Fig. 9.2. Recent data has shown a high prevalence of insulin resistance and glucose intolerance in humans with PAH [18, 21], corroborating the animal data. Thus, PAH-associated BMPR2 dysfunction appears to be linked to insulin resistance in both animal models and human patients.

Adipokines and PAH

A second important feature of obesity is increased generation of adipokines. Adipose cells actively secrete cytokines (so-called adipokines) and play a role not just in the local microenvironment where fat is present but also in the circulating hormonal milieu [37]. Several adipokines have been postulated to have pulmonary vascular-specific effects including adiponectin, ghrelin, and leptin [38–42]. Adiponectin is a particularly attractive mediator of the adipokine effect on PH. The obese adiponectin-deficient mice spontaneously develop mild PH, and adiponectin overexpression can reverse animal models of PH [38, 42]. Similarly, in mice with ApoE deficiency, adiponectin levels were found to be higher in female mice, where lower pulmonary vascular pressures were found [35, 36]. Rosiglitazone therapy in male ApoE-deficient mice reduces adiponectin levels and pulmonary pressure [36]. Adiponectin inhibits PDGF, a potent mitogen for pulmonary artery smooth muscle cells, which serves as a potential mechanistic link for the adverse effects of deficiency of adiponectin on the pulmonary vasculature. In total, these data suggest a protective role for adiponectin in pulmonary vascular disease; however, these animal findings have not been correlated in human disease to date.

Dyslipidemia, Insulin Resistance, and PAH

Dyslipidemia is another potential underlying mechanism linking obesity, metabolic syndrome, and pulmonary vascular disease. Some animal data, however, suggest that the important feature of the metabolic syndrome and obesity on the pulmonary vasculature is insulin resistance rather than dyslipidemia. ApoE-deficient mice fed a high-fat diet developed elevated triglycerides and total cholesterol, and a portion developed PH. However, in these mice, the presence of lipid derangement correlated poorly with the presence of PH, whereas it tracks closely with the presence of insulin resistance [35]. Although there is data suggesting that the HMG CoA reductase inhibitor simvastatin is protective in some rodent models of PH, these effects appear to be mediated through anti-inflammatory statin effects, not lowering of plasma lipid concentrations [43, 44]. Finally, although human PAH patients have been shown to have low HDL cholesterol compared with control patients matched for cardiovascular risk factors and lower levels correlated with worse survival in PAH [45], interventions in PAH using HMG CoA reductase therapy have not been successful [46]. These animal and human data point to a lesser role for dyslipidemia in promotion of pulmonary vascular disease and a greater role for insulin resistance.

Oxidant Injury and PAH

There may be other features of obesity and metabolic syndrome that promote pulmonary vascular disease, in particular, oxidant injury which has been well studied in both PH [47, 48] and obesity. However, it is presently unknown if oxidative stress in PH is exacerbated by obesity [20]. Further studies of these links are warranted.

Human Data Linking PAH and Obesity

Despite these strong animal data, it remains unknown if obesity alone can contribute to the development of PAH. We and others have previously published that obesity is commonly present in PAH patients [19, 21], but a causal role in humans is not established. Recently, Burger and colleagues compared BMI data from a US registry of PAH patients with normative values from the National Health and Nutrition Examination Survey (NHANES) and found that there was no difference in average BMI between PAH patients and the NHANES cohort [49]. However, there were higher percentages of obese patients (BMI>30) in the PAH cohort, suggesting a correlation between the two conditions [49].

Pulmonary Venous Hypertension

Obesity, with or without coronary artery disease from underlying diabetes mellitus and systemic hypertension, is a risk factor for HFPEF which is increasingly identified as a cause of pulmonary venous hypertension (WHO group 2) through elevated left atrial pressure and transmission of this pressure to the pulmonary arteries [23, 24]. We have observed that when two or more features of the metabolic syndrome are present, patients with PH, without evidence of systolic LV dysfunction, are substantially more likely (OR 30.7, CI 3.6–260.0) to have PVH than PAH after a thorough evaluation [19]. These same risk factors can also contribute to systolic left ventricular failure and subsequent pulmonary venous hypertension. In addition, either type of left ventricular dysfunction can be associated with a reactive component of PH and the development of markedly elevated PAP [19, 50].

Obesity Hypoventilation Syndrome (OHS)

OHS is a type of alveolar hypoventilation and is well described in the literature [51]. The pathogenesis of this syndrome (explored in depth in Chap. 6) underlies several of the mechanisms responsible for the development of PH associated with obesity. Hypercapnia and hypoxia are hallmarks of OHS, and both can contribute directly to PH through vasoconstriction of the pulmonary vasculature.

Hypercapnia

Numerous studies, dating back over 50 years, have demonstrated that acute hypercapnia in normal subjects causes pulmonary vasoconstriction with increases in pulmonary artery pressure and pulmonary vascular resistance [52–54]. Whether elevated levels of CO_2 or the acidosis that accompanies acute hypercapnia is the main factor responsible for vasoconstriction is unclear. Administration of bicarbonate to increase pH in studies of normal subjects exposed to elevated CO_2 as well as patients with chronic lung disease and chronic hypercapnia reported both improvement and worsening of PH in different patients [52]. In addition, patients with OHS develop a compensatory metabolic alkalosis so that their acidosis in general is mild. One study did find a correlation with chronic hypercapnia and PH in a small group of patients [54]. However, just how much chronic hypercapnia contributes to sustained pulmonary vasoconstriction and PH is not known.

Hypoxia

Hypoxia is one of the most potent stimulus for pulmonary vasoconstriction and was first described by von Euler and Liljestrand in 1946 [55]. It plays an important role in the development of PH in diverse lung diseases including emphysema and interstitial lung disease [56]. In obese patients, excess weight increases the respiratory system load and the work of breathing (up to three times control) [57] and is associated with respiratory muscle weakness [58] with a resultant decrease in expiratory reserve volume and maximum voluntary ventilation, ventilation-perfusion mismatching, and hypoxia [59–62]. In addition, as the term implies, patients with OHS have a depressed ventilatory drive contributing to both hypercapnia and hypoxia [63]. Interestingly, at least in animal models, hypercapnia may mitigate the vasoconstrictive effects of hypoxia, muddling somewhat the role of hypoxia in the development of PH in obese patients [64]. This is supported by the fact that not all patients with OHS develop PH. Other factors undoubtedly contribute to PH including sleep apnea, left heart dysfunction, and the metabolic syndrome.

Sleep-Disordered Breathing

Obesity is strongly associated with sleep-disordered breathing (SDB) [65], another subcategory of group 3 PH. However, studies on the role of obesity in the development of PH from sleep-disordered are conflicting. In addition, in the absence of parenchymal lung disease, most often chronic obstructive pulmonary disease (COPD), PH seen in SDB is generally mild (mPAP of 20–30 mmHg) [66]. Two studies have reported an elevated BMI in patients with obstructive sleep apnea (OSA) who develop PH compared to those that did not develop PH, and one of these studies demonstrated a significant correlation of PAP with BMI, Fig. 9.3. However, in the larger of the two studies involving 220 consecutive patients diagnosed with OSA, higher BMI fell out as a factor for the development of PH in multiple regression analysis [67, 68]. Conversely, three studies examining PH in OSA [69–71] and one evaluating RV function in OSA found no correlation with BMI [72]. Confounding several of these studies is the inclusion of patients with COPD [68, 69], the strong association of PH with PVH [70], or the inability to exclude PVH as a cause of PH due to lack of direct hemodynamic measurements [72] or no measurement of pulmonary wedge pressure [69]. Further, PH was defined as a mean pulmonary artery pressure of >20 mmHg which would be considered normal in the WHO classification of PH. Few, if any, patients had PH of >25 mmHg in the absence of daytime hypoxia.

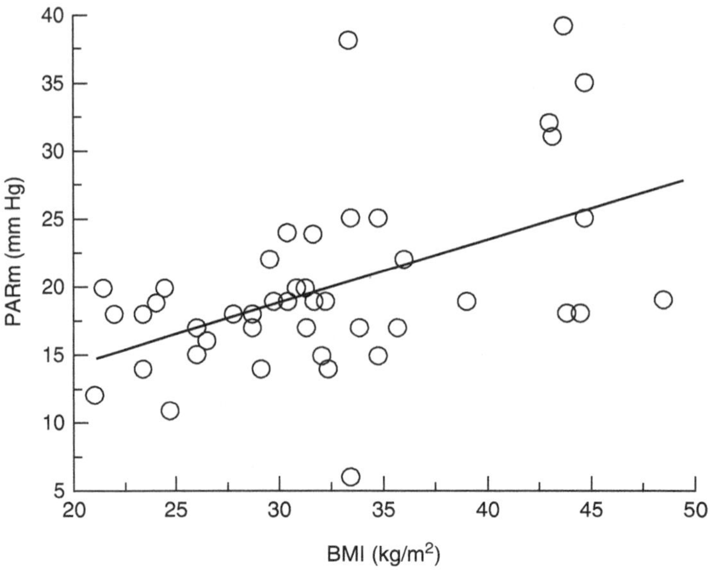

Fig. 9.3 Correlation between mean pulmonary artery pressure and body mass index. $r=0.50$, $p=0.0006$, PAPm = mean pulmonary artery pressure, BMI = body mass index (Reprinted with permission from Bady et al. [91])

Patients with OHS appear to have a higher risk for OSA and for the development of PH associated with OSA than patients with obesity alone. Studies have shown a prevalence of OHS between 10% and 20% in obese patients with OSA and increases with higher BMI [51]. Between 74% and 88% of OHS patients have been reported to have OSA [73, 74]. In one study, PH was found significantly more often in patients with OHS than without, 58% versus 9%, respectively, although it was for the most part mild with a mPAP of 23 ± 10 mmHg [74]. The OHS patients were also morbidly obese with a BMI of 40 ± 8 kg/m^2. They had mild restriction on pulmonary function testing; significantly greater desaturation at night and at baseline, not only compared to OSA patients but a group of OSA patients with COPD as well; and, by definition, a higher $PaCO_2$ compared to the other two groups.

These studies raise the issue of the degree of obesity in terms of a risk factor for PH. The variation in BMI in different studies is substantial, and it may be that mild obesity is much less of a risk factor for PH than morbid obesity. However, this has not been well evaluated. Overall, it appears that obesity, particularly morbid obesity and OHS, in conjunction with OSA, is a risk factor for the development of at least mild PH. However, the studies are difficult to interpret, and other factors such as the metabolic syndrome or HFPEF likely contribute to the development of PH. This is an area that requires significantly more study.

Implications of Obesity for the Diagnosis and Management of Pulmonary Hypertension

Diagnostic Considerations

PH frequently has a nonspecific presentation including insidious onset of dyspnea, symptoms and signs of right heart failure, and, in advanced disease, exertional chest pain and syncope. There are several published guidelines for the evaluation of suspected PH [1, 2]. Many features of this diagnostic evaluation are affected by obesity.

Often, the first diagnostic test in the evaluation of PH is a transthoracic echocardiogram. There are many limitations to this study posed by obesity including difficulty with viewing the right ventricle through subcutaneous fat, challenges with proper windowing of tricuspid regurgitation to determine right ventricular systolic pressure, and increased intravascular volume that can make Doppler-derived indices of ventricular filling less accurate [26, 75–77].

A major obstacle that obesity presents to diagnostic evaluation of PH are the weight limits to testing apparatus, e.g., weight limits to the table for ventilation-perfusion scan, computed tomography scan, pulmonary angiography, and right heart catheterization. This is of particular concern in the evaluation of possible chronic thromboembolic PH, an important diagnosis to make as this is a potentially curative as opposed to other forms of PH. Although obesity is known to be a risk factor for acute thromboembolic disease [78], analysis of risk factors for chronic thromboembolic PH has not shown that obesity plays a role in development of this complication [79].

Although PVH is the most likely etiology of PH in obesity patients, PAH is not infrequently diagnosed. Therapy for PAH is markedly different from management of group 2 or 3 disease, and PAH-specific therapy is not known to be less efficacious than in the nonobese patients. Therefore, a diagnosis should be pursued when clinically appropriate. In patients with a high index of suspicion for PAH after noninvasive testing or in whom there is an unclear diagnosis, right heart catheterization (RHC) is indicated. RHC is mandatory for definitive diagnosis of PH and in differentiating PAH from PVH. In addition, in patients diagnosed with PAH, RHC allows for determination of vasoreactivity by administration of a short-acting pulmonary vasodilator such as nitric oxide as well as poor prognostic features such as elevated right atrial pressure or low cardiac index to aid in determination of therapeutic recommendations [80].

Obesity may complicate several aspects of right heart catheterization, including challenges with intravenous access and weight limitations of the procedure table, but the major complication obesity presents is the determination of an accurate surrogate for left atrial pressure. A central feature of understanding pulmonary vascular pathophysiology is knowledge of left atrial pressure. Pulmonary artery occlusion pressure is the most commonly used surrogate for left atrial pressure, but left ventricular end-diastolic pressure may be used in the absence of mitral stenosis and in our experience is less affected by respiratory variation in obese individuals.

In markedly obese patients, major respiratory effects on pulmonary artery occlusion pressure tracings, due to large changes in pleural pressure with breathing, are common, and it may be difficult to discern the proper location to determine the occlusion pressure. Given that there may be a discrepancy between pulmonary artery occlusion pressure and left ventricular end-diastolic pressure when the two are simultaneously measured [81], we often recommend that severely obese patients have measurement of left ventricular end-diastolic pressure if possible to ensure correct diagnosis.

In some patients with morbid obesity, weight may preclude several aspects of diagnostic testing including ventilation-perfusion scanning, good quality echocardiography, and right heart catheterization. In general, these patients have such severe exercise limitations related to their obesity that therapy for PAH is unlikely to be helpful in the absence of weight loss. We do not recommend empiric therapy aimed at PAH (e.g., phosphodiesterase five inhibitors, endothelin receptor antagonists, or prostaglandins) for such individuals; rather, we advise nutritional consultation, weight loss, cardiac rehabilitation, and reassessment if their weight drops to such a point where they may undergo diagnostic testing. In patients with repeated thromboembolic events, lifelong anticoagulation would be warranted in any case, so this therapy may be recommended.

Disease-Specific Recommendations

When PVH is diagnosed, therapy is aimed at the cause of left atrial hypertension, as shown in Fig. 9.1, and reduction in left atrial pressure will concomitantly lower pulmonary artery pressure. Weight loss is likely to be beneficial in management of both systolic and non-systolic heart failure. Discussion of the mechanisms is outside the scope of this chapter.

Treatment Aimed Directly at PAH

Therapeutic response to PAH-specific medications is not known to be dependent on weight. Thus, standard treatment algorithms can be followed [1, 2]. If patients have an acute response to vasodilators administered during right heart catheterization, they should be treated with calcium channel blockers [82]. This finding is rare, however, and most patients will be treated with either oral medications, such as an endothelin receptor antagonist or a phosphodiesterase inhibitor, or a non-enteral prostaglandin dependent on disease severity and patient characteristics. There are no contraindications to any of these therapies based on weight; however, occasionally prostaglandin infusion therapy may be difficult in the severely obese. Prostaglandins may be administered by intermittent inhalations or by continuous intravenous or subcutaneous infusion. Inhalational therapy is not complicated by weight, but occasionally morbidly obese individuals will have difficulty with maintenance of intravenous lines. Nonetheless, we have recommended and continue to use continuous infusion prostaglandin therapy in obese as well as nonobese patients.

Treatment Aimed at Weight Loss

A critical management recommendation in obese patients with PAH is weight loss. Patients have limited ability to augment cardiac output during exercise due to pulmonary vascular limitations; therefore, lower body mass may allow less requirement for blood flow and increase exercise capacity even without substantial improvement in PAH. Cardiopulmonary rehabilitation has been shown to improve 6-min walk distance in PAH [83], and we routinely recommend this therapy to all of our patients, regardless of weight. Improved exercise may aid in augmentation of weight loss, additionally. As insulin resistance and occult diabetes are common in PAH regardless of body mass [18, 21], routine screening for prediabetes and diabetes is indicated. PAH substantially increases surgical risk with anything more than minor procedures; thus, bariatric surgery is not currently recommended for obese patients with PAH even with the knowledge that adipokines, insulin resistance, and possibly dyslipidemia may play a role in promotion of pulmonary vascular injury. There has been a single report of dramatic improvement in a patient with PAH after bariatric surgery [84], but further study is warranted before this procedure can even be considered safe in patients with PAH.

Treatment of OSA

Mainstays of treatment of OHS and OSA are weight loss, positive airway pressure (PAP) therapy, and supplemental oxygen. Improvement in pulmonary function tests has been shown following weight loss with a significant improvement in forced expiratory volume in 1 s and forced vital capacity [85, 86], patients with the highest BMI demonstrating the greatest percent improvement [85]. Other studies have shown improvement in lung volumes [86, 87] and respiratory muscle strength [87]. Positive airway pressure therapy improves PH in patients with OSA, but this was measured by echocardiography only, and both the PH and the improvement were mild [88, 89]. Whether improvement in OSA or improvement in other factors such as HFPEF accounts for the change is uncertain. Supplemental oxygen has been shown in numerous studies in a variety of respiratory disorders to improve PH and should be prescribed for patients with OHS or OSA who exhibit desaturation. Medroxyprogesterone, a respiratory stimulant, has been used in OHS, but there are not large controlled trials, and there may be no improvement or even worsening of dyspnea in patients who cannot normalize their PCO_2 with voluntary ventilation [51]. Finally, tracheostomy may be helpful in patients with OHS who are intolerant of or do not improve with positive airway pressure [51].

Assessment of Treatment

In PAH, it may be very difficult to determine response to therapy in patients who have a major exercise limitation related to their weight. Six-minute walk test and

New York Heart Association functional class are the most readily available determinants of response to therapy; however, these tests may be heavily influenced by weight. The 6-min walk test is affected by body mass index [90], and percent predicted values may be more useful for patients with a BMI of 35 kg/m^2 or greater. Functional class may be heavily influenced by weight-related activity limitations, and thus it is difficult to discern if therapy has improved symptoms. In such cases, greater reliance on echocardiography or even invasive hemodynamics may be warranted.

Conclusions

There is long-standing data on the role of hypoxia and hypercapnia related to OHS and SDB in obesity, but now there is also mounting evidence that obesity and related adipokines, insulin resistance, and dyslipidemia may contribute to development of PAH as well. With rising rates of obesity, these findings and their implications for human pulmonary vascular disease are of major importance. Further studies of the risk of PAH with obesity, the role of bariatric surgery in alteration of pulmonary vascular disease, and the complex interaction of hypercarbia and hypoxia on pulmonary vascular disease development will enhance our ability to treat, and perhaps prevent, PH in obese patients.

References

1. Badesch DB, Champion HC, Sanchez MA, Hoeper MM, Loyd JE, Manes A, et al. Diagnosis and assessment of pulmonary arterial hypertension. J Am Coll Cardiol. 2009;54(1 Suppl): S55–66.
2. McLaughlin VV, Archer SL, Badesch DB, Barst RJ, Farber HW, Lindner JR, et al. ACCF/AHA 2009 expert consensus document on pulmonary hypertension a report of the American College of Cardiology Foundation Task Force on Expert Consensus Documents and the American Heart Association developed in collaboration with the American College of Chest Physicians; American Thoracic Society, Inc.; and the Pulmonary Hypertension Association. J Am Coll Cardiol. 2009;53(17):1573–619.
3. Tuder RM, Marecki JC, Richter A, Fijalkowska I, Flores S. Pathology of pulmonary hypertension. Clin Chest Med. 2007;28(1):23–42. vii.
4. Morrell NW, Adnot S, Archer SL, Dupuis J, Jones PL, MacLean MR, et al. Cellular and molecular basis of pulmonary arterial hypertension. J Am Coll Cardiol. 2009;54(1 Suppl):S20–31.
5. Giaid A, Saleh D, Yanagisawa M, Forbes RD. Endothelin-1 immunoreactivity and mRNA in the transplanted human heart. Transplantation. 1995;59(9):1308–13.
6. Newman JH, Wheeler L, Lane KB, Loyd E, Gaddipati R, Phillips 3rd JA, et al. Mutation in the gene for bone morphogenetic protein receptor II as a cause of primary pulmonary hypertension in a large kindred. N Engl J Med. 2001;345(5):319–24.
7. Christman BW, McPherson CD, Newman JH, King GA, Bernard GR, Groves BM, et al. An imbalance between the excretion of thromboxane and prostacyclin metabolites in pulmonary hypertension. N Engl J Med. 1992;327(2):70–5.
8. Champion HC, Bivalacqua TJ, D'Souza FM, Ortiz LA, Jeter JR, Toyoda K, et al. Gene transfer of endothelial nitric oxide synthase to the lung of the mouse in vivo. Effect on agonist-induced and flow-mediated vascular responses. Circ Res. 1999;84(12):1422–32.

9. Sitbon O, Brenot F, Denjean A, Bergeron A, Parent F, Azarian R, et al. Inhaled nitric oxide as a screening vasodilator agent in primary pulmonary hypertension. A dose-response study and comparison with prostacyclin. Am J Respir Crit Care Med. 1995;151(2 Pt 1):384–9.
10. Barst RJ, Gibbs JS, Ghofrani HA, Hoeper MM, McLaughlin VV, Rubin LJ, et al. Updated evidence-based treatment algorithm in pulmonary arterial hypertension. J Am Coll Cardiol. 2009;54(1 Suppl):S78–84.
11. Humbert M, Sitbon O, Chaouat A, Bertocchi M, Habib G, Gressin V, et al. Survival in patients with idiopathic, familial, and anorexigen-associated pulmonary arterial hypertension in the modern management era. Circulation. 2010;122(2):156–63.
12. Simonneau G, Robbins IM, Beghetti M, Channick RN, Delcroix M, Denton CP, et al. Updated clinical classification of pulmonary hypertension. J Am Coll Cardiol. 2009;54(1 Suppl):S43–54.
13. McLaughlin VV, Shillington A, Rich S. Survival in primary pulmonary hypertension: the impact of epoprostenol therapy. Circulation. 2002;106(12):1477–82.
14. Hemnes AR, Zaiman A, Champion HC. PDE5A inhibition attenuates bleomycin-induced pulmonary fibrosis and pulmonary hypertension through inhibition of ROS Generation and RhoA/Rho kinase Activation. Am J Physiol Lung Cell Mol Physiol. 2008;294(1):L24–33.
15. Nadrous HF, Pellikka PA, Krowka MJ, Swanson KL, Chaowalit N, Decker PA, et al. Pulmonary hypertension in patients with idiopathic pulmonary fibrosis. Chest. 2005;128(4):2393–9.
16. Dickens C. The Pickwick papers. London: Chapman and Hall; 1837.
17. Alberti KG, Eckel RH, Grundy SM, Zimmet PZ, Cleeman JI, Donato KA, et al. Harmonizing the metabolic syndrome: a joint interim statement of the international diabetes federation task force on epidemiology and prevention; National heart, lung, and blood institute; American heart association; World heart federation; International atherosclerosis society; and International association for the study of obesity. Circulation. 2009;120(16):1640–5.
18. Zamanian RT, Hansmann G, Snook S, Lilienfeld D, Rappaport KM, Reaven GM, et al. Insulin resistance in pulmonary arterial hypertension. Eur Respir J. 2009;33(2):318–24.
19. Robbins IM, Newman JH, Johnson RF, Hemnes AR, Fremont RD, Piana RN, et al. Association of the metabolic syndrome with pulmonary venous hypertension. Chest. 2009;136(1):31–6.
20. Pugh ME, Hemnes AR. Metabolic and hormonal derangements in pulmonary hypertension: from mouse to man. Int J Clin Pract Suppl. 2010;64(168):5–13.
21. Pugh ME, Robbins IM, Rice TW, West J, Newman JH, Hemnes AR. Unrecognized glucose intolerance is common in pulmonary arterial hypertension. J Heart Lung Transplant. 2011;30(8):904–11.
22. Guglin M, Khan H. Pulmonary hypertension in heart failure. J Card Fail. 2010;16(6):461–74.
23. McMurray JJ, Carson PE, Komajda M, McKelvie R, Zile MR, Ptaszynska A, et al. Heart failure with preserved ejection fraction: clinical characteristics of 4133 patients enrolled in the I-PRESERVE trial. Eur J Heart Fail. 2008;10(2):149–56.
24. Borlaug BA, Paulus WJ. Heart failure with preserved ejection fraction: pathophysiology, diagnosis, and treatment. Eur Heart J. 2011;32(6):670–9.
25. Thenappan T, Shah SJ, Gomberg-Maitland M, Collander B, Vallakati A, Shroff P, et al. Clinical characteristics of pulmonary hypertension in patients with heart failure and preserved ejection fraction. Circ Heart Fail. 2011;4(3):257–65.
26. Poirier P, Giles TD, Bray GA, Hong Y, Stern JS, Pi-Sunyer FX, et al. Obesity and cardiovascular disease: pathophysiology, evaluation, and effect of weight loss: an update of the 1997 American Heart Association Scientific Statement on Obesity and Heart Disease from the Obesity Committee of the Council on Nutrition, Physical Activity, and Metabolism. Circulation. 2006; 113(6):898–918.
27. Hamid R, Cogan JD, Hedges LK, Austin E, Phillips 3rd JA, Newman JH, et al. Penetrance of pulmonary arterial hypertension is modulated by the expression of normal BMPR2 allele. Hum Mutat. 2009;30(4):649–54.
28. Machado RD, Pauciulo MW, Thomson JR, Lane KB, Morgan NV, Wheeler L, et al. BMPR2 haploinsufficiency as the inherited molecular mechanism for primary pulmonary hypertension. Am J Hum Genet. 2001;68(1):92–102.
29. Du L, Sullivan CC, Chu D, Cho AJ, Kido M, Wolf PL, et al. Signaling molecules in nonfamilial pulmonary hypertension. N Engl J Med. 2003;348(6):500–9.

30. Lane KB, Machado RD, Pauciulo MW, Thomson JR, Phillips 3rd JA, Loyd JE, et al. Heterozygous germline mutations in BMPR2, encoding a TGF-beta receptor, cause familial primary pulmonary hypertension. The International PPH Consortium. Nat Genet. 2000;26(1):81–4.
31. Itoh T, Nagaya N, Ishibashi-Ueda H, Kyotani S, Oya H, Sakamaki F, et al. Increased plasma monocyte chemoattractant protein-1 level in idiopathic pulmonary arterial hypertension. Respirology. 2006;11(2):158–63.
32. Farber HW, Loscalzo J. Pulmonary arterial hypertension. N Engl J Med. 2004;351(16):1655–65.
33. Ameshima S, Golpon H, Cool CD, Chan D, Vandivier RW, Gardai SJ, et al. Peroxisome proliferator-activated receptor gamma (PPARgamma) expression is decreased in pulmonary hypertension and affects endothelial cell growth. Circ Res. 2003;92(10):1162–9.
34. Geraci MW, Moore M, Gesell T, Yeager ME, Alger L, Golpon H, et al. Gene expression patterns in the lungs of patients with primary pulmonary hypertension: a gene microarray analysis. Circ Res. 2001;88(6):555–62.
35. Hansmann G, Wagner RA, Schellong S, Perez VA, Urashima T, Wang L, et al. Pulmonary arterial hypertension is linked to insulin resistance and reversed by peroxisome proliferator-activated receptor-gamma activation. Circulation. 2007;115(10):1275–84.
36. Hansmann G, de Jesus Perez VA, Alastalo TP, Alvira CM, Guignabert C, Bekker JM, et al. An antiproliferative BMP-2/PPARgamma/apoE axis in human and murine SMCs and its role in pulmonary hypertension. J Clin Invest. 2008;118(5):1846–57.
37. Trayhurn P, Bing C, Wood IS. Adipose tissue and adipokines – energy regulation from the human perspective. J Nutr. 2006;136(7 Suppl):1935S–9.
38. Summer R, Fiack CA, Ikeda Y, Sato K, Dwyer D, Ouchi N, et al. Adiponectin deficiency: a model of pulmonary hypertension associated with pulmonary vascular disease. Am J Physiol Lung Cell Mol Physiol. 2009;297(3):L432–8.
39. Hansmann G, Rabinovitch M. The protective role of adiponectin in pulmonary vascular disease. Am J Physiol Lung Cell Mol Physiol. 2010;298(1):L1–2.
40. Maruna P, Lindner J, Kubzova KM. Leptin and soluble leptin receptor changes after pulmonary endarterectomy: relations to cortisol and cytokine network. Physiol Res. 2009;58(4):569–76.
41. Medoff BD, Okamoto Y, Leyton P, Weng M, Sandall BP, Raher MJ, et al. Adiponectin deficiency increases allergic airway inflammation and pulmonary vascular remodeling. Am J Respir Cell Mol Biol. 2009;41(4):397–406.
42. Weng M, Raher MJ, Leyton P, Combs TP, Scherer PE, Bloch KD, et al. Adiponectin decreases pulmonary arterial remodeling in mouse models of pulmonary hypertension. Am J Respir Cell Mol Biol. 2010;45:340–7.
43. Girgis RE, Li D, Zhan X, Garcia JG, Tuder RM, Hassoun PM, et al. Attenuation of chronic hypoxic pulmonary hypertension by simvastatin. Am J Physiol Heart Circ Physiol. 2003;285(3):H938–45.
44. Girgis RE, Mozammel S, Champion HC, Li D, Peng X, Shimoda L, et al. Regression of chronic hypoxic pulmonary hypertension by simvastatin. Am J Physiol Lung Cell Mol Physiol. 2007;292(5):L1105–10.
45. Heresi GA, Aytekin M, Newman J, Didonato J, Dweik RA. Plasma levels of high-density lipoprotein cholesterol and outcomes in pulmonary arterial hypertension. Am J Respir Crit Care Med. 2010;182(5):661–8.
46. Kawut SM, Bagiella E, Lederer DJ, Shimbo D, Horn EM, Roberts KE, et al. Randomized clinical trial of aspirin and simvastatin for pulmonary arterial hypertension: ASA-STAT. Circulation. 2011;123(25):2985–93.
47. Robbins IM, Morrow JD, Christman BW. Oxidant stress but not thromboxane decreases with epoprostenol therapy. Free Radic Biol Med. 2005;38(5):568–74.
48. Nozik-Grayck E, Suliman HB, Majka S, Albietz J, Van Rheen Z, Roush K, et al. Lung EC-SOD overexpression attenuates hypoxic induction of Egr-1 and chronic hypoxic pulmonary vascular remodeling. Am J Physiol Lung Cell Mol Physiol. 2008;295(3):L422–30.

49. Burger CD, Foreman AJ, Miller DP, Safford RE, McGoon MD, Badesch DB. Comparison of body habitus in patients with pulmonary arterial hypertension enrolled in the registry to evaluate early and long-term PAH disease management with normative values from the national health and nutrition examination survey. Mayo Clin Proc. 2011;86(2):105–12.
50. Butler J, Chomsky DB, Wilson JR. Pulmonary hypertension and exercise intolerance in patients with heart failure. J Am Coll Cardiol. 1999;34(6):1802–6.
51. Mokhlesi B. Obesity hypoventilation syndrome: a state-of-the-art review. Respir Care. 2010;55(10):1347–62.
52. Kilburn KH, Asmundsson T, Britt RC, Cardon R. Effects of breathing 10 per cent carbon dioxide on the pulmonary circulation of human subjects. Circulation. 1969;39(5):639–53.
53. Fishman AP, Fritts Jr HW, Cournand A. Effects of breathing carbon dioxide upon the pulmonary circulation. Circulation. 1960;22:220–5.
54. Krieger J, Sforza E, Apprill M, Lampert E, Weitzenblum E, Ratomaharo J. Pulmonary hypertension, hypoxemia, and hypercapnia in obstructive sleep apnea patients. Chest. 1989;96(4):729–37.
55. Von Euler UaLG. Observations on the pulmonary artery pressure in the cat. Acta Physiol Scand. 1946;12:301–20.
56. Ghofrani HA, Voswinckel R, Reichenberger F, Weissmann N, Schermuly RT, Seeger W, et al. Hypoxia- and non-hypoxia-related pulmonary hypertension – established and new therapies. Cardiovasc Res. 2006;72(1):30–40.
57. Sharp JT, Henry JP, Sweany SK, Meadows WR, Pietras RJ. The total work of breathing in normal and obese men. J Clin Invest. 1964;43:728–39.
58. Kelly TM, Jensen RL, Elliott CG, Crapo RO. Maximum respiratory pressures in morbidly obese subjects. Respiration. 1988;54(2):73–7.
59. Holley HS, Milic-Emili J, Becklake MR, Bates DV. Regional distribution of pulmonary ventilation and perfusion in obesity. J Clin Invest. 1967;46(4):475–81.
60. Barrera F, Reidenberg MM, Winters WL, Hungspreugs S. Ventilation-perfusion relationships in the obese patient. J Appl Physiol. 1969;26(4):420–6.
61. Vaughan RW, Cork RC, Hollander D. The effect of massive weight loss on arterial oxygenation and pulmonary function tests. Anesthesiology. 1981;54(4):325–8.
62. Ladosky W, Botelho MA, Albuquerque Jr JP. Chest mechanics in morbidly obese non-hypoventilated patients. Respir Med. 2001;95(4):281–6.
63. Leech J, Onal E, Aronson R, Lopata M. Voluntary hyperventilation in obesity hypoventilation. Chest. 1991;100(5):1334–8.
64. Zwillich CW, Sutton FD, Pierson DJ, Greagh EM, Weil JV. Decreased hypoxic ventilatory drive in the obesity-hypoventilation syndrome. Am J Med. 1975;59(3):343–8.
65. Young T, Palta M, Dempsey J, Skatrud J, Weber S, Badr S. The occurrence of sleep-disordered breathing among middle-aged adults. N Engl J Med. 1993;328(17):1230–5.
66. Sajkov D, McEvoy RD. Obstructive sleep apnea and pulmonary hypertension. Prog Cardiovasc Dis. 2009;51(5):363–70.
67. Bady E, Achkar A, Pascal S, Orvoen-Frija E, Laaban JP. Pulmonary arterial hypertension in patients with sleep apnoea syndrome. Thorax. 2000;55(11):934–9.
68. Chaouat A, Weitzenblum E, Krieger J, Oswald M, Kessler R. Pulmonary hemodynamics in the obstructive sleep apnea syndrome. Results in 220 consecutive patients. Chest. 1996; 109(2):380–6.
69. Laks L, Lehrhaft B, Grunstein RR, Sullivan CE. Pulmonary hypertension in obstructive sleep apnoea. Eur Respir J. 1995;8(4):537–41.
70. Sanner BM, Doberauer C, Konermann M, Sturm A, Zidek W. Pulmonary hypertension in patients with obstructive sleep apnea syndrome. Arch Intern Med. 1997;157(21):2483–7.
71. Sajkov D, Wang T, Saunders NA, Bune AJ, Neill AM, Douglas MR. Daytime pulmonary hemodynamics in patients with obstructive sleep apnea without lung disease. Am J Respir Crit Care Med. 1999;159(5 Pt 1):1518–26.

72. Sanner BM, Konermann M, Sturm A, Muller HJ, Zidek W. Right ventricular dysfunction in patients with obstructive sleep apnoea syndrome. Eur Respir J. 1997;10(9):2079–83.
73. Sugerman HJ, Fairman RP, Sood RK, Engle K, Wolfe L, Kellum JM. Long-term effects of gastric surgery for treating respiratory insufficiency of obesity. Am J Clin Nutr. 1992;55 (2 Suppl):597S–601.
74. Kessler R, Chaouat A, Schinkewitch P, Faller M, Casel S, Krieger J, et al. The obesity-hypoventilation syndrome revisited: a prospective study of 34 consecutive cases. Chest. 2001; 120(2):369–76.
75. de Simone G, Daniels SR, Devereux RB, Meyer RA, Roman MJ, de Divitiis O, et al. Left ventricular mass and body size in normotensive children and adults: assessment of allometric relations and impact of overweight. J Am Coll Cardiol. 1992;20(5):1251–60.
76. Lauer MS, Anderson KM, Larson MG, Levy D. A new method for indexing left ventricular mass for differences in body size. Am J Cardiol. 1994;74(5):487–91.
77. Poirier P, Giles TD, Bray GA, Hong Y, Stern JS, Pi-Sunyer FX, et al. Obesity and cardiovascular disease: pathophysiology, evaluation, and effect of weight loss. Arterioscler Thromb Vasc Biol. 2006;26(5):968–76.
78. Tapson VF. Acute pulmonary embolism. N Engl J Med. 2008;358(10):1037–52.
79. Bonderman D, Wilkens H, Wakounig S, Schafers HJ, Jansa P, Lindner J, et al. Risk factors for chronic thromboembolic pulmonary hypertension. Eur Respir J. 2009;33(2):325–31.
80. Hemnes AR, Forfia PR, Champion HC. Assessment of pulmonary vasculature and right heart by invasive haemodynamics and echocardiography. Int J Clin Pract Suppl. 2009;162:4–19.
81. Halpern SD, Taichman DB. Misclassification of pulmonary hypertension due to reliance on pulmonary capillary wedge pressure rather than left ventricular end-diastolic pressure. Chest. 2009;136(1):37–43.
82. Sitbon O, Humbert M, Jais X, Ioos V, Hamid AM, Provencher S, et al. Long-term response to calcium channel blockers in idiopathic pulmonary arterial hypertension. Circulation. 2005;111(23):3105–11.
83. Mereles D, Ehlken N, Kreuscher S, Ghofrani S, Hoeper MM, Halank M, et al. Exercise and respiratory training improve exercise capacity and quality of life in patients with severe chronic pulmonary hypertension. Circulation. 2006;114(14):1482–9.
84. Mathier MA, Zhang J, Ramanathan RC. Dramatic functional improvement following bariatric surgery in a patient with pulmonary arterial hypertension and morbid obesity. Chest. 2008;133(3):789–92.
85. Santana AN, Souza R, Martins AP, Macedo F, Rascovski A, Salge JM. The effect of massive weight loss on pulmonary function of morbid obese patients. Respir Med. 2006;100(6): 1100–4.
86. Ray CS, Sue DY, Bray G, Hansen JE, Wasserman K. Effects of obesity on respiratory function. Am Rev Respir Dis. 1983;128(3):501–6.
87. Weiner P, Waizman J, Weiner M, Rabner M, Magadle R, Zamir D. Influence of excessive weight loss after gastroplasty for morbid obesity on respiratory muscle performance. Thorax. 1998;53(1):39–42.
88. Sajkov D, Wang T, Saunders NA, Bune AJ, McEvoy RD. Continuous positive airway pressure treatment improves pulmonary hemodynamics in patients with obstructive sleep apnea. Am J Respir Crit Care Med. 2002;165(2):152–8.
89. Arias MA, Garcia-Rio F, Alonso-Fernandez A, Martinez I, Villamor J. Pulmonary hypertension in obstructive sleep apnoea: effects of continuous positive airway pressure: a randomized, controlled cross-over study. Eur Heart J. 2006;27(9):1106–13.
90. Enright PL, Sherrill DL. Reference equations for the six-minute walk in healthy adults. Am J Respir Crit Care Med. 1998;158(5 Pt 1):1384–7.
91. Bady E, Achkar A, Pascal S, Orvoen-Frija E, Laaban JP. Pulmonary arterial hypertension in patients with sleep apnoea syndrome. Thorax. 2000;55:934–9.

Chapter 10
Obesity and Acute Lung Injury

Renee D. Stapleton and Benjamin T. Suratt

Abstract Acute lung injury (ALI) is a common clinical inflammatory syndrome associated with severe acute hypoxemic respiratory with a case fatality of 30–40%. Although counterintuitive, several studies now suggest that the survival of obese and extremely obese critically ill patients with ALI (as well as obese critically ill patients in general) is equal to or better than their lean critically ill counterparts. The mechanisms underlying these findings are not yet clear but may be related to obesity-associated alterations of the host inflammatory response or to decreased susceptibility to ventilator-induced lung injury in these patients. Despite possible survival benefits afforded by obesity in ALI, studies do suggest that obese patients may have longer durations of ventilation and ICU stays. This information is important for clinicians to consider when discussing prognosis and expectations with critically ill patients and their families.

Keywords Acute lung injury • ARDS • Obesity • Diabetes • Dyslipidemia • Leptin • Mechanical ventilation • Outcomes • Survival

Objectives

- Understand the clinical outcomes of obese patients with acute lung injury
- Describe the pathogenesis of acute lung injury and how it may be altered by obesity

R.D. Stapleton, M.D., Ph.D.
Department of Medicine, Division of Pulmonary and Critical Care Medicine,
University of Vermont College of Medicine,
149 Beaumont Avenue HSRF 222, Burlington, VT 05405, USA
e-mail: renee.stapleton@uvm.edu

B.T. Suratt, M.D. (✉)
Department of Medicine, Division of Pulmonary and Critical Care Medicine, University of Vermont College of Medicine, 89 Beaumont Avenue Given E407A, Burlington, VT 05405, USA
e-mail: benjamin.suratt@uvm.edu

A.E. Dixon and E.M. Clerisme-Beaty (eds.), *Obesity and Lung Disease: A Guide to Management*, Respiratory Medicine, DOI 10.1007/978-1-62703-053-3_10,

- Discuss potential impact of obesity on ventilator-induced lung injury
- Discuss strategies for management of obese critically ill ventilated patients

Introduction

Acute lung injury (ALI) is a clinical syndrome defined by bilateral pulmonary infiltrates and severe acute hypoxemic respiratory that is not caused by heart failure [1]. ALI is common in critical illness, with 200,000 US cases of ALI per year and a case fatality of 30–40% in the USA [2, 3]. The prevalence of obesity and extreme obesity has been steadily increasing in developed countries for many years, with dire public health consequences including increased all-cause mortality [4]. However, in critically ill patients including those with ALI, a decade of observational evidence now suggests that obese and extremely obese patients may have lower mortality rates than normal weight patients. Therefore, although obese patients may have increased morbidity related to the intensive care unit (ICU) including increased ICU and hospital lengths of stay (LOS), contrary to what might be assumed by clinicians, the survival of obese and extremely obese critically ill patients is equal to or better than their lean critically ill counterparts. The mechanisms for these findings are not yet clear, but recent biologic data may begin to provide an explanation.

The aims of this chapter are twofold. First, the literature regarding the epidemiology of obesity and ALI will be reviewed. Subsequently, potential biologic mechanisms that may explain the clinical findings of improved survival in critically ill obese patients will be discussed.

Clinical Outcomes of ALI in Obese Patients

ALI and its more severe form, the acute respiratory distress syndrome (ARDS), are common severe complications of pulmonary or systemic injury, resulting in severe acute hypoxemic respiratory failure [1]. There are approximately 200,000 cases of ALI per year in the USA, and the public health impact is tremendous [2]. ALI results in 3.6 million annual hospital days and substantial mortality with nearly 40% of ALI patients dying [2, 3, 5, 6]. Additionally, survivors experience significant morbidity with reduced health-related quality of life and musculoskeletal, cognitive, and psychological function [7, 8]. The most common risk factor for ALI is sepsis, and patients whose risk is sepsis have considerably worse outcomes than patients with other risk factors [2, 9].

The devastating manifestations of ALI result from a complex cascade that includes massive activation of the proinflammatory response [10, 11]. Activated macrophages release cytokines such as interleukin (IL)-1β (beta), IL-6, IL-8, and tumor necrosis factor (TNF)-α (alpha), which activate neutrophils that then produce proteases, oxidants, and lipid mediators that perpetuate the lung injury cycle [12].

Only one ALI-specific therapy has been found to improve survival. In a large randomized controlled trial (RCT) performed by the National Heart, Lung, and Blood Institute Acute Respiratory Distress Syndrome Network (NHLBI ARDS Network), low tidal volume ventilation decreased mortality with an absolute reduction of 8.8% [13]. A better understanding of ALI pathogenesis is therefore urgently needed to enable research into novel therapies for this devastating syndrome.

The prevalence of obesity, especially extreme obesity (BMI ≥40 kg/m^2), has been rapidly increasing for the past two decades in the USA and other developed countries [4]. Over one third of the American population is obese, and over 5% is extremely obese [14]. The public health consequences of this rise in obesity are considerable, as obesity is associated with increased all-cause mortality in both men and women [4].

Studies in ALI and General Critical Illness

Several years ago, evidence began to emerge describing outcomes of obese and extremely obese critically ill patients. Several observational studies have since reported that survival in obese and extremely obese critically ill patients may be paradoxically improved compared to normal weight critically ill patients [15–20], while other studies have reported that mortality in the obese and extremely obese is at least as good as that of critically ill lean patients [20–30]. The majority of these reports have included general medical, surgical, and trauma ICU patients; only three prior studies have specifically focused on acute lung injury, and these are summarized in Table 10.1 [18, 25, 26].

The first ALI study was a secondary analysis of 807 patients enrolled in a randomized controlled trial of traditional versus low tidal volumes conducted by the National Heart, Lung, and Blood Institute ARDS Network [25]. Underweight patients were not examined, and severely obese patients (BMI > 40 kg/m^2) comprised a small percentage (4.7%) of the study group because the parent study excluded patients with a weight-to-height ratio of more than 1.0 kg/cm. BMI data were also missing for 6.1% of participants. In both adjusted and unadjusted analyses, no significant differences between normal weight and obese patients were found in 28-day or 180-day mortality, rate of unassisted ventilation by day 28, or ventilator-free days between normal weight and obese patients. Other morbidity outcomes, such as ICU length of stay, were not reported.

Subsequent to this research, an observational study utilizing Project Impact® (a subscription database operated by the Society of Critical Care Medicine designed to measure and describe the care of ICU patients) data to further explore outcomes in 1,488 critically ill obese patients with ALI was published [18]. Participants were included if the admission diagnosis was consistent with ALI, BMI on admission could be calculated, and mechanical ventilation was initiated within 24 h of ICU admission. Underweight patients in this group had a higher adjusted mortality than normal weight patients. Unadjusted hospital mortality was significantly associated with BMI, with the highest mortality seen in underweight patients (54.6%), and the lowest in extremely

Table 10.1 Summary of published studies of clinical outcomes in obese critically Ill patients with acute lung injury

	O'Brien et al. [25]	O'Brien et al. [18]	Morris et al. [26]
Participants	807	1,488	825
Design	Secondary analysis of data from ARDS Network RCT	Cohort study using Project Impact database	Secondary analysis of prospectively collected data from King County Lung Injury Project
ALI definition	AECC	Diagnosis codes from database	AECC
Primary outcome	28-day mortality	Hospital mortality	Hospital mortality
Findings of adjusted analyses	Not significantly different between obese and normal weight patients	Significantly decreased odds of death in obese compared with normal weight patients	Not significantly different between obese and normal weight patients
Secondary outcomes	Ventilator-free days, achievement of unassisted ventilation, 180-day mortality	ICU LOS, hospital LOS, discharge location	Duration of mechanical ventilation, ICU length of stay, hospital length of stay, discharge location
Findings of adjusted analyses	Not significantly different between obese and normal weight patients	Not significantly different between obese and normal weight patients	Significantly longer duration of mechanical ventilation, ICU LOS, and hospital LOS in severely obese survivors compared with normal weight patients. Severely obese patients also more likely to be discharged to a rehabilitation or skilled nursing facility than to home

RCT randomized controlled trial, *ARDS* acute respiratory distress syndrome, *ALI* acute lung injury, *AECC* American-European Consensus Conference

obese patients (29.0%). After statistical adjustment for age, gender, race, Simplified Acute Physiology Score, admission condition, patient origin, preexisting diseases/ conditions, and ICU processes of care, patients in all obese categories had a decreased risk of death relative to normal weight patients. However, this difference was statistically significant only in the obese group with BMI 30–39.9 kg/m^2. ICU and hospital LOS and discharge location did not differ by BMI category.

The third and most recent study to examine patients with ALI was an analysis of data from 825 participants in the King County Lung Injury Project in Seattle, where all hospitalized patients in and around King County were screened for the presence of ALI from April 1999 to July 2000 [26]. Because this study used population-based data, the results are likely generalizable to all ALI patients. Similar to the prior study, crude mortality was highest in underweight patients and decreased with increasing BMI. Unadjusted analyses revealed no statistically significant differences in mortality between the overweight, obese, or extremely obese groups when compared to normal weight patients. Severely obese patients (BMI > 40 kg/m^2) who survived had longer duration of mechanical ventilation, ICU LOS, and hospital LOS than normal weight patients, and they were more likely to be discharged to a rehabilitation or skilled nursing facility than to home.

In addition to these individual studies, three recent meta-analyses of outcomes in critically ill obese patients have been published [31–33]. The first included 62,045 patients from 14 studies and concluded that hospital mortality was significantly lower in obese patients with BMI ≥30 kg/m^2 than in normal weight patients (RR 0.83, 95% CI 0.74–0.92). However, obese patients also had significantly longer duration of mechanical ventilation (1.48 days, 95% CI 0.07–2.89; $p = .04$) and ICU LOS (1.08 days, 95% CI 0.27–1.88; $p = .009$) [31]. The second meta-analysis included 22 studies totaling 88,051 patients [32]. There was no difference in ICU mortality between normal weight and obese patients, but obese patients had a significantly lower hospital mortality (RR = 0.76 with 95% CI 0.59–0.92). In contrast to the prior meta-analysis, this study found that when data were aggregated, there was no association between BMI and duration of mechanical ventilation or ICU LOS. The third meta-analysis included patients from 23 studies and found that mortality was significantly lower in the overweight (OR 0.91, 95% CI 0.84–0.98) and obese (OR 0.82, 95% CI 0.68–0.98) groups, but there was no difference in survival among severely obese compared with normal weight patients [33]. Differences between the results of these three meta-analyses can be explained by their inclusion of different studies, but the overall results indicate that obese critically ill patients likely have a survival advantage compared with normal weight patients in the ICU.

Since publication of the above meta-analyses, an additional report focusing on outcomes in extremely obese patients has been published [20]. The authors analyzed data from a multicenter international observational study of ICU nutrition practices occurring in 355 ICUs in 33 countries during 2007–2009. Patients included in the parent study were adults more than 17 years old who were mechanically ventilated and in the ICU for at least 72 h. Of the 8,813 patients included, 3,490 were normal weight, 2,604 were overweight (BMI 25–29.9 kg/m^2), 1,772 were obese (BMI 30–39.9 kg/m^2), 348 had BMI 40–49.9 kg/m^2, 118 had BMI 50–59.9 kg/m^2, and 58 had BMI ≥60 kg/m^2. Adjusted analyses found that overweight (OR 0.80, 95%CI 0.71–0.90) and obese (OR 0.73, 95%CI 0.64–0.84) patients had significantly reduced mortality compared with normal weight patients. There was also a notable trend toward improved survival in the extremely obese group (BMI ≥40 kg/m^2) with the odds of death equal to 0.87

(95% CI 0.69–1.09, $p=0.07$) compared with normal weight patients. Adjusted results also demonstrated that obese and extremely obese patients who survive have longer durations of mechanical ventilation and ICU LOS, with the most severely obese patients (BMI ≥60 kg/m^2) also having longer hospital LOS.

In summary, current evidence suggests that overweight, obese, and extremely obese critically ill patients have lower mortality compared to normal weight patients, but their morbidity including ICU length of stay and duration of mechanical ventilation is likely higher. The three published studies of obese patients with ALI suggest that increased BMI may be associated with a greater risk of developing ALI [34], but paradoxically does not increase mortality, and may in fact be protective [18, 25, 26].

Limitations of Prior Investigations

There are several limitations to prior studies in outcomes in critically ill patients with and without ALI. First, BMI has been used in all studies as the measure of obesity, but it may not accurately reflect obesity syndromes compared with other measurements, such as waist circumference [35]. Furthermore, measurement of BMI may be altered by intravenous fluid administration in ICU patients before weight is obtained or erroneous assessment of height in supine critically ill patients [36]. Third, a tool for assessing severity of illness specifically in obese patients does not exist, and current assessment tools, including APACHE and SAPS [37, 38], may not accurately reflect mortality risk in obese patients due to unknown factors that may be specific to the obese population. Fourth, processes of care for obese and extremely obese patients in different hospitals and ICUs are likely to be highly variable and may bias results, either toward improved or worse outcomes for obese patients. Finally, diagnosing ALI and assessing the degree of critical illness in extremely obese patients can be very difficult (e.g., measuring noninvasive blood pressure measurements [39] or interpreting of chest radiographs), thus leading to misclassification and incorrect case ascertainment, although many studies report an improvement in outcomes in the overweight and obese groups where such misclassification is less likely [40]. Additionally, one recent study of a cohort of 1,795 critically ill patients at risk for ARDS found that increasing BMI was significantly associated with the subsequent development of ARDS. However, this increased risk was due to a greater incidence of hypoxemic respiratory failure and not a greater incidence of bilateral pulmonary infiltrates on chest radiograph, thus suggesting that misinterpretation of chest radiographs in obese patients is not responsible for incorrect ascertainment [34].

Possible Explanation of Findings

Results of the above clinical studies have now prompted interest in investigating mechanisms by which obesity may influence ICU outcomes. Reasons for increased duration of mechanical ventilation and ICU LOS in obese patients with ALI observed in some studies may be due to physiologic factors that lead to longer duration of care but do not increase mortality. For example, lung derecruitment due to the weight of the abdomen and chest wall and provider reluctance to extubate an extremely obese patient may contribute to longer duration of ventilation [41].

However, explanations of why survival in obese patients with ALI is at least as good as, if not better than, that in normal weight patients are less clear. Obesity may be somehow protective in ALI, but the mechanisms by which that might occur have not been elucidated. A recent study found that obese patients with ALI have lower levels of several proinflammatory cytokines (IL-6, IL-8, and surfactant protein D) that are known to be increased in ALI and to be associated with increased mortality [40], thus suggesting that innate immunity and the inflammatory response may be altered in obesity.

Biologic Relationship of Obesity and ALI

Obesity and the Pathogenesis of ALI

Despite decades of research, the pathogenesis of ALI remains incompletely understood. Following an inciting event, alveolar macrophage activation, pulmonary recruitment of neutrophils, and alveolar endothelial and epithelial injury are thought to be central factors in both the onset and progression of this syndrome, which is also then promulgated by ventilator-induced lung injury (VILI) (Fig. 10.1) [11, 12, 42–45]. In accordance with such a schema, increases in both airspace neutrophilia and plasma cytokine levels, including TNF-α (alpha), IL-1β (beta), IL-6, and IL-8, have been shown to correlate with increased morbidity and mortality from this disease [43, 44, 46–48].

It is increasingly recognized that ALI pathogenesis and hence outcome may be influenced by host factors, including genetic polymorphisms and comorbid conditions [12, 45]. In this light, the clinical evidence that obesity may have an ameliorative effect on ALI and critical care outcomes suggests obesity may be one such factor. Such an interaction would be surprising, as obesity is itself believed to be an inflammatory state with baseline increased circulating neutrophil levels [49, 50], elevations in blood TNF-α (alpha), IL-1β (beta), IL-6, and IL-8 [51, 52], and innate immune cell activation [53–55] with endothelial injury [56–58], perhaps predictive of inflammatory synergy between the obese state and ALI. Nevertheless, it has recently been reported that plasma IL-6 and IL-8 *fall* with rising BMI in ALI patients [40], indicating that although obesity may increase the risk of *developing* ALI [34], perhaps through preexisting vascular injury, it may paradoxically have an *attenuating* effect on ALI-associated inflammation and hence the progression of the disease.

Although human studies examining the effects of obesity on ALI pathophysiology are scarce, recent reports in animal models suggest that such models may recapitulate the clinical effects of obesity, allowing further dissection of the underlying

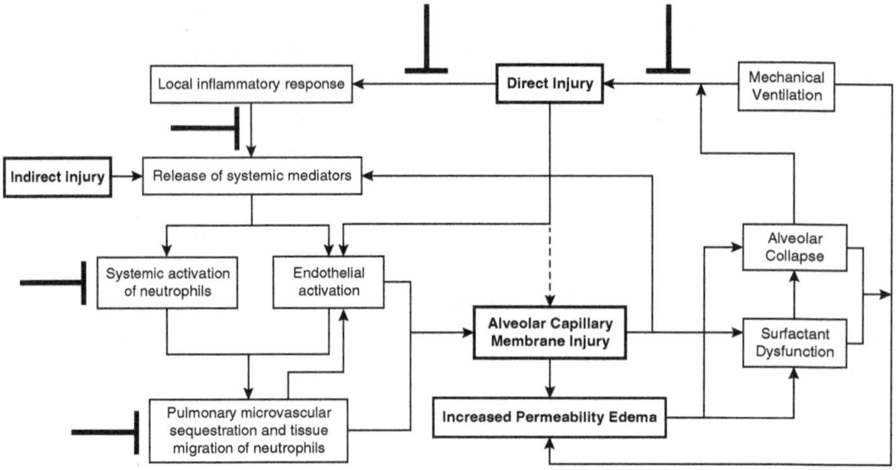

Fig. 10.1 Pathophysiologic mechanisms of acute lung injury and the possible effects of obesity. In this schematized view of the pathophysiologic pathways of ALI/ARDS, direct injuries to the lung damage the alveolar capillary membrane (ACM) and initiate local and subsequently systemic inflammatory cascades, which may be dampened by the effects of obesity and the metabolic syndrome (⊥). Indirect injuries initiate the pathophysiologic pathways of ALI/ARDS primarily through release of systemic cytokines. Following both direct and indirect initiators of ALI/ARDS, the release of systemic inflammatory mediators activates circulating neutrophils and the vascular endothelium of the lung, leading to pulmonary microvascular sequestration of neutrophils and inflammatory injury to the ACM. Although obesity may promote vascular injury in ALI, it appears to attenuate cytokine release and neutrophil activation. This injury is critical in the failure of alveolar/capillary membrane barrier function and flooding of the alveoli with proteinaceous edema fluid. Both ACM injury and alveolar edema cause surfactant loss and dysfunction, which promote alveolar instability and collapse, driving further edema formation and alveolar injury, particularly in the setting of mechanical ventilation, which also may be attenuated in the setting of obesity (Adapted with permission from Suratt and Parsons [45])

mechanisms. Most animal studies examining obesity-associated effects on pulmonary immunity and inflammation have focused on models of asthma and pneumonia, and, as detailed elsewhere in this volume, although some forms of airway inflammation appear to be amplified by obesity [59], the response to pneumonia is blunted [60–62], suggesting that the inflammatory response in the alveoli (the site of ALI) is impaired. In the few published reports examining obesity's effects on acute lung injury models, obese mice and rats demonstrate reduced inflammation, lung injury, and mortality from LPS-, hyperoxia-, and ozone-induced ALI [63–66], although in the case of ozone exposure, findings are mixed and appear to vary with the acuity of exposure [66–68]. To date, investigators have primarily examined spontaneously obese, genetically mutant leptin-*deficient* mice (ob/ob; Lep^{ob}), and leptin-*resistant* mice (db/db; $Lepr^{db}$) and rats (Zucker; $Lepr^{fa}$), yet one of these reports [66] also examined the effects of the potentially more clinically relevant diet-induced obesity and found similar attenuation in inflammation and lung injury.

Obesity, the Metabolic Syndrome, and the Inflammatory Response in ALI

Given the systemic abnormalities associated with obesity and the accompanying metabolic syndrome, obesity's effects on the pathogenesis of ALI almost certainly reflect interaction between multiple facets of the obese state. Although few reports focus on obesity itself, a growing literature examines the effects of the metabolic syndrome on ALI pathogenesis and outcome. The most extensively investigated element of the metabolic syndrome in this regard is diabetes.

Diabetes has been shown to be associated with a reduced risk of developing ALI in three large clinical studies of high-risk patients including those with sepsis, aspiration, trauma, and massive transfusion [69–71], with an adjusted odds ratio ranging from 0.33 to 0.58 [72]. Although this protective effect is reproducible in animal models of diabetes [63, 73–75], the underlying mechanisms remain unclear. Diabetes is associated with impaired innate immune response [76, 77], which although believed to drive the increased risk of infection in diabetics [78], might conversely attenuate inappropriate inflammatory states such as ALI. Evidence supporting roles for either hyperglycemia or insulin resistance in the attenuation of ALI is conflicting, and recently attention has focused on the possibility that this protective effect may be related to the systemic actions of diabetic *therapies*, such as exogenous insulin and PPAR-γ (gamma) agonists [72].

Comparable studies investigating dyslipidemia and its effects on ALI risk and pathogenesis have not yet been published. However, as with obesity in general, dyslipidemia is associated with baseline elevations in circulating neutrophil levels in both humans and mouse models, often in the absence of accompanying obesity [79–82]. Persistent activation of both monocytes and neutrophils is described in dyslipidemic states, accompanied by endothelial injury [83], and may be driven by direct effects of lipid species on leukocytes [84, 85]. Yet, in this setting, there appear to be defects in neutrophil and monocyte function [86, 87], and recently animal models of hypercholesterolemia without obesity have suggested that the development of LPS-induced ALI is blunted [88]. Whether such defects might reflect tonic activation of the innate immune system with "desensitization" to acute stimuli or other effects of the dyslipidemic state is not yet known.

Another significant feature of the metabolic syndrome and obesity in general is the dysregulation of adipokine release and response. Although initially described as hormone-like signaling molecules released by adipose tissue and involved in metabolic homeostasis, adipokines such as leptin, adiponectin, and visfatin have recently been shown to have quite protean effects including modulation of both innate and adaptive immune systems [89, 90]. The best studied of these molecules is leptin, which was originally described as a regulator of appetite. Leptin has been shown to be important in the marrow development of the myelomonocytic lineages [91, 92] and to serve as an activation and survival signal for neutrophils in the periphery [93–95]. Interestingly, leptin also appears to act as a neutrophil chemoattractant

[96–98] and may be released by the injured lung [99, 100], while serum levels of leptin are elevated in critical illness [101–103], together suggesting a possible role for leptin in the development of ALI.

How leptin's effects on innate immune function may be altered in obesity is poorly understood. Obesity is typically accompanied by a state of hyperleptinemic leptin resistance in which leptin response is blunted despite high circulating levels of this cytokine, presumably due to receptor desensitization. Elevated leptin levels in patients with end-stage renal disease have been implicated in the neutrophil dysfunction that accompanies that state [98], while animal models of aleptinemia and leptin resistance suggest that the development of hyperoxic ALI is blunted in this setting [64, 65]. Whether hyperleptinemia and leptin resistance may affect the development of human ALI has not yet been addressed.

In reviewing the literature describing the many effects of the metabolic syndrome, it is important to emphasize that both human and, with rare exceptions, animal studies examining "discrete" elements of the metabolic syndrome have not examined these in isolation of obesity or the other facets of the syndrome. For instance, none of the reported clinical studies on diabetes and ALI included BMI as a confounding variable, and the db/db mouse model, although used in various studies to specifically examine leptin resistance, diabetes, or obesity, is also noted to be extremely dyslipidemic. Thus, it remains unclear which elements of obesity and the metabolic syndrome may be operative in the majority of reported findings.

Obese Pulmonary Mechanics: VILI Attenuated?

One further possibility that must be considered when examining the potential interaction between obesity and ALI focuses on the biomechanical effects of obesity. As detailed elsewhere in this volume, obese individuals manifest altered pulmonary mechanics compared to lean individuals, at baseline and when mechanically ventilated. Obese patients with ARDS demonstrate similar changes, with a combination of reduced chest wall and lung compliance leading to a lower FRC and consequently atelectasis, increased airways resistance and closure, and ventilation/perfusion mismatch [104, 105]. Although these changes likely underlie obesity-associated delays in liberation from mechanical ventilation, how such alterations might be protective in ALI is unclear.

It is possible that the combination of lower respiratory system compliance and higher airways resistance, which yield atelectasis and higher static and dynamic airway pressures for a given tidal volume, may prompt clinicians to selectively increase PEEP and decrease tidal volumes in the obese, thus mimicking or accentuating a protective low tidal volume strategy. However, it has been shown that obese ALI patients are typically ventilated at *higher* tidal volumes (cc/kg ideal body weight) than normal weight patients [25, 26], indicating that, in light of comparable to improved survival in the obese, mechanical ventilation (even at higher tidal volumes) may be better tolerated in these patients. Furthermore, although overall mortality in the RCT of low tidal volume ventilation in ALI was not different between lean and obese patients [25], data from this study suggest that obese patients may have tolerated higher tidal volumes (12 cc/kg IBW) better than did lean patients. The relative reduction in mortality attributable to lower tidal volumes (6 cc/kg IBW) in the overall cohort was 30%, yet when stratified into normal, overweight, and obese BMI categories, the relative reductions in mortality between high and low tidal volume arms of the study were 42%, 27%, and 12%, respectively, although this finding did not reach statistical significance. Thus, obese patients may be less susceptible to VILI. Whether this might be related to the mechanical interaction between obese patients and ventilation or an additional manifestation of attenuated inflammatory response in obese ALI has yet to be examined.

Clinical Recommendations

Caring for critically ill obese and severely obese patients in a clinical setting can be challenging. Like all ICU patients, special attention should be paid to prevention of infection with measures such as the use of a checklist during central line insertion to prevent central line-associated blood stream infection [106] and semirecumbent positioning to prevent ventilator-associated pneumonia [107]. Prior studies have also suggested that obese patients who are mechanically ventilated receive tidal volumes early in their ICU course substantially greater than the 6 cc/kg predicted body weight shown to improve survival [13, 26, 40]. ICU clinicians should therefore be conscientious when choosing tidal volumes in obese patients. Furthermore, the recumbent position leads to increased atelectasis and greater mechanical loading of the diaphragm in obesity, contributing to hypoxia and difficulty weaning. Therefore, consideration should be given to positioning obese patients as upright as safely possible and transitioning to chair during weans, both of which have been shown to improve mechanics in these patients [108]. Lastly, the pharmacokinetics and pharmacodynamics of many drugs commonly used in critical illness are substantially altered in obese and severely obese patients compared with those of normal weight (e.g., heparin and benzodiazepines); attention to detail when using these medicines is important.

Conclusions

Survival in the general population is j-shaped, with increased mortality in underweight people, lowest mortality in patients with a BMI near 25 kg/m^2, and increasing mortality rates in overweight, obese, and extremely obese patients [4]. Evidence in critically ill patients, however, suggests that overweight, obese, and extremely obese patients have lower mortality compared to normal weight patients. The limited studies of obese patients with ALI published to date show that rising BMI may increase the risk for the development of ALI [34], but paradoxically does not increase mortality from this disease, and may in fact be protective [18, 25, 26]. Health professionals may assume that obese patients have worse survival and morbidity due to presumed difficulties of caring for such critically ill patients including transport, body positioning, intravascular access, diagnostic imaging, and ventilator weaning. While the literature does suggest that obese patients may have longer durations of ventilation and ICU lengths of stay, their survival is at least as good as normal weight patients. This information is important for clinicians to recognize when discussing prognosis and expectations with critically ill patients and their families.

References

1. Bernard GR, Artigas A, Brigham KL, Carlet J, Falke K, Hudson L, et al. The American-European Consensus Conference on ARDS. Definitions, mechanisms, relevant outcomes, and clinical trial coordination. Am J Respir Crit Care Med. 1994;149(3 Pt 1):818–24.
2. Rubenfeld GD, Caldwell E, Peabody E, Weaver J, Martin DP, Neff M, et al. Incidence and outcomes of acute lung injury. N Engl J Med. 2005;353(16):1685–93.
3. Stapleton RD, Wang BM, Hudson LD, Rubenfeld GD, Caldwell ES, Steinberg KP. Causes and timing of death in patients with ARDS. Chest. 2005;128(2):525–32.
4. Adams KF, Schatzkin A, Harris TB, Kipnis V, Mouw T, Ballard-Barbash R, et al. Overweight, obesity, and mortality in a large prospective cohort of persons 50 to 71 years old. N Engl J Med. 2006;355(8):763–78.
5. Milberg JA, Davis DR, Steinberg KP, Hudson LD. Improved survival of patients with acute respiratory distress syndrome (ARDS): 1983–1993. JAMA. 1995;273(4):306–9.
6. Abel SJ, Finney SJ, Brett SJ, Keogh BF, Morgan CJ, Evans TW. Reduced mortality in association with the acute respiratory distress syndrome (ARDS). Thorax. 1998;53(4):292–4.
7. Rubenfeld GD, Herridge MS. Epidemiology and outcomes of acute lung injury. Chest. 2007;131(2):554–62.
8. Dowdy DW, Eid MP, Dennison CR, Mendez-Tellez PA, Herridge MS, Guallar E, et al. Quality of life after acute respiratory distress syndrome: a meta-analysis. Intensive Care Med. 2006;32(8):1115–24.
9. Hudson LD, Milberg JA, Anardi D, Maunder RJ. Clinical risks for development of the acute respiratory distress syndrome. Am J Respir Crit Care Med. 1995;151(2 Pt 1):293–301.
10. Weiland JE, Davis WB, Holter JF, Mohammed JR, Dorinsky PM, Gadek JE. Lung neutrophils in the adult respiratory distress syndrome. Clinical and pathophysiologic significance. Am Rev Respir Dis. 1986;133(2):218–25.
11. Tate RM, Repine JE. Neutrophils and the adult respiratory distress syndrome. Am Rev Respir Dis. 1983;128(3):552–9.
12. Ware LB, Matthay MA. The acute respiratory distress syndrome. N Engl J Med. 2000;342(18):1334–49.
13. The Acute Respiratory Distress Syndrome Network. Ventilation with lower tidal volumes as compared with traditional tidal volumes for acute lung injury and the acute respiratory distress syndrome. N Engl J Med. 2000;342(18):1301–8.
14. Flegal KM, Carroll MD, Ogden CL, Curtin LR. Prevalence and trends in obesity among US adults, 1999–2008. JAMA. 2010;303(3):235–41.
15. Finkielman JD, Gajic O, Afessa B. Underweight is independently associated with mortality in post-operative and non-operative patients admitted to the intensive care unit: a retrospective study. BMC Emerg Med. 2004;4(1):3.

16. Garrouste-Orgeas M, Troche G, Azoulay E, Caubel A, de Lassence A, Cheval C, et al. Body mass index. An additional prognostic factor in ICU patients. Intensive Care Med. 2004; 30(3):437–43.
17. Aldawood A, Arabi Y, Dabbagh O. Association of obesity with increased mortality in the critically ill patient. Anaesth Intensive Care. 2006;34(5):629–33.
18. O'Brien Jr JM, Phillips GS, Ali NA, Lucarelli M, Marsh CB, Lemeshow S. Body mass index is independently associated with hospital mortality in mechanically ventilated adults with acute lung injury. Crit Care Med. 2006;34(3):738–44.
19. Peake SL, Moran JL, Ghelani DR, Lloyd AJ, Walker MJ. The effect of obesity on 12-month survival following admission to intensive care: a prospective study. Crit Care Med. 2006;34(12):2929–39.
20. Martino JL, Stapleton RD, Wang M, Day AG, Cahill NE, Dixon AE, et al. Extreme obesity and outcomes in critically ill patients. Chest. 2011;140:1198–206.
21. Marik P, Doyle H, Varon J. Is obesity protective during critical illness? An analysis of a National ICU database. Crit Care Shock. 2003;6:156–62.
22. Tremblay A, Bandi V. Impact of body mass index on outcomes following critical care. Chest. 2003;123(4):1202–7.
23. Smith RL, Chong TW, Hedrick TL, Hughes MG, Evans HL, McElearney ST, et al. Does body mass index affect infection-related outcomes in the intensive care unit? Surg Infect (Larchmt). 2007;8(6):581–8.
24. Newell MA, Bard MR, Goettler CE, Toschlog EA, Schenarts PJ, Sagraves SG, et al. Body mass index and outcomes in critically injured blunt trauma patients: weighing the impact. J Am Coll Surg. 2007;204(5):1056–61. discussion 62–4.
25. O'Brien Jr JM, Welsh CH, Fish RH, Ancukiewicz M, Kramer AM. Excess body weight is not independently associated with outcome in mechanically ventilated patients with acute lung injury. Ann Intern Med. 2004;140(5):338–45.
26. Morris AE, Stapleton RD, Rubenfeld GD, Hudson LD, Caldwell E, Steinberg KP. The association between body mass index and clinical outcomes in acute lung injury. Chest. 2007; 131(2):342–8.
27. Alban RF, Lyass S, Margulies DR, Shabot MM. Obesity does not affect mortality after trauma. Am Surg. 2006;72(10):966–9.
28. Brown CV, Rhee P, Neville AL, Sangthong B, Salim A, Demetriades D. Obesity and traumatic brain injury. J Trauma. 2006;61(3):572–6.
29. Ciesla DJ, Moore EE, Johnson JL, Burch JM, Cothren CC, Sauaia A. Obesity increases risk of organ failure after severe trauma. J Am Coll Surg. 2006;203(4):539–45.
30. Ray DE, Matchett SC, Baker K, Wasser T, Young MJ. The effect of body mass index on patient outcomes in a medical ICU. Chest. 2005;127(6):2125–31.
31. Akinnusi ME, Pineda LA, El Solh AA. Effect of obesity on intensive care morbidity and mortality: a meta-analysis. Crit Care Med. 2008;36(1):151–8.
32. Hogue Jr CW, Stearns JD, Colantuoni E, Robinson KA, Stierer T, Mitter N, et al. The impact of obesity on outcomes after critical illness: a meta-analysis. Intensive Care Med. 2009;35(7): 1152–70.
33. Oliveros H, Villamor E. Obesity and mortality in critically ill adults: a systematic review and meta-analysis. Obesity (Silver Spring). 2008;16(3):515–21.
34. Gong MN, Bajwa EK, Thompson BT, Christiani DC. Body mass index is associated with the development of acute respiratory distress syndrome. Thorax. 2010;65(1):44–50.
35. National Institutes of Health. Clinical guidelines on the identification, evaluation, and treatment of overweight and obesity in adults – the evidence report. Obes Res. 1998;6(Suppl 2):51S–209.
36. McCallister JW, Adkins EJ, O'Brien Jr JM. Obesity and acute lung injury. Clin Chest Med. 2009;30(3):495–508. viii.
37. Knaus WA, Draper EA, Wagner DP, Zimmerman JE. APACHE II: a severity of disease classification system. Crit Care Med. 1985;13(10):818–29.

38. Le Gall JR, Lemeshow S, Saulnier F. A new Simplified Acute Physiology Score (SAPS II) based on a European/North American multicenter study. JAMA. 1993;270(24):2957–63.
39. Maxwell MH, Waks AU, Schroth PC, Karam M, Dornfeld LP. Error in blood-pressure measurement due to incorrect cuff size in obese patients. Lancet. 1982;2(8288):33–6.
40. Stapleton RD, Dixon AE, Parsons PE, Ware LB, Suratt BT. The association between BMI and plasma cytokine levels in patients with acute lung injury. Chest. 2010;138(3):568–77.
41. Walz JM, Zayaruzny M, Heard SO. Airway management in critical illness. Chest. 2007;131(2):608–20.
42. Moraes TJ, Chow CW, Downey GP. Proteases and lung injury. Crit Care Med. 2003;31 (4 Suppl):S189–94.
43. Baughman RP, Gunther KL, Rashkin MC, Keeton DA, Pattishall EN. Changes in the inflammatory response of the lung during acute respiratory distress syndrome: prognostic indicators. Am J Respir Crit Care Med. 1996;154(1):76–81.
44. Goodman RB, Strieter RM, Martin DP, Steinberg KP, Milberg JA, Maunder RJ, et al. Inflammatory cytokines in patients with persistence of the acute respiratory distress syndrome. Am J Respir Crit Care Med. 1996;154(3 Pt 1):602–11.
45. Suratt BT, Parsons PE. Mechanisms of acute lung injury/acute respiratory distress syndrome. Clin Chest Med. 2006;27(4):579–89.
46. Meduri GU, Headley S, Kohler G, Stentz F, Tolley E, Umberger R, et al. Persistent elevation of inflammatory cytokines predicts a poor outcome in ARDS. Plasma IL-1 beta and IL-6 levels are consistent and efficient predictors of outcome over time. Chest. 1995;107(4): 1062–73.
47. Parsons PE, Eisner MD, Thompson BT, Matthay MA, Ancukiewicz M, Bernard GR, et al. Lower tidal volume ventilation and plasma cytokine markers of inflammation in patients with acute lung injury. Crit Care Med. 2005;33(1):1–6.
48. Ware LB. Prognostic determinants of acute respiratory distress syndrome in adults: impact on clinical trial design. Crit Care Med. 2005;33(3 Suppl):S217–22.
49. Kim JA, Park HS. White blood cell count and abdominal fat distribution in female obese adolescents. Metabolism. 2008;57(10):1375–9.
50. Desai MY, Dalal D, Santos RD, Carvalho JA, Nasir K, Blumenthal RS. Association of body mass index, metabolic syndrome, and leukocyte count. Am J Cardiol. 2006;97(6):835–8.
51. Ramos EJ, Xu Y, Romanova I, Middleton F, Chen C, Quinn R, et al. Is obesity an inflammatory disease? Surgery. 2003;134(2):329–35.
52. Yudkin JS. Adipose tissue, insulin action and vascular disease: inflammatory signals. Int J Obes Relat Metab Disord. 2003;27(Suppl 3):S25–8.
53. Cottam DR, Schaefer PA, Shaftan GW, Velcu L, Angus LD. Effect of surgically induced weight loss on leukocyte indicators of chronic inflammation in morbid obesity. Obes Surg. 2002;12(3):335–42.
54. Cottam DR, Schaefer PA, Fahmy D, Shaftan GW, Angus LD. The effect of obesity on neutrophil Fc receptors and adhesion molecules (CD16, CD11b, CD62L). Obes Surg. 2002;12(2): 230–5.
55. Nijhuis J, Rensen SS, Slaats Y, van Dielen FM, Buurman WA, Greve JW. Neutrophil activation in morbid obesity, chronic activation of acute inflammation. Obesity (Silver Spring). 2009;17(11):2014–8.
56. Blann AD, Bushell D, Davies A, Faragher EB, Miller JP, McCollum CN. von Willebrand factor, the endothelium and obesity. Int J Obes Relat Metab Disord. 1993;17(12):723–5.
57. van Harmelen V, Eriksson A, Astrom G, Wahlen K, Naslund E, Karpe F, et al. Vascular peptide endothelin-1 links fat accumulation with alterations of visceral adipocyte lipolysis. Diabetes. 2008;57(2):378–86.
58. Pontiroli AE, Frige F, Paganelli M, Folli F. In morbid obesity, metabolic abnormalities and adhesion molecules correlate with visceral fat, not with subcutaneous fat: effect of weight loss through surgery. Obes Surg. 2009;19(6):745–50.
59. Shore SA. Obesity and asthma: lessons from animal models. J Appl Physiol. 2007;102(2): 516–28.

60. Ikejima S, Sasaki S, Sashinami H, Mori F, Ogawa Y, Nakamura T, et al. Impairment of host resistance to *Listeria monocytogenes* infection in liver of db/db and ob/ob mice. Diabetes. 2005;54(1):182–9.
61. Hsu A, Aronoff DM, Phipps J, Goel D, Mancuso P. Leptin improves pulmonary bacterial clearance and survival in ob/ob mice during pneumococcal pneumonia. Clin Exp Immunol. 2007;150(2):332–9.
62. Mancuso P, Gottschalk A, Phare SM, Peters-Golden M, Lukacs NW, Huffnagle GB. Leptin-deficient mice exhibit impaired host defense in Gram-negative pneumonia. J Immunol. 2002;168(8):4018–24.
63. Wright JK, Nwariaku FN, Clark J, Falck JC, Rogers T, Turnage RH. Effect of diabetes mellitus on endotoxin-induced lung injury. Arch Surg. 1999;134(12):1354–8.
64. Bellmeyer A, Martino JM, Chandel NS, Scott Budinger GR, Dean DA, Mutlu GM. Leptin resistance protects mice from hyperoxia-induced acute lung injury. Am J Respir Crit Care Med. 2007;175(6):587–94.
65. Barazzone-Argiroffo C, Muzzin P, Donati YR, Kan CD, Aubert ML, Piguet PF. Hyperoxia increases leptin production: a mechanism mediated through endogenous elevation of corticosterone. Am J Physiol Lung Cell Mol Physiol. 2001;281(5):L1150–6.
66. Shore SA, Lang JE, Kasahara DI, Lu FL, Verbout NG, Si H, et al. Pulmonary responses to subacute ozone exposure in obese vs. lean mice. J Appl Physiol. 2009;107(5):1445–52.
67. Lu FL, Johnston RA, Flynt L, Theman TA, Terry RD, Schwartzman IN, et al. Increased pulmonary responses to acute ozone exposure in obese db/db mice. Am J Physiol Lung Cell Mol Physiol. 2006;290(5):L856–65.
68. Johnston RA, Theman TA, Lu FL, Terry RD, Williams ES, Shore SA. Diet-induced obesity causes innate airway hyperresponsiveness to methacholine and enhances ozone-induced pulmonary inflammation. J Appl Physiol. 2008;104(6):1727–35.
69. Moss M, Guidot DM, Steinberg KP, Duhon GF, Treece P, Wolken R, et al. Diabetic patients have a decreased incidence of acute respiratory distress syndrome. Crit Care Med. 2000;28(7):2187–92.
70. Gong MN, Thompson BT, Williams P, Pothier L, Boyce PD, Christiani DC. Clinical predictors of and mortality in acute respiratory distress syndrome: potential role of red cell transfusion. Crit Care Med. 2005;33(6):1191–8.
71. Iscimen R, Cartin-Ceba R, Yilmaz M, Khan H, Hubmayr RD, Afessa B, et al. Risk factors for the development of acute lung injury in patients with septic shock: an observational cohort study. Crit Care Med. 2008;36(5):1518–22.
72. Honiden S, Gong MN. Diabetes, insulin, and development of acute lung injury. Crit Care Med. 2009;37(8):2455–64.
73. Boichot E, Sannomiya P, Escofier N, Germain N, Fortes ZB, Lagente V. Endotoxin-induced acute lung injury in rats. Role of insulin. Pulm Pharmacol Ther. 1999;12(5):285–90.
74. Alba-Loureiro TC, Martins EF, Landgraf RG, Jancar S, Curi R, Sannomiya P. Role of insulin on PGE2 generation during LPS-induced lung inflammation in rats. Life Sci. 2006;78(6):578–85.
75. de Oliveira Martins J, Meyer-Pflug AR, Alba-Loureiro TC, Melbostad H, Costa da Cruz JW, Coimbra R, et al. Modulation of lipopolysaccharide-induced acute lung inflammation: role of insulin. Shock. 2006;25(3):260–6.
76. Alba-Loureiro TC, Munhoz CD, Martins JO, Cerchiaro GA, Scavone C, Curi R, et al. Neutrophil function and metabolism in individuals with diabetes mellitus. Braz J Med Biol Res. 2007;40(8):1037–44.
77. Moreno-Navarrete JM, Fernandez-Real JM. Antimicrobial-sensing proteins in obesity and type 2 diabetes: the buffering efficiency hypothesis. Diabetes Care. 2011;34(Suppl 2):S335–41.
78. Moutschen MP, Scheen AJ, Lefebvre PJ. Impaired immune responses in diabetes mellitus: analysis of the factors and mechanisms involved. Relevance to the increased susceptibility of diabetic patients to specific infections. Diabete Metab. 1992;18(3):187–201.

79. Huang ZS, Chien KL, Yang CY, Tsai KS, Wang CH. Peripheral differential leukocyte counts in humans vary with hyperlipidemia, smoking, and body mass index. Lipids. 2001; 36(3):237–45.
80. Giugliano G, Brevetti G, Lanero S, Schiano V, Laurenzano E, Chiariello M. Leukocyte count in peripheral arterial disease: a simple, reliable, inexpensive approach to cardiovascular risk prediction. Atherosclerosis. 2010;210(1):288–93.
81. Gomes AL, Carvalho T, Serpa J, Torre C, Dias S. Hypercholesterolemia promotes bone marrow cell mobilization by perturbing the SDF-1:CXCR4 axis. Blood. 2010;115(19): 3886–94.
82. Drechsler M, Megens RT, van Zandvoort M, Weber C, Soehnlein O. Hyperlipidemia-triggered neutrophilia promotes early atherosclerosis. Circulation. 2010;122(18):1837–45.
83. Hansson GK, Libby P. The immune response in atherosclerosis: a double-edged sword. Nat Rev Immunol. 2006;6(7):508–19.
84. Kopprasch S, Leonhardt W, Pietzsch J, Kuhne H. Hypochlorite-modified low-density lipoprotein stimulates human polymorphonuclear leukocytes for enhanced production of reactive oxygen metabolites, enzyme secretion, and adhesion to endothelial cells. Atherosclerosis. 1998;136(2):315–24.
85. Lehr HA, Krombach F, Munzing S, Bodlaj R, Glaubitt SI, Seiffge D, et al. In vitro effects of oxidized low density lipoprotein on CD11b/CD18 and L-selectin presentation on neutrophils and monocytes with relevance for the in vivo situation. Am J Pathol. 1995;146(1): 218–27.
86. Porreca E, Sergi R, Baccante G, Reale M, Orsini L, Febbo CD, et al. Peripheral blood mononuclear cell production of interleukin-8 and IL-8-dependent neutrophil function in hypercholesterolemic patients. Atherosclerosis. 1999;146(2):345–50.
87. Stragliotto E, Camera M, Postiglione A, Sirtori M, Di Minno G, Tremoli E. Functionally abnormal monocytes in hypercholesterolemia. Arterioscler Thromb. 1993;13(6):944–50.
88. Madenspacher JH, Draper DW, Smoak KA, Li H, Griffiths GL, Suratt BT, et al. Dyslipidemia induces opposing effects on intrapulmonary and extrapulmonary host defense through divergent TLR response phenotypes. J Immunol. 2010;185(3):1660–9.
89. Fantuzzi G. Adipose tissue, adipokines, and inflammation. J Allergy Clin Immunol. 2005; 115(5):911–9. quiz 20.
90. La Cava A, Matarese G. The weight of leptin in immunity. Nat Rev Immunol. 2004;4(5): 371–9.
91. Umemoto Y, Tsuji K, Yang FC, Ebihara Y, Kaneko A, Furukawa S, et al. Leptin stimulates the proliferation of murine myelocytic and primitive hematopoietic progenitor cells. Blood. 1997;90(9):3438–43.
92. Claycombe K, King LE, Fraker PJ. A role for leptin in sustaining lymphopoiesis and myelopoiesis. Proc Natl Acad Sci USA. 2008;105(6):2017–21.
93. Moore SI, Huffnagle GB, Chen GH, White ES, Mancuso P. Leptin modulates neutrophil phagocytosis of *Klebsiella pneumoniae*. Infect Immun. 2003;71(7):4182–5.
94. Caldefie-Chezet F, Poulin A, Tridon A, Sion B, Vasson MP. Leptin: a potential regulator of polymorphonuclear neutrophil bactericidal action? J Leukoc Biol. 2001;69(3):414–8.
95. Bruno A, Conus S, Schmid I, Simon HU. Apoptotic pathways are inhibited by leptin receptor activation in neutrophils. J Immunol. 2005;174(12):8090–6.
96. Ottonello L, Gnerre P, Bertolotto M, Mancini M, Dapino P, Russo R, et al. Leptin as a uremic toxin interferes with neutrophil chemotaxis. J Am Soc Nephrol. 2004;15(9): 2366–72.
97. Caldefie-Chezet F, Poulin A, Vasson MP. Leptin regulates functional capacities of polymorphonuclear neutrophils. Free Radic Res. 2003;37(8):809–14.
98. Montecucco F, Bianchi G, Gnerre P, Bertolotto M, Dallegri F, Ottonello L. Induction of neutrophil chemotaxis by leptin: crucial role for p38 and Src kinases. Ann N Y Acad Sci. 2006;1069: 463–71.
99. Bruno A, Chanez P, Chiappara G, Siena L, Giammanco S, Gjomarkaj M, et al. Does leptin play a cytokine-like role within the airways of COPD patients? Eur Respir J. 2005;26(3):398–405.

100. Vernooy JH, Drummen NE, van Suylen RJ, Cloots RH, Moller GM, Bracke KR, et al. Enhanced pulmonary leptin expression in patients with severe COPD and asymptomatic smokers. Thorax. 2009;64(1):26–32.
101. Torpy DJ, Bornstein SR, Chrousos GP. Leptin and interleukin-6 in sepsis. Horm Metab Res. 1998;30(12):726–9.
102. Arnalich F, Lopez J, Codoceo R, Jim nez M, Madero R, Montiel C. Relationship of plasma leptin to plasma cytokines and human survival in sepsis and septic shock. J Infect Dis. 1999;180(3):908–11.
103. Yousef AA, Amr YM, Suliman GA. The diagnostic value of serum leptin monitoring and its correlation with tumor necrosis factor-alpha in critically ill patients: a prospective observational study. Crit Care. 2010;14(2):R33.
104. Gattinoni L, Chiumello D, Carlesso E, Valenza F. Bench-to-bedside review: chest wall elastance in acute lung injury/acute respiratory distress syndrome patients. Crit Care. 2004;8(5):350–5.
105. Hess DR, Bigatello LM. The chest wall in acute lung injury/acute respiratory distress syndrome. Curr Opin Crit Care. 2008;14(1):94–102.
106. Berenholtz SM, Pronovost PJ, Lipsett PA, Hobson D, Earsing K, Farley JE, et al. Eliminating catheter-related bloodstream infections in the intensive care unit. Crit Care Med. 2004;32(10):2014–20.
107. Drakulovic MB, Torres A, Bauer TT, Nicolas JM, Nogue S, Ferrer M. Supine body position as a risk factor for nosocomial pneumonia in mechanically ventilated patients: a randomised trial. Lancet. 1999;354(9193):1851–8.
108. Burns SM, Egloff MB, Ryan B, Carpenter R, Burns JE. Effect of body position on spontaneous respiratory rate and tidal volume in patients with obesity, abdominal distension and ascites. Am J Crit Care. 1994;3(2):102–6.

Chapter 11
Mechanical Ventilation of Patients with Severe Obesity

Mikhail Litinski, Robert L. Owens, and Atul Malhotra

Abstract In recent years, obesity has become endemic in developed countries. Medical care of the obese patient is extremely challenging, especially critically ill obese individuals. The challenge of providing medical care to obese patients is multifactorial and stems from difficulty performing diagnostic and therapeutic procedures, difficulty providing logistical support, and the necessity of extrapolating data usually obtained from the study of leaner populations. Obesity affects respiratory physiology and also predisposes to obstructive sleep apnea (OSA) and obesity hypoventilation syndrome (OHS). As a result, patients with obesity may be at higher risk for respiratory failure and greater duration of mechanical ventilation.

Keywords Obesity • Mechanical ventilation • Mechanical ventilation • Obstructive sleep apnea • Obesity hypoventilation syndrome • Pulmonary function test • Positive end-expiratory pressure • Acute respiratory distress syndrome • Weaning from mechanical ventilation

M. Litinski, M.D. (✉)
Department of Surgery, Saint Barnabas Medical Center,
94 Old Short Hills Road, Livingston, NJ 07039, USA
e-mail: mlitinski@barnabashealth.org

R.L. Owens, M.D.
Divisions of Sleep and Pulmonary and Critical Care Medicine, Brigham and Women's Hospital, 221 Longwood Avenue, BLI 035Q, Boston, MA 02115, USA
e-mail: rowens@partners.org

A. Malhotra, M.D.
Department of Medicine, Brigham and Women's Hospital and Harvard Medical School, 75 Francis Street, Boston, MA 02115, USA
e-mail: amalhotra1@partners.org

A.E. Dixon and E.M. Clerisme-Beaty (eds.), *Obesity and Lung Disease: A Guide to Management*, Respiratory Medicine, DOI 10.1007/978-1-62703-053-3_11,

Objectives

- Review the effects of obesity on lung function and upper airway mechanics.
- Describe the mechanisms of benefit of CPAP/NIPPV in obesity.
- Review strategies to minimize intubation and postintubation complications in obese patients.
- Describe strategies for mechanical ventilation in obese patients.

Introduction

In recent years, obesity has emerged as one of the most prevalent epidemics in developed countries [1]. Obesity has a multitude of associated pathological consequences and places afflicted individuals at high risk for medical and surgical complications. Obese patients in the intensive care unit (ICU) may suffer prolonged duration of mechanical ventilation and ICU length of stay [2]. In response, medical societies have created management recommendations for patients with obesity based on existing data and expert opinion where data are sparse [3]. The goal of this chapter is to summarize the physiological consequences of obesity to enable the practioner to avoid complications of mechanical ventilation and to optimize management of obesity-related conditions, such as obstructive sleep apnea (OSA) and obesity hypoventilation syndrome (OHS). Individualizing therapy based on these physiological principles holds promise for the future as clinical trials are ongoing using this approach.

Influence of Obesity on Lung Function

Obesity is defined as body mass index (BMI) greater than 30 kg/m^2. Obesity alters respiratory physiology in a number of unfavorable ways, including decreased lung volumes, increased airway resistance, decreased total respiratory system compliance, and decreased gas exchange. Moreover, upper airway physiology is also affected. As will be discussed below, obesity is also the dominant risk factor for OSA, and both obesity and OSA are generally necessary to develop obesity hypoventilation syndrome (OHS) [4, 5]. Thus, before discussing mechanical ventilation in such patients, an understanding of obesity-related physiological changes is critical.

Lung Volumes

The three factors that determine lung volume at any given point of the respiratory cycle are respiratory muscle activity, and chest wall and lung tissue recoil forces. In morbidly obese subjects, the chest wall has decreased outward recoil due to

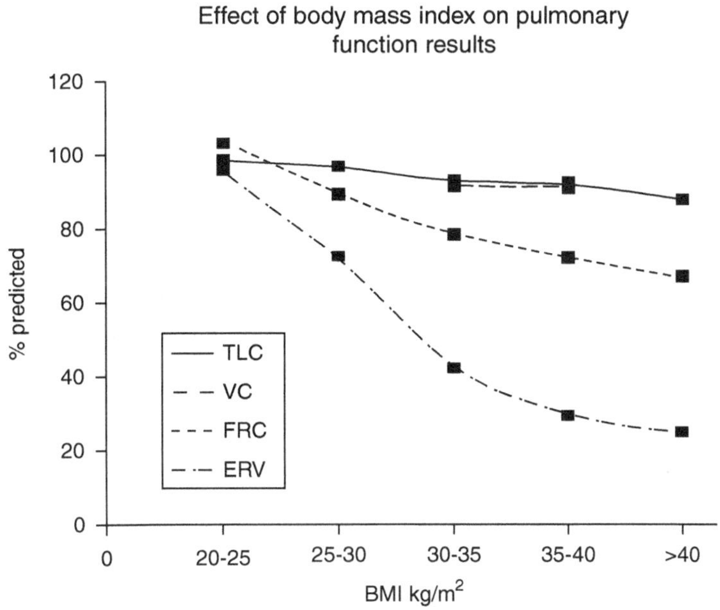

Fig. 11.1 Effect of body mass index on pulmonary function results (Adapted from Berger et al. [8])

greater weight, leading to decreased functional residual capacity (FRC). FRC is comprised of expiratory reserve volume (ERV), the maximum volume that can be exhaled with the use of respiratory muscles after normal exhalation, and residual volume (RV), the gas that stays in the lungs after ERV is expelled. In severely obese individuals, ERV may be substantially reduced causing FRC to approach residual volume [6]. However, in relatively healthy obese individuals, total lung capacity (TLC) and vital capacity (VC) are less vulnerable to the effects of obesity (Fig. 11.1), with TLC being reduced only in the extremes of obesity. This pattern of reduced FRC with relatively preserved RV is in contrast to pulmonary parenchymal causes of restriction (e.g., fibrosis) in which RV and FRC are both reduced. Thus, the combination of severely decreased ERV and normal or only modestly decreased TLC and VC on lung volume testing is the expected change in obese patients.

Resistance, Compliance, and Lung Function

In addition to gross changes in lung volume, obesity also causes changes in airflow. For example, airway resistance is inversely related to airway size, which is a function of lung volume. As lung volume decreases, airway resistance increases precipitously according to the Poiseuille equation (in which resistance increases with decreases in airway radius by the fourth or fifth power, depending on laminar or turbulent flow).

Moreover, increased chest weight can cause elevated pleural pressures, which can lead to atelectasis and airway closure even during tidal breathing [7]. These abnormalities can in turn lead to V/Q mismatch and shunt, yielding hypoxemia.

Obesity, the Upper Airway, and Obstructive Sleep Apnea

OSA is characterized by recurrent collapse of the upper airway during sleep, leading to intermittent hypoxemia and sleep fragmentation. Obesity is the key risk factor for OSA. Although the exact mechanism(s) is not known, one possible explanation is anatomical compromise of the pharyngeal airway due to increased peripharyngeal fat deposition. In this model, increased fat deposition increases the extraluminal pressure, increasing the tendency for airway collapse. During wakefulness, OSA patients are able to offset this increased collapsibility by increased activity of pharyngeal dilator muscles. However, during sleep (or anesthesia), dilator muscle activity falls and repetitive apnea becomes evident. CPAP is effective in eliminating obstructive events since it acts as a pneumatic splint to prevent collapse of the upper airway by raising its transmural pressure.

Obesity Hypoventilation Syndrome

OHS is another syndrome associated with obesity. Because the vast majority (>90%) of OHS patients have concomitant OSA, many people consider these two conditions to be a spectrum of one disease. OHS is defined by hypoventilation ($P_{CO2}>45$ mmHg) in the setting of obesity (BMI>30 kg/m^2) without other underlying cause such as parenchymal lung disease or neuromuscular abnormality. OHS patients have increased work of breathing for the reasons listed above: increased upper and lower airway resistance and mass loading of the chest wall and abdomen.

Some data suggest that hypoventilation occurs during sleep with gradual retention of CO_2 over time: the ventilatory response is inadequate for the accumulation of CO_2 such that gradual elevations in serum bicarbonate and daytime $PaCO_2$ eventually occur [8]. Although this is the classical explanation for OHS, several other interesting hypotheses deserve mention. An alternative hypothesis is that OSA may cause hypoxic or inflammatory injury that leads to respiratory muscle dysfunction. OHS may also be a result of decreased drive to breathe since OHS patients demonstrate impaired central respiratory drive, including diminished responsiveness to hypoxic and hypercapnic stimuli, although it is not clear if this finding is a cause or result of OHS [9, 10]. Of interest is that many patients with OHS often present with acute on chronic respiratory failure to the intensive care unit [11]. Lastly, more recent data suggest that obese individuals exhibit resistance to leptin at a receptor level. Leptin was first described as a hormone secreted by adipose tissue and primarily involved in regulation of appetite [12]. More recently, it has been appreciated that leptin also has a role in regulation of ventilation. For example, leptin infusion increases minute ventilation in leptin-deficient mice, even before there has been any change in weight [13]. In humans, serum leptin is a better predictor of hypoventilation than BMI, and treatment of OHS can lead to reductions in serum leptin [14, 15]. However, further data are clearly needed.

Physiological Effects of CPAP/NIPPV

Noninvasive ventilation is increasingly used in clinical practice and counteracts many of the physiological effects of obesity. Continuous positive airway pressure (CPAP) can be applied over the nose or nose and mouth. CPAP can counterbalance the collapsing forces acting on the upper airway and acts as a pneumatic splint. Additionally, application of positive pressure increases FRC, which prevents lower airway closure and atelectasis. Cumulatively, these effects improve oxygenation. In addition to positive expiratory pressure, NIPPV also applies a driving pressure during spontaneous inspiration which augments the effect of inspiratory muscle activity. Thus, bi-level PAP can be used to increase ventilation and decrease work of breathing. NIPPV can be delivered via a bi-level PAP device or via a critical care mechanical ventilator – some devices have features of both. On more advanced machines, various independent variables can be manipulated, including pressure – or volume-targeted modes, trigger sensitivity, inspiratory time, rise time, etc.

A new mode of NIPPV was developed combining features of pressure-targeted and volume-cycled ventilation. Average volume-assured pressure support (AVAPS) is able to adjust pressure support to deliver a fixed average tidal volume. The role of AVAPS in the management of OHS or respiratory failure is being evaluated, with some data suggesting potential benefit in small cohorts [16].

Management of Obese Patients Before and During Intubation

Recognizing an ever growing number of patients suffering from obesity-related comorbidities, the American Society of Anesthesiologists published guidelines on perioperative management of patients with OSA [17]. A focus of these recommendations was to minimize complications during intubation and to avoid prolonged mechanical ventilation and extubation failures. The principles of perioperative management in the morbidly obese were: preoperative diagnosing of OSA, use of CPAP in perioperative period, use of regional rather than general anesthesia whenever possible, meticulous reversal of neuromuscular blockade, use of lateral rather than supine positioning, and extended close monitoring in the postoperative period (see Table 11.1). While most of these ASA recommendations require rigorous corroboration, we believe that they reflect sound physiological principles. For example, lateral posture may well improve end-expiratory lung volume, upper

Table 11.1 Summary of measures which can be undertaken to minimize respiratory complications in patients with OSA in perioperative period (Adopted from ref [17])

Preoperative preparation	Intraoperative management	Postoperative management
1. Establish the diagnosis of OSA 2. Preoperative initiation of CPAP or NIV	1. Local anesthesia and peripheral nerve block should be used where applicable	1. Use of NSAIDs as opioid sparing medication for post-op analgesia when feasible
3. If unable to tolerate CPAP or NIV preoperatively, alternative treatment for OSA should be initiated (weight loss, oral devices, etc.)	2. Ventilation should be continuously monitored throughout the entire procedure when moderate sedation or greater levels of sedation used	2. Utilization of CPAP or NIV in patients who were using it preoperatively as soon as possible after the surgery 3. Use supplemental oxygen to avoid hypoxemia
4. Difficult airway management algorithm resources available	3. General anesthesia with secured airway preferred over deep sedation without secured airway 4. Patients with OSA should be extubated while awake whenever feasible 5. Full reversal of neuromuscular blockade should be ascertained before extubation 6. Extubation should performed in nonsupine position	4. Avoid supine position during sleep if possible

airway patency and collapsibility, result in improved gas exchange, and may reduce aspiration risk. Also, medications used for sedation and anesthesia frequently compromise upper airway motor control in addition to their effects on respiratory pump muscles. Thus, postextubation patients both in the OR and in the ICU may be at particularly high risk of upper airway compromise. Upper airway compromise may also have important clinical consequences. In a case–control study design, Gupta et al. showed that patients with unrecognized OSA have a higher rate of postoperative complications after knee and hip replacement surgery than those who were treated with PAP prior to the procedure [18]. Complications included increased length of ICU stay, cardiac events, and reintubation. While safety comparison trials of regional and general anesthesia are lacking to the best of our knowledge in obese subjects, use of regional anesthesia appears to be safer as it offers less pronounced hemodynamic and respiratory suppressive effects [19]. In regard to the different positions during surgical procedures in obese individuals and its physiological effect on cardiopulmonary system, a thorough review is available; however, specific studies to address this question are lacking [20].

Obesity and Intubation

To answer specific questions regarding morbidity and mortality conferred by severe obesity and its comorbidities in the perioperative period, the Longitudinal Assessment of Bariatric Surgery Consortium group examined perioperative risk factors in a prospective, multicenter observational study of patients undergoing bariatric surgery. Using a composite endpoint of death, need for reintervention, and thromboembolism, the authors found that comorbid OSA was associated independently with a significantly higher rate of postoperative complications [21]. Thus, preoperative screening for OSA and perioperative CPAP use have been advocated, although as of yet there are no compelling clinical trial data to confirm the wisdom of this approach. Definitive data on perioperative risk of obesity and sleep apnea are difficult to acquire given the low incidence of serious complications with modern anesthesia. In addition anesthesiologists may adapt their clinical practice to manage patients with obesity and suspected OSA. For example, Mallampati score and neck circumference are important factors in anesthetic assessment, but may also be markers of OSA [22]. Thus, the current standard of care may already manage OSA patients adequately, although further data are certainly required.

Securing the airway in the obese patient can be challenging, even for the most experienced anesthetist. Obesity has been shown in some studies to be a risk factor for having a difficult airway, defined as problems with therapeutic manipulations of the airway (i.e., bag-mask ventilation, direct laryngoscopy and endotracheal intubation, need for surgical airway) [23–25]. As such, establishing an airway in an obese patient may be difficult, and success is often based on a correct initial risk assessment and a well-thought-out induction plan.

Endotracheal (ET) intubation is recommended as the most secure artificial airway. Several factors may complicate endotracheal intubation in obese patients. During preparation for ET intubation, obesity may complicate bag-mask ventilation by several mechanisms. First, excess soft tissue can make bag-mask ventilation difficult. Using a 2-person technique during bag-mask ventilation has been shown to improve ventilation, probably by minimizing air leak [26]. Use of nasal trumpets and oral airways may also be helpful. Second, reduced FRC contributes to rapid oxygen desaturation. Reverse Trendelenburg positioning during bag-mask ventilation may alleviate this situation to some degree, improving upper airway patency and chest wall mechanics, thus increasing FRC and oxygen reserve. Using preoxygenation with near 100% oxygen concentration may provide additional oxygen reserve in preparation for ET intubation, although whether preoxygenation increases resorptive atelectasis in obese patients is unclear. Third, obesity may be an independent risk factor for difficult intubation as a result of limited neck mobility, mouth opening, and tracheal as well as hypopharyngeal anatomy distortion. Several studies have been conducted to identify the position of obese patients that would allow optimal visualization of the vocal cords. The "ramp position" with head elevated appeared to be superior to sniffing and supine positions [27, 28]. While rapid sequence intubation is not contraindicated in obese patients, its use in obesity should be done with caution, due to the possibility of the "can't intubate, can't ventilate" scenario. For obese patients, an awake fiberoptic intubation is preferred since it avoids neuromuscular blockade and may use only minimal or moderate sedation. The pharmacodynamics and pharmacokinetics of neuromuscular blocking (NMB) agents as well as sedatives and analgesics may be altered in obese individuals due to increases in the glomerular filtration rate and volume of distribution [29].

Mechanical Ventilation in Obese Patients

Once intubated, the initial selection of the parameters for mechanical ventilation in obese patients may be a challenging task due to alterations of pulmonary physiology in this patient population. For example, commonly used initial positive end-expiratory pressure (PEEP) settings may allow alveolar derecruitment and contribute to hypoxemia. Understanding the impact of obesity on the chest wall is critical in this regard.

Transpulmonary Versus Plateau Pressure for Selecting Ventilator Setting in Obese Patients

Although airway pressure is commonly used as a convenient measure, the critical pressure in terms of barotrauma and atelectasis is the transpulmonary pressure. Transpulmonary pressure is the difference between airway and pleural pressure. The transpulmonary pressure has been confirmed as the relevant physiological measurement in experiments in which the chest wall was cast [30, 31]. In these experiments, a high P_{plat} alone did not cause lung overdistension and injury, so long as the pleural pressures were also elevated. Although pleural pressure effects may be negligible in healthy, lean individuals, in severely obese patients, pleural pressure effects may be quite pronounced due to the weight of the chest wall and abdomen. Pleural pressure can be estimated by esophageal manometry which when situated in the lower third of esophagus gives an approximate estimate of midthoracic pleural pressure. Use of pleural pressure estimates can provide reassurance against overdistension during inspiration by keeping peak inflation transpulmonary pressure below 25 cmH_2O (see Fig. 11.2) [32, 33].

Role of PEEP in Preventing Complications of Mechanical Ventilation in Obese Patients

In addition, during the expiratory phase of the respiratory cycle, elevated pleural pressure in obese individuals may promote atelectasis in the dependent areas (e.g., posterior segments). This situation creates areas of heterogeneity within the

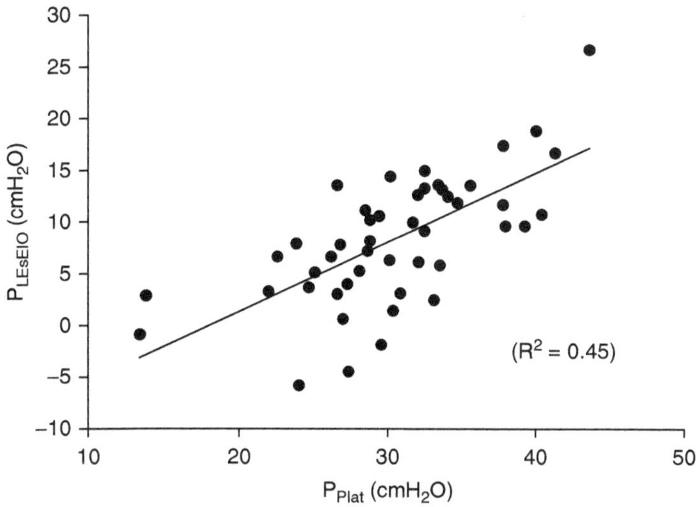

Fig. 11.2 Plateau pressure (Pplat) is an imperfect surrogate for inspiratory transpulmonary pressure (PLEsEIO). Some patients with higher pleural pressure will have high Pplat even with a low transpulmonary pressure (Adapted from Loring et al. [35])

lung tissue even in the absence of prominent lung injury. Previous studies have estimated that the effective pressure gradient between atelectatic and normal lung regions may reach >100 cmH_2O even when the applied airway pressure does not exceed 30 cmH_2O due to high shear forces at the junctions of normal and abnormal lung [34]. This scenario may contribute to so-called atelectrauma in which repetitive alveolar collapse has been postulated to contribute to lung injury and systemic inflammation.

One of the ways to alleviate the above pathophysiological phenomenon is to promote lung homogeneity by applying appropriate PEEP, which can prevent alveolar collapse at end-exhalation and thus keep alveoli open throughout the respiratory cycle. Adequate PEEP should decrease areas of atelectasis and heterogeneity, improving gas exchange and decreasing the risk for shear force injury resulting from repetition of the opening and closing of atelectatic alveoli during respiratory cycle. However, it is important to use the appropriate level of PEEP, as suboptimal levels will not fully prevent derecruitment, and excessive levels may promote overdistension and hemodynamic compromise. Obese patients may require high PEEP levels to offset the effect of high pleural pressure at the end of expiration. That is, with typical initial ventilator settings, the end-expiratory transpulmonary pressure could be negative (see Fig. 11.3) [35]. Given the unpredictability of obesity effects on respiratory mechanics, we favor an individualized physiological approach to mechanical ventilation, rather than "one size fits all" [36]. Titrating PEEP to a positive end-expiratory transpulmonary pressure can lead to improved gas exchange [32]. Although measurement of esophageal pressure may be beneficial, the strategy is lacking definitive data and outcome data are still emerging. Therefore, in clinical

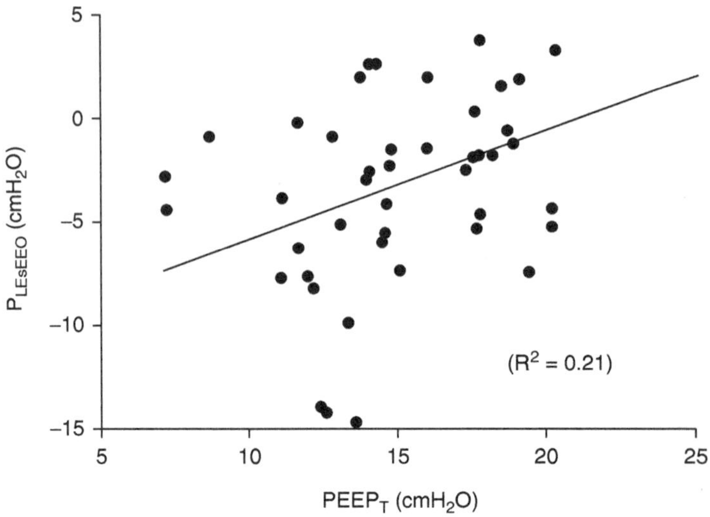

Fig. 11.3 Even modest level of extrinsic PEEP may not prevent a negative transpulmonary pressure at end-expiration in those with high pleural pressure. PEEP positive end-expiratory pressure, PEEPT extrinsic PEEP, PLEsEEO transpulmonary pressure estimated by esophageal manometry at end-expiration (Adapted from Loring et al. [35])

practice, titration of ventilator settings based on gas exchange is commonly used due to its simplicity. A variety of methods have been discussed in terms of PEEP titration including the pressure/volume curve, the so-called stress index, and imaging techniques, among others. One of the early attempts to identify best strategy of mechanical ventilation in ARDS patients, undertaken by Amato et al., used the lower inflection point of the respiratory pressure-volume curve to set PEEP. In combination with other lung protective strategies, this method for setting PEEP was associated with improved survival compared to a conventional mechanical ventilatory approach [37]. The ideal method of PEEP titration however remains unclear. Caramez et al., tried to answer this question by using an animal model of ARDS. The authors compared the relationship of nine variables to the "open-lung PEEP" value, represented in the study by the PEEP at the best dynamic tidal respiratory compliance. Various estimates of optimal PEEP based on mechanics or gas exchange all yielded similar values [38].

Effect of PEEP Applied during Mechanical Ventilation on Respiratory Parameters

Clinically, there have been three very large randomized trials of the effect of low vs. high PEEP on mortality in ARDS, with applied PEEP levels set based on oxygenation tables rather than lung mechanics [39–41]. All of the trials showed improved compliance, gas exchange, and decreased FiO_2 requirements in the high PEEP groups, although there was no effect on mortality. Unfortunately none of the above studies were designed to assess the impact of body weight on respiratory mechanics or PEEP settings. Regardless, in our experience, BMI is a poor predictor of end-expiratory esophageal pressure in the critically ill, emphasizing the need for physiological measurements rather than estimates based on demographics. A recently published trial assessed the potential benefits of titrating PEEP adjusted for pleural pressure compared with PEEP titration based on ARDS network recommendations. Both groups received low tidal volume ventilation and were heavily sedated or paralyzed. This trial showed improved oxygenation, respiratory compliance, and a trend toward improved survival in the transpulmonary pressure directed group [32]. Obese patients may potentially be at special advantage for individualized ventilator settings as pleural pressure is often elevated (although unpredictably) in this patient population. Pleural pressure elevations in critically ill patients with obesity are a function of intra-abdominal pressures, which are often elevated but, again, highly variable. Malbrain conducted a prevalence study of intra-abdominal hypertension in 97 critically ill patients in 13 ICUs. While no difference was found between intra-abdominal pressure (IAP) in surgical and medical patients, patients with higher BMI demonstrated significantly higher IAP. Other factors including fluid accumulation can raise intra-abdominal pressure, and thus obesity alone is unlikely to be a method to guide therapy. However, BMI was the only independent predictor of IAP in a multivariate analysis. Larger randomized trials, which would specifically include obese individuals with sophisticated physiological measurements, are needed to shed light on this subject [42]. Another source of variability is the degree to which elevated abdominal pressures are transmitted to the thorax [43].

Another important aspect of mechanical ventilation in obese patients is the concept of predicted body weight. The ARDS Network trial showed that ventilation of ARDS patients with tidal volume of 6 ml/kg of *predicted* body weight has survival benefit over ventilation with tidal volume of 12 ml/kg [44]. Lung volume is proportional to height (and influenced by sex and race) but not to weight. Calculating tidal volume based on actual body weight may lead to alveolar overdistension and barotrauma.

Weaning Obese Individuals from Mechanical Ventilation: The Role of NIPPV

The process of weaning patients from mechanical ventilation should be considered as soon as possible to avoid morbidity and mortality associated with prolonged intubation [45]. Obese patients may be at high risk for failure of liberation from mechanical ventilation for several reasons. Even in normal weight individuals, in the immediate postextubation period, patients may have impaired central ventilatory drive and protective airway reflexes due to general anesthesia or sedation. These sedative agents might accumulate in adipose tissue and be

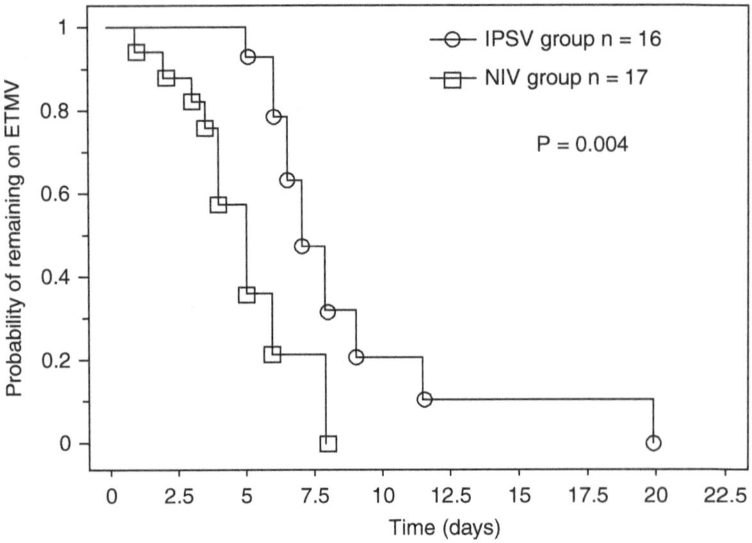

Fig. 11.4 Cumulative probability of remaining on endotracheal mechanical ventilation (ETMV) in the invasive pressure support ventilation (IPSV) and the noninvasive ventilation (NV) weaning group (From Girault et al. [49]; reprinted with permission of the American Thoracic Society. Copyright © 2011 American Thoracic Society)

slower to clear in obese patients. Prolonged endotracheal intubation may potentially lead to impairment of pharyngeal protective mechanisms and contribute to upper airway compromise postextubation in those patients already predisposed to upper airway collapse. The endotracheal tube may irritate the pharyngeal mucosa which could compromise the integrity of upper airway mechanoreceptors critical to mediating the negative pressure reflex [46]. Not surprisingly, obesity has been noted to be a risk factor for failed fast-track extubation in patients after coronary bypass surgery and abdominal aortic aneurysm repair [47, 48].

Using NIPPV in the early postextubation period may help to overcome the aforementioned difficulties in liberation from mechanical ventilation in obese patients. Girault et al. evaluated 53 consecutive patients in a prospective randomized controlled trial who presented with acute on chronic respiratory failure and who required initial endotracheal intubation [49]. All patients failed T-piece trials, even though they met simple criteria for readiness for extubation, including demonstrating a rapid shallow breathing index (RSBI) less than 105 breaths/l. Utilization of NIPPV early after extubation significantly reduced the duration of invasive mechanical ventilation and was successful in preventing reintubation (Fig. 11.4). No effect of BMI was reported on either of the above outcomes. Based on the notion that larger end-expiratory lung volume may improve upper airway patency in obese individuals with OSA, reverse Trendelenburg position may also be a helpful adjunct to NIPPV in the early postextubation period in obese individuals [50].

Conclusion

The obesity pandemic has raised important challenges for society, including respiratory and critical care physicians. Mechanical ventilation of critically ill obese patients requires detailed knowledge of pulmonary pathophysiology, patient-ventilator interaction, and the modulating effect of obesity. Despite substantial advances made in these areas recently, numerous questions remained unanswered. The best strategy to avoid ventilator-induced lung injury, including barotrauma and atelectrauma, in obese patients remains to be proven. Another remaining question concerns the best way to identify optimal PEEP to avoid atelectrauma and maintain optimal alveolar recruitment. We would advocate for further research into the individualized care of the obese patient, possibly using esophageal manometry, and the role of NIPPV.

References

1. McTigue K, Larson JC, Valoski A, Burke G, Kotchen J, Lewis CE, et al. Mortality and cardiac and vascular outcomes in extremely obese women. JAMA. 2006;296(1):79–86.
2. Akinnusi ME, Pineda LA, El Solh AA. Effect of obesity on intensive care morbidity and mortality: a meta-analysis. Crit Care Med. 2008;36(1):151–8.
3. Dixon AE, Holguin F, Sood A, Salome CM, Pratley RE, Beuther DA, et al. An official American thoracic society workshop report: obesity and asthma. Proc Am Thorac Soc. 2010;7(5):325–35.
4. Eckert DJ, Malhotra A. Pathophysiology of adult obstructive sleep apnea. Proc Am Thorac Soc. 2008;5(2):144–53.
5. Koenig SM. Pulmonary complications of obesity. Am J Med Sci. 2001;321(4):249–79.
6. Biring MS, Lewis MI, Liu JT, Mohsenifar Z. Pulmonary physiologic changes of morbid obesity. Am J Med Sci. 1999;318(5):293–7.
7. Rubinstein I, Zamel N, DuBarry L, Hoffstein V. Airflow limitation in morbidly obese, nonsmoking men. Ann Intern Med. 1990;112(11):828–32.
8. Berger KI, Norman RG, Ayappa I, Oppenheimer BW, Rapoport DM, Goldring RM. Potential mechanism for transition between acute hypercapnia during sleep to chronic hypercapnia during wakefulness in obstructive sleep apnea. Adv Exp Med Biol. 2008;605:431–6.
9. Zwillich CW, Sutton FD, Pierson DJ, Greagh EM, Weil JV. Decreased hypoxic ventilatory drive in the obesity-hypoventilation syndrome. Am J Med. 1975;59(3):343–8.
10. Sampson MG, Grassino K. Neuromechanical properties in obese patients during carbon dioxide rebreathing. Am J Med. 1983;75(1):81–90.
11. Lee WY, Mokhlesi B. Diagnosis and management of obesity hypoventilation syndrome in the ICU. Crit Care Clin. 2008;24(3):533–49. vii.
12. Mantzoros CS. The role of leptin in human obesity and disease: a review of current evidence. Ann Intern Med. 1999;130(8):671–80.
13. O'Donnell CP, Schaub CD, Haines AS, Berkowitz DE, Tankersley CG, Schwartz AR, et al. Leptin prevents respiratory depression in obesity. Am J Respir Crit Care Med. 1999;159 (5 Pt 1):1477–84.
14. Yee BJ, Cheung J, Phipps P, Banerjee D, Piper AJ, Grunstein RR. Treatment of obesity hypoventilation syndrome and serum leptin. Respiration. 2006;73(2):209–12.
15. Phipps PR, Starritt E, Caterson I, Grunstein RR. Association of serum leptin with hypoventilation in human obesity. Thorax. 2002;57(1):75–6.
16. Storre JH, Seuthe B, Fiechter R, Milioglou S, Dreher M, Sorichter S, et al. Average volume-assured pressure support in obesity hypoventilation: a randomized crossover trial. Chest. 2006; 130(3):815–21.

17. Gross JB, Bachenberg KL, Benumof JL, Caplan RA, Connis RT, Cote CJ, et al. Practice guidelines for the perioperative management of patients with obstructive sleep apnea: a report by the American Society of Anesthesiologists Task Force on perioperative management of patients with obstructive sleep apnea. Anesthesiology. 2006;104(5):1081–93. quiz 117–8.
18. Gupta RM, Parvizi J, Hanssen AD, Gay PC. Postoperative complications in patients with obstructive sleep apnea syndrome undergoing hip or knee replacement: a case–control study. Mayo Clin Proc. 2001;76(9):897–905.
19. Passannante AN, Tielborg M. Anesthetic management of patients with obesity with and without sleep apnea. Clin Chest Med. 2009;30(3):569–79.
20. Brodsky JB. Positioning the morbidly obese patient for anesthesia. Obes Surg. 2002;12(6):751–8.
21. Flum DR, Belle SH, King WC, Wahed AS, Berk P, Chapman W, et al. Perioperative safety in the longitudinal assessment of bariatric surgery. N Engl J Med. 2009;361(5):445–54.
22. Davies RJ, Stradling JR. The relationship between neck circumference, radiographic pharyngeal anatomy, and the obstructive sleep apnoea syndrome. Eur Respir J. 1990;3(5):509–14.
23. Adams JP, Murphy PG. Obesity in anaesthesia and intensive care. Br J Anaesth. 2000;85(1): 91–108.
24. Fox GS, Whalley DG, Bevan DR. Anaesthesia for the morbidly obese. Experience with 110 patients. Br J Anaesth. 1981;53(8):811–6.
25. Juvin P, Lavaut E, Dupont H, Lefevre P, Demetriou M, Dumoulin JL, et al. Difficult tracheal intubation is more common in obese than in lean patients. Anesth Analg. 2003;97(2):595–600.
26. Davidovic L, LaCovey D, Pitetti RD. Comparison of 1- versus 2-person bag-valve-mask techniques for manikin ventilation of infants and children. Ann Emerg Med. 2005;46(1):37–42.
27. Collins JS, Lemmens HJ, Brodsky JB, Brock-Utne JG, Levitan RM. Laryngoscopy and morbid obesity: a comparison of the "sniff" and "ramped" positions. Obes Surg. 2004;14(9):1171–5.
28. Lee BJ, Kang JM, Kim DO. Laryngeal exposure during laryngoscopy is better in the 25 degrees back-up position than in the supine position. Br J Anaesth. 2007;99(4):581–6.
29. Chagnac A, Weinstein T, Korzets A, Ramadan E, Hirsch J, Gafter U. Glomerular hemodynamics in severe obesity. Am J Physiol. 2000;278(5):F817–22.
30. Hernandez LA, Peevy KJ, Moise AA, Parker JC. Chest wall restriction limits high airway pressure-induced lung injury in young rabbits. J Appl Physiol. 1989;66(5):2364–8.
31. Dreyfuss D, Saumon G. Ventilator-induced lung injury: lessons from experimental studies. Am J Respir Crit Care Med. 1998;157(1):294–323.
32. Talmor D, Sarge T, Malhotra A, O'Donnell CR, Ritz R, Lisbon A, et al. Mechanical ventilation guided by esophageal pressure in acute lung injury. N Engl J Med. 2008;359(20):2095–104.
33. Pelosi P, Chiumello D, Calvi E, Taccone P, Bottino N, Panigada M, et al. Effects of different continuous positive airway pressure devices and periodic hyperinflations on respiratory function. Crit Care Med. 2001;29(9):1683–9.
34. Mead J, Takishima T, Leith D. Stress distribution in lungs: a model of pulmonary elasticity. J Appl Physiol. 1970;28(5):596–608.
35. Loring SH, O'Donnell CR, Behazin N, Malhotra A, Sarge T, Ritz R, et al. Esophageal pressures in acute lung injury: do they represent artifact or useful information about transpulmonary pressure, chest wall mechanics, and lung stress? J Appl Physiol. 2010;108(3):515–22.
36. Malhotra A. Low-tidal-volume ventilation in the acute respiratory distress syndrome. N Engl J Med. 2007;357(11):1113–20.
37. Amato MB, Barbas CS, Medeiros DM, Magaldi RB, Schettino GP, Lorenzi-Filho G, et al. Effect of a protective-ventilation strategy on mortality in the acute respiratory distress syndrome. N Engl J Med. 1998;338(6):347–54.
38. Caramez MP, Kacmarek RM, Helmy M, Miyoshi E, Malhotra A, Amato MB, et al. A comparison of methods to identify open-lung PEEP. Intensive Care Med. 2009;35(4):740–7.
39. Brower RG, Lanken PN, MacIntyre N, Matthay MA, Morris A, Ancukiewicz M, et al. Higher versus lower positive end-expiratory pressures in patients with the acute respiratory distress syndrome. N Engl J Med. 2004;351(4):327–36.
40. Meade MO, Cook DJ, Guyatt GH, Slutsky AS, Arabi YM, Cooper DJ, et al. Ventilation strategy using low tidal volumes, recruitment maneuvers, and high positive end-expiratory pressure for

acute lung injury and acute respiratory distress syndrome: a randomized controlled trial. JAMA. 2008;299(6):637–45.
41. Mercat A, Richard JC, Vielle B, Jaber S, Osman D, Diehl JL, et al. Positive end-expiratory pressure setting in adults with acute lung injury and acute respiratory distress syndrome: a randomized controlled trial. JAMA. 2008;299(6):646–55.
42. Malbrain ML, Chiumello D, Pelosi P, Wilmer A, Brienza N, Malcangi V, et al. Prevalence of intra-abdominal hypertension in critically ill patients: a multicentre epidemiological study. Intensive Care Med. 2004;30(5):822–9.
43. Owens RL, Harris RS, Malhotra A. Is the way to man's heart (and lung) through the abdomen? Crit Care (Lond). 2009;13(6):199.
44. The Acute Respiratory Distress Syndrome Network. Ventilation with lower tidal volumes as compared with traditional tidal volumes for acute lung injury and the acute respiratory distress syndrome. N Engl J Med. 2000;342(18):1301–8.
45. Heyland DK, Cook DJ, Griffith L, Keenan SP, Brun-Buisson C. The attributable morbidity and mortality of ventilator-associated pneumonia in the critically ill patient. The Canadian Critical Trials Group. Am J Respir Crit Care Med. 1999;159(4 Pt 1):1249–56.
46. Horner RL, Innes JA, Holden HB, Guz A. Afferent pathway(s) for pharyngeal dilator reflex to negative pressure in man: a study using upper airway anaesthesia. J Physiol. 1991;436: 31–44.
47. Parlow JL, Ahn R, Milne B. Obesity is a risk factor for failure of "fast track" extubation following coronary artery bypass surgery. Can J Anaesth. 2006;53(3):288–94.
48. Borracci RA, Dayan R, Rubio M, Axelrud G, Ochoa G, Rodriguez LD. Operating room extubation (ultra fast-track anesthesia) in patients undergoing on-pump and off-pump cardiac surgery. Arch Cardiol Mex. 2006;76(4):383–9.
49. Girault C, Daudenthun I, Chevron V, Tamion F, Leroy J, Bonmarchand G. Noninvasive ventilation as a systematic extubation and weaning technique in acute-on-chronic respiratory failure: a prospective, randomized controlled study. Am J Respir Crit Care Med. 1999;160(1):86–92.
50. Heinzer RC, Stanchina ML, Malhotra A, Fogel RB, Patel SR, Jordan AS, et al. Lung volume and continuous positive airway pressure requirements in obstructive sleep apnea. Am J Respir Crit Care Med. 2005;172(1):114–7.

Chapter 12
Obesity and Lung Health in Children

Jason E. Lang

Abstract Obesity among children has increased dramatically and has received considerable recent public health attention. The impact of obesity on lung health has become a recognized problem worldwide and an area of intense research. Obese children and adolescents are at greater risk for asthma, impaired lung mechanics, sleep-disordered breathing, and obesity hypoventilation syndrome. This chapter will discuss our current understanding of these conditions and will explore the possible mechanisms underlying the increased asthma risk among obese children. Obesity may influence the phenotypic characteristics of asthma. For example, obese children with asthma may have more difficulty achieving symptom control. We will explore the current knowledge of how obesity in childhood affects the complex disease characteristics of asthma.

Keywords Obesity • Overweight • Asthma • Lung function • Adipokine • Montelukast • Obesity hypoventilation • Obstructive sleep apnea

Objectives

- Review the impact of obesity on lung function in otherwise healthychildren.
- Understand the association and possible mechanisms linking obesitywith asthma development.
- Examine the current data on how obesity affects the asthma endotypeand management in children.
- Review how obesity affects sleep-disordered breathing andhypoventilation in children.

J.E. Lang, M.D. (✉)
Department of Pulmonology, Allergy & Immunology, Center for Pharmacogenomics & Translational Research, Mayo Clinic College of Medicine, Nemours Children's Clinic, 807 Children's Way, Jacksonville, FL 32207, USA
e-mail: jelang@nemours.org

A.E. Dixon and E.M. Clerisme-Beaty (eds.), *Obesity and Lung Disease: A Guide to Management*, Respiratory Medicine, DOI 10.1007/978-1-62703-053-3_12,

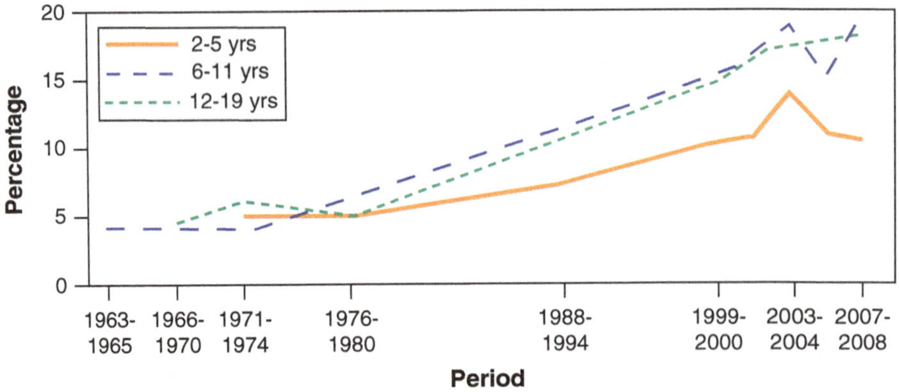

Fig. 12.1 Prevalence of obesity during childhood by age group – United States, 1963–2008. Obesity is defined as a body mass index ≥ 95th percentile for age and gender. (Taken from MMWR [159])

Introduction

Obesity is a serious public health problem among children. Obesity rates have increased dramatically among adults in past decades; however, the acceleration of obesity rates has been greatest among children [1, 2] (Fig. 12.1). Pediatric obesity is also not a problem limited to North America (Table 12.1). Worldwide, there are now more than 40 million children below the age of 5 who are overweight or obese [3, 4]. As the prevalence of obesity in children has risen, so has several obesity-related comorbidities – most notably diabetes, hypertension, and dyslipidemia. Obesity in children also negatively affects respiratory health and in ways that are often distinct from adults.

This chapter will address obesity's effect on respiratory health in otherwise healthy children. We will also discuss the link between obesity and both asthma risk and asthma phenotype – and how these relationships may be modified by other individual factors such as age, gender, and race. Obesity refers to an excessive amount of body fat. The nomenclature for pediatric obesity used by most experts is based on age and gender-based normative data involving the body mass index (BMI) [2, 5–7]. *Overweight* refers to a BMI above the 85th percentile of age – and gender-matched children, while *obesity* refers to a BMI > 95th percentile [8]. Though it is the most commonly accepted indicator of adiposity (fatness) in children above 2 years of age, body mass index (BMI) serves only as a surrogate because it measures the relationship between weight and height. Because BMI percentile and BMI z-scores both overestimate adiposity in shorter and more muscular children, BMI-based markers used in statistical analyses may obscure important relationships between adiposity and respiratory outcomes. There is some evidence that alternate measures that focus on actual total body fat (such as dual X-ray absorptiometry (DEXA) or air-displacement plethysmography) may be more useful. Since BMI-based measures in children

Table 12.1 International prevalences of childhood overweight

Country	Prevalence, %	Ages sampled	Source
Brazil [160]	27.6	10–17	Barbiero SM, Public Health Nutr (2009)
Italy [161]	33.4	9–13	Lazzeri G, J Prev Med Hyg (2008)
Japan [162]	20	6–13	Nakano, J Med Invest (2010)
Kuwait [163]	30.9	10–14	Al-Isa, Eur J Clin Nutr (2004)
New Zealand [164]	31	5–14	Utter J, Int J Pediatr Obes (2007)
Saudi Arabia [165]	34	5–18	El Mouzan MI, Ann Saudi Med (2010)
United Arab Emirates [166]	35.2	5–17	Malik Obes Rev (2007)
USA [2]	34.3	12–19	Odgen, JAMA (2006)

Overweight most commonly defined as a body mass index ≥ 85th percentile for age and gender

are greatly affected by skeletal muscle development and somatic growth, we may not be able to fully understand the effects of obesity on the respiratory system until more data exist utilizing more precise measures of adiposity.

Obesity and Respiratory Function in Healthy Children

Even among otherwise healthy children, obesity is associated with impaired respiratory function. Though some studies that examine the relationship between obesity and lung function focus specifically on pubertal or prepubertal cohorts, it is yet unclear how much age modifies the effect of obesity. It is possible that age and other individual factors such as sex, atopy status, and race may be important to consider in assessing the effect of obesity. However, to date, consistent patterns of effect modification have yet to become evident and may require very large cohorts to avoid false associations (type 1 errors). Among prepubescent children, obesity has been associated with greater chest symptoms such as breathlessness and cough [9] and greater objectively defined exercise-induced bronchospasm [10]. The exact cause of these findings is unclear. Compared with adults, the relationship between obesity and spirometric lung volumes in children is less consistent in the literature. Obesity has been associated with increased [11], decreased [12], and unchanged [9] spirometric lung volumes. There is also some evidence for an association between obesity in boys and airflow obstruction, and between obesity in girls and reduced vital capacity [12]. Airflow obstruction (represented by reduced FEV_1/FVC) has been a more consistent finding among obese children [11, 12] often with normal or even increased vital capacity. Age, pubertal status, and ethnicity may also be obesity effect modifying factors on lung function. For example, among obese Mexican–American youths, adolescents had a much stronger association with airflow obstruction compared to their school-age counterparts [11]. However, in a separate study looking at airway reactivity and symptom reporting, obese school-age children had greater exercise-induced airway reactivity [10] and chest symptoms [13].

Among otherwise healthy adolescents, evidence exists for obesity-related reductions in spirometric lung volumes and increases in airflow obstruction [11, 14–16]. These associations were present using surrogate measures of adiposity including BMI z-score, BMI percentile, DEXA total body fat percent, waist-height ratio, and skin-fold measures. Li and colleagues found that a significant percent of obese adolescents displayed reduced functional residual capacity, residual volume, and diffusing capacity for carbon monoxide (DLCO), but not airflow obstruction [17]. Li found the above changes in lung function only when determining obesity status using DEXA (and not when using BMI). Non-asthmatic obese adolescents, similar to younger children, may be more likely to have exercise-induced airway hyperreactivity [15, 18]. These studies involve small samples; however, at least some of these exercise-induced spirometry changes appear to result from airflow obstruction and not solely obesity-related muscle fatigue [18].

Explanations for these obesity-related patterns of lung dysfunction include occult asthma, restrictive lung and chest wall disease, respiratory muscle weakness, and lung growth alterations related to obesity. Alterations in the pattern of growth and development that associate with obesity may make up a set of confounding processes that impact the risk of reduced airway caliber. The lack of consistency in lung function changes noted above may stem from effect modification related to sex, race, socioeconomics, genetics, and specific obesity-related comorbidities. Much more analysis is required, involving larger samples that can adjust for these possible effect modifiers and that more accurately measure adiposity.

Obesity and Asthma Risk in Children

Like obesity, asthma has also increased in prevalence in recent decades, raising the question of a possible causal link between obesity and asthma. Many cross-sectional studies have documented an association between obesity and asthma. Cross-sectional analytic studies are valuable to establish associations and for hypothesis generation; however, they are inadequate for evaluating temporality or cause-effect relationships. Instead, longitudinal studies can better assess the sequence of risks and disease. More than 15 longitudinal cohort studies have been conducted in adults and children. When lean and obese non-asthmatics are followed prospectively, obese participants, almost universally, develop asthma at a higher rate. Obesity clearly increases the risk for new asthma diagnosis in adults [19–26] and children [27–33], though the precise nature of the association remains controversial [34–39].

Longitudinal Cohort Studies

Assessing risk for asthma requires prospectively following an at-risk cohort (e.g., obese) and a non at-risk cohort (e.g., nonobese) for the development of the condition in question (asthma) and cannot rely on cross-sectional or case–control studies [40]. The current literature includes several high-quality cohort studies among diverse populations that have assessed the risk of incident asthma among lean and obese children [27–33]. These studies involve children of varying age, geography, socioeconomic status, and race/ethnicity. Across the span of pediatric ages, overweight status appears to increase the risk for incident asthma. Although the risk ratios vary among studies, obesity appears to roughly double the risk for new asthma in children [28, 30, 31]. Though some reports suggest that obesity-related asthma risk may be stronger among adult females, there is not a consistent gender effect in children. Importantly, obesity-related asthma risk also does not appear to be mediated through atopy [27–29, 32]. Alterations in the rate of growth, distinct from obesity status itself, may also influence asthma risk in children. Gold found that extremes in the *change* in body mass index (BMI) and *low* baseline BMI were associated with asthma risk [30], further suggesting that alterations in growth patterns (not just obesity status itself) may be a substantial root cause for the obesity-asthma link. Additionally, it is not clear if aberrant growth (obesity or underweight) mediates the development of asthma, or instead aberrant growth and asthma stem from the same root cause and merely signify a noncausal association (Fig. 12.2).

Since asthma lacks a precise set of diagnostic criteria and evidence exists for overdiagnosis of asthma in some groups [41, 42], it would be rational to hypothesize that obesity-related breathlessness and exertional dyspnea might contribute to overdiagnosis of asthma and result in an erroneous epidemiologic (obesity-asthma) link. However, erroneous asthma diagnosis is unlikely to explain all of the increased asthma risk. Castro-Rodriguez et al. reported increased objective markers of true asthma (peak flow variability and responsiveness to bronchodilator) in overweight girls compared with lean girls [29]. We also evaluated lean and obese children referred to a pediatric specialty asthma clinic in order to determine whether high BMI percentile among referrals was associated with misdiagnosis of asthma or if obese referrals had significantly different objective measures of asthma compared to lean referrals [41]. We found a good diagnostic correlation between referring physicians and asthma specialists that was not affected by BMI. Among patients diagnosed to have asthma by a specialist, a greater BMI percentile was associated with significantly reduced FEV_1, FEF25 – 75, and FEV_1/FVC. We concluded that in general physicians do not erroneously diagnose asthma in children due to overweight status. Similar conclusions have been made among adults [42].

Possible Etiologies

The etiology underlying the increased asthma risk among obese children is unknown. Several theories exist that have been detailed previously [35, 43, 44] and are

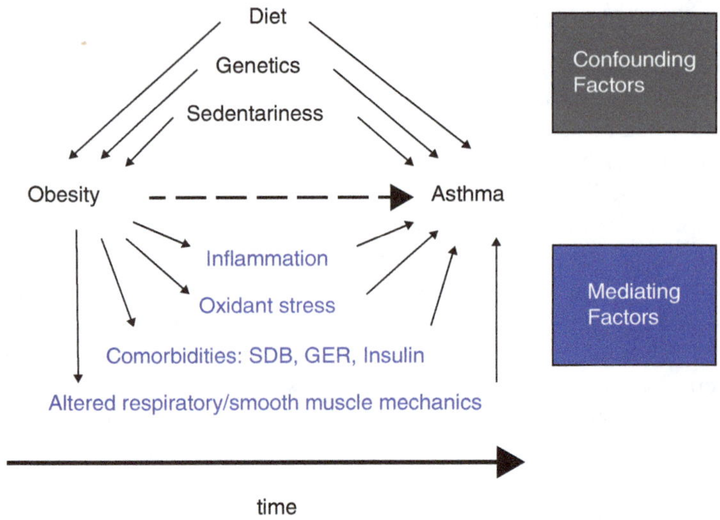

Fig. 12.2 Model of commonly proposed obesity-asthma mechanisms. This schema depicts possible etiologic mechanisms when obesity antedates asthma. The mechanisms are divided into confounders (when the factor is etiologically associated with both conditions) and mediators (when obesity acts through a separate *mediating* factor that leads to asthma). Each mechanism has some supporting evidence though it is likely that more than one mechanism is truly present in the obesity-asthma link. *SDB* sleep-disordered breathing, *GER* gastroesophageal reflux

addressed in the respective chapters by Drs. Salome and Shore in this text. These theories involve mediating factors stemming from the obese state, leading to the characteristics of asthma. These include abnormal circulating inflammation and oxidant stress, chest restriction with airway narrowing, and obesity-related comorbidities (Fig. 12.2). Assessing lung inflammation and responses in children remains challenging and limited by current technologies. Studies in children involving bronchodilator responsiveness, bronchoconstricting agonists (e.g., methacholine challenge), and airway inflammatory markers have yet to show a consistent pattern of obesity-related hyperresponsiveness. Therefore, discussions about the etiology of obesity-related asthma in children remain speculative. Other factors that may contribute to asthma risk among the obese that require more investigation include the possible confounding factors of diet, sedentariness, and shared genetics.

Dietary Factors

Unhealthy lifestyle factors related to obesity (such as a fatty diet or reduced physical activity) may play a role in asthma risk. For example, the typical "Western" high-fat diet contains up to 25-fold more omega-6 (n-6) polyunsaturated fatty acids

(PUFA) than omega-3 (n-3) PUFAs. n-6 PUFAs are found in eggs and most vegetable oils (such as corn oil) that are now commonly used in cooking in many developed countries, while n-3 PUFAs are contained in cold water fish (such as salmon, herring, tuna), mussels, and flaxseeds. The current 25:1 n-6-to-n-3 ratio is much higher than the < 2:1 ratio that was typical during the majority of human evolution [45–47]. A typical high-fat "Western" diet with abundant n-6 PUFA promotes and maintains a low leukocyte plasma membrane n-3/n-6 PUFA ratio and appears to increase cellular expression of 5-lipoxygenase pathway products (such as leukotrienes), TNFα, and other molecules important in asthma pathogenesis [48–51], and also increases free radical generation [52–55]. High dietary fat has been associated with obesity, asthma risk [56–58], and particular asthma characteristics such as airway reactivity [59]. A lower dietary and inflammatory cell n-6/n-3 PUFA ratio has been associated with improvements in asthma outcomes [60–64]. Interestingly, a "Mediterranean" diet that has more n-3 fatty acids and antioxidants appears to protect from recurrent wheezing in young children [65].

Importantly, obese individuals (including children) on average consume more n-6 dietary PUFAs and have a reduced dietary n-3/n-6 ratio in their diet compared to leans [66]. Not surprisingly, obese adolescents do appear to have lower serum n-3 PUFA (especially docosahexaenoic acid (DHA)) and lower n-3/n-6 PUFA serum levels compared to lean adolescents [67], suggesting that abnormal n-3 PUFA metabolism seen in the obese state may contribute to elevated asthma risk. Recently, Wood and colleagues showed that high-fat intake in healthy and asthmatic adults can lead to both greater inflammation in the airway and diminished lung function following bronchodilator administration [68]. These observations suggest that a high-fat diet, consumed chronically, may have a significant impact on the development of both obesity and asthma.

Sedentariness

A second lifestyle factor that is an important consideration in the obesity-asthma link is physical activity. Children who are overweight sustain less routine physical exertion than their lean counterparts [69]. Some reports suggest that physical activity may be important in reducing asthma risk [70] and reducing asthma symptoms [71–73], though other reports have not corroborated these findings [29, 65]. Lucas et al. have raised the concern that past cohort studies may not have been able to adequately adjust for reduced physical activity. If so, it is possible that reduced activity in combination with other obesity-related factors may be contributing to increased asthma incidence [36]. Indeed, repeated exercise promotes hyperventilation, cyclic airway smooth muscle stretch, and bronchodilation. In vitro studies suggest that exercise-related cyclic respiratory epithelial compression may improve both airway caliber and clearance [74]. Fredberg and others have pointed out that airway smooth muscle stretch that results from deep breathing is among the most effective bronchodilators [75, 76] and methods for maintaining airway patency. It is very possible that frequent exercise and exhaustive play during childhood (which has been shown to be reduced in obese children) [77, 78] plays a protective role in avoiding the development of asthma. More studies are needed to determine if, and to what degree, activity level is a confounding covariate in the obesity-asthma risk relationship. Regardless, most experts strongly suggest frequent exercise for optimal lung and cardiovascular health in children, especially in children with asthma or obesity.

Shared Genetics

Lastly, it would also be rational to hypothesize that the obesity-asthma link stems from common genetic origins [44, 79]. It is likely that genes contributing to one multifactorial complex disease probably also contribute directly or indirectly to other complex diseases. Our current genetic understanding has resulted from discovering associations between obesity and asthma phenotypes and candidate gene variants. For example, several promising genomic areas that contain genes connected with both obesity and asthma (5q23-32, 6p21-23, 11q13, and 12q13-24) have been identified [34, 43, 44, 79–82]. Only five genes have polymorphisms that have been associated with both obesity and asthma [83, 84]. These include the following genes: β2-adrenergic receptor gene (ADRB2), TNFα, lymphotoxin-α (LTA), vitamin D receptor (VDR), and protein kinase C-α (PRKCA). Further interrogation of these and other genetic loci is needed among cohorts with and without obesity and with and without asthma in order to better understand the nature of the obesity-asthma link.

Fetal Programming

Lastly, considering that the rise of asthma and particularly obesity has been so precipitous over recent decades, it is rationale to consider other contributors besides just changes in genetics or postnatal exposures. One consideration should be fetal programming, that is, unfavorable exposures during gestation that induces alterations in organ development and somatic growth that lead to lasting changes and risk for later disease. Through both epidemiologic and experimental evidence, it is clear that the fetus becomes exposed to the antigens and cytokines of the maternal environment. Other contributing factors might include total placenta nourishment; transplacental passage of antigens, cytokines, sex hormones, and macro – and micronutrient during organogenesis; intrauterine space restriction; and amniotic fluid antigens and cytokines. Nutritional factors in particular have been associated with both abnormal acceleration and deceleration of fetal growth, both of which have been associated with the conditions of obesity and asthma.

It is possible that more than one of the several mechanisms mentioned above (or mechanisms not yet considered) may act to increase asthma risk in the obese.

Obesity and Asthma Phenotype in Children

Currently, there is not a consensus about whether obese asthma constitutes a distinct phenotype in children. Here, we will explore important phenotypic factors including overall severity, atopy status, oxidation, and inflammation in the airway, lung mechanics, and response to rescue and controller asthma therapy to assess the current state of knowledge.

Severity

The current data do not conclusively suggest that obese children with asthma experience greater disease severity. Asthma *severity* describes the intrinsic intensity of the disease process (symptoms), the patient's functional impairment, the risk of a severe exacerbation, and the level of daily preventive treatment needed to control the disease [85].

Impairment

Several reports suggest that asthma-related impairment is more severe among obese children [86–94] while others have found no real difference [95–100]. Two large population-based studies have reported greater asthma severity among obese asthmatics based on either patient symptom reporting or physician reporting of diagnostic severity [87, 92]. Though these results come from well-designed epidemiologic studies (e.g., NHANES, ISAAC), they reflect either patient reporting or provider diagnoses, rather than objective measures of asthma and these findings may be vulnerable to differential misclassification bias. Obese asthmatic children and adults do generally report reduced asthma-related quality of life compared to normal weight asthmatics [86, 93, 101, 102]. However, when well-phenotyped pediatric cohorts are examined using objective measurements to detect a possible effect of obesity on disease severity, very little difference in asthma severity can be found [95, 100, 103]. Recently, we described a cohort of school-age children and adolescents with generally mild asthma [104]. The obese adolescents had very similar symptom reporting compared to their nonobese counterparts, while the 6–11-year-old obese asthmatics had *improved* asthma symptoms compared to leans. We have found similar results among a highly characterized pediatric cohort with poorly controlled asthma (Lang, unpublished).

Risk

Asthma severity in the urgent care setting has been assessed among obese children in four recent reports [90, 91, 96, 97]. Obesity was associated with a significantly higher rate of hospitalization (34 % vs. 25 %) [91]. However, asthma severity using the Modified Pulmonary Index Score (heart rate, respiratory rate, oximetry, wheezing presence, prolonged expiratory phase, and accessory muscle use) was the same in obese versus lean asthmatics. Ginde and colleagues, using a similar index score, also saw no greater asthma severity among obese children in the setting of acute disease [96]. These discrepancies may be due to the heterogeneous nature of obese asthma, modifying covariates (gender, age, race, and age of asthma onset), or severity misclassification bias on the part of providers. Luder found that obese asthmatics were more likely to be on a greater number of asthma medications [94], while Vargas did not [89]. We evaluated 10,291 lean and obese children diagnosed with asthma at four Nemours Children's Clinics pediatric asthma clinics over a 10-year period. We found a small but statistically significant increase in odds for severe asthma diagnosis and advanced treatment (EPR-3 treatment step 5 or higher) in obese versus lean children with asthma (Lang, unpublished). However, obese children with asthma seen in our clinic were not more likely to be experiencing an exacerbation. Overall, though obese children may report greater symptoms (impairment domain), little data suggest that obese children with asthma are at higher risk for severe exacerbation (risk domain).

The other major domain influencing asthma severity is the level of therapy required to control symptoms. Data suggest that obese asthmatics are at least as hard to control as their lean counterparts, and in some adult reports, are less responsive to conventional therapies [90, 91, 103, 105–109]. Evidence suggests that this reduced treatment efficacy may be rooted in true glucocorticosteroid resistance [105]. Recently, Forno and colleagues showed that obese children may also be less responsive to inhaled corticosteroids [110]. Corticosteroid resistance among obese asthmatic children could explain some reports of greater symptoms and greater disease severity.

Lung Function

Obese adult asthmatics generally have similar lung function (or modest reductions in vital capacity) and bronchodilator response compared to lean asthmatics [103, 111]. Fewer studies have reported spirometric outcomes in lean and obese children with asthma. Unlike in adults, obesity in children does not appear to reduce vital capacity or total lung capacity substantially [86, 93, 95, 98], and in some reports, may be associated with greater lung volumes and capacity [14]. However, obese children with asthma may have a mild obstructive impairment in airway flows [16, 41, 94, 100, 104], though this has not been a universal finding [9, 86, 95, 98].

Airways hyperresponsiveness (AHR) denotes excessive constriction triggered by innocuous stimuli and is an important phenotypic component of true asthma. Both AHR and the response to bronchodilator correlate with airway inflammation [112–114] and help assess asthma control and risk of future exacerbation. Obese children with asthma appear to have similar responsiveness to bronchoprovocation compared to lean asthmatic children [86]. Additionally, obese children with asthma appear to have similar or even reduced response to bronchodilators [9, 93, 100] compared to lean asthmatic children. These results provide some evidence that obesity-related risk for new asthma and possible increases in asthma severity are not due to increases in traditional airway inflammation. Instead, it seems more likely that obesity-related symptoms in children are related to greater airflow obstruction from mechanical effects.

Atopy

Though there are some reports of obesity being a risk factor for atopy among adolescent girls [39, 115, 116], obesity does not appear to consistently increase the risk for atopy. An NHANES III analysis of children 4–17 years of age showed a stepwise increase in prevalence of asthma with increasing BMI that did not include a similar increase in atopy (measured by skin prick testing) [117]. A second large sample of European children answering an ISAAC-based survey demonstrated an association between obesity and asthma, but not between obesity and atopy [118]. Overall, more investigation is needed into the relationship between obesity and atopy because it is possible that the current lack of consistency in the literature may be due to effect modification by regional exposures [119], gender, and age [115, 120].

Airway Inflammation

The measurement of airway inflammation in the obese asthmatic patient is an area in need of further study. Currently, there is little evidence that obesity leads to greater allergic airway inflammation in children. Exhaled nitric oxide levels (a surrogate of eosinophilic inflammation) among obese asthmatic children may be the same or even reduced compared to similar leans [121–125]. A few studies in adult obese asthmatics have shown reduced eosinophilic inflammation compared with similar leans [101, 102]. Obese asthmatic children did not have elevated airway LTB_4 [121]. Recent adult studies suggest that obesity may enhance neutrophilic airway inflammation [126] and systemic leukotriene production [127], though this has not been evaluated in children. The discovery of neutrophilic inflammation in obese asthmatics is consistent with findings of reduced corticosteroids efficacy in this group, since inhaled steroids are generally ineffective against neutrophilic inflammation.

Leukotriene production is important in asthma pathogenesis [128, 129] and may be upregulated in patients with obesity [127, 130]. There is preliminary evidence that genes, more common among the obese, may affect upregulate leukotriene pathway. We previously determined the allele frequencies of the addition/deletion promoter polymorphism in the ALOX5 gene among a population of lean and obese asthmatics undergoing a clinical trial [131, 132]. The relative risk of obesity in individuals carrying the variant allele is 2.04 compared to carriers of the wild type ($p=0.0165$) (Lang, unpublished). It is rational to hypothesize that obese, non-asthmatic persons may be at enhanced risk for incident asthma due in part to greater upregulation of the leukotriene pathway [131, 133]. Lastly, whereas increasing obesity appears to reduce response to inhaled corticosteroids, montelukast (a leukotriene receptor antagonist) appears to have a stable effect with increasing BMI [134].

Table 12.2 Summary of phenotypic observations in the obese asthmatic child

Characteristic	Traditional phenotype	Obese phenotype
Severity	–	Greater asthma symptoms, reduced QOL
Onset	Early onset	Early onset; delayed onset also common
Atopy	Very common	May be less common
Airway inflammation	Eosinophilic, elevated FENO	More data needed; may be mixed with greater neutrophilic component/ reduced FENO
Lung function	Episodic airway obstruction; variable remodeling	Normal FVC, variable reduction in FEV1/FVC
Bronchodilator response	Very common	Common; slightly reduced compared to leans
Bronchoprovocation/AHR	Present	Present
Airflow perception	–	Greater in children; reduced in adults
Response to therapy	Steroid resistance rare	Steroid resistance may be more common; LTRA may be helpful
Common comorbidities	Allergic rhinitis, eczema, sinusitis, anxiety, GER	Hyperinsulinemia, elevated triglycerides, LDL; anxiety/depression, GER
Resolution	–	Weight loss improves asthma control

QOL quality of life, *FENO* fractional exhalation nitric oxide, *FVC* forced vital capacity, *FEV* forced expiratory volume, *LTRA* leukotriene receptor antagonist, *GER* gastroesophageal reflux, *LDL* low-density lipoprotein

Asthma and obesity are conditions involving excess oxidative stress. Asthmatics have increased airway 8-isoprostane, a marker of arachidonic acid oxidation. Reactive oxygen species within the airway reacts with normal enzymes causing impaired airway function and inflammation. Airway 8-isoprostane is elevated in adult asthmatics who are obese [135]. Excess oxidative stress and injury is possibly a second mechanism making the obese-asthma phenotype less responsive to inhaled corticosteroid therapy. Though the exact nature of the obese-asthma phenotype in children is far from clear, some patterns are emerging (Table 12.2).

The Obese Asthmatic Child: Management Considerations

Weight Loss

Studies in adults have evaluated asthma outcomes following weight loss [136–139]. The most consistent findings involve improved spirometric lung volumes, asthma symptom reporting, and reduced nonspecific symptoms of breathlessness and exercise intolerance. It is difficult to decipher general improvements in cardiorespiratory health following weight loss from asthma-specific improvements. Though the impact of weight loss in obese children with asthma has not been adequately studied, weight loss is an Evidence B recommendation of the EPR-3 [85]. It is rational to expect similar improvements in symptom control and lung volumes among children as that seen in adults. Exercise and other lifestyle intervention remains an important area of future research for obese children with asthma.

Medications

Current research does not support major deviations from current GINA and NHLBI EPR-3 guidelines when considering the management of the obese asthmatic child. Recent studies may provide some focused guidance to the clinician caring for an obese asthmatic child. Evidence suggests that obesity may blunt the response to some controller therapies (inhaled corticosteroids [105, 107, 134] and low-dose theophylline [103]). In fact, a recent report suggests a possible genetic explanation for this pattern of reduced steroid response that may also be coupled with enhanced montelukast response [140]. These findings in conjunction with evidence of superior adherence [141] suggest that montelukast may be particularly useful in the obese asthmatic population.

Since much of the impairment domain of asthma control involves subjective assessment and quality of life issues, attention to obesity-related sequelae that may interact with asthma symptoms remains critically important. Though empiric treatment for "silent" gastroesophageal reflux so far does not seem warranted [142], some obese patients with gastroesophageal reflux and cough may improve with antireflux medications. Clinicians should maintain a high index of suspicion for certain obesity-related conditions such as sleep-disordered breathing and metabolic syndrome. Lastly, depression with anxiety is associated with both obesity and asthma and is commonly overlooked. For these reasons, some children with obese asthma may need more intensive self-management education and help with adherence/concordance. Since mood can affect self-mastery, a jointly designed home asthma plan that considers all of the patient's comorbidities may be most effective.

The most universally effective management plan for obese children with persistent asthma continues to involve weight loss, daily exercise, a balanced low-fat diet, and repeated asthma education regarding inhaler technique and trigger avoidance. Pharmacologic controller therapy with inhaled corticosteroids and leukotriene modifiers should be first-line therapies. Response heterogeneity likely exists among obese asthmatics as it does among lean asthmatics. This means that among moderate asthmatics, a significant portion of patients will show a clear response preference to one of the following choices: ICS-LABA, or ICS plus montelukast, or to a higher dose of ICS alone [143]. Because of the flat dose–response curve and steroid resistance seen among obese asthmatics, preference toward ICS plus montelukast for stepup therapy may be warranted. Regardless of the stepup therapy chosen, close follow-up is critically important in order to reiterate proper inhaler techniques, weight-control, low-fat diet, daily exercise, and monitoring of asthma symptoms and medication side effects.

Sleep-Disordered Breathing and Obesity Hypoventilation Syndrome

Obese children are at considerably elevated risk for developing obstructive hypoventilation and obstructive sleep apnea (OSA) [144]. Traditionally, OSA in children stems from either tonsillar hypertrophy or craniomandibular anomalies. However, with the increasing prevalence of obesity among children, more cases of childhood OSA appear to stem from obesity. In children, the odds of OSA among the obese may be as high as 500 % that of nonobese children. Obesity likely leads to OSA from crowding of the pharyngeal airway leading to reduced caliber and greater collapsibility. One recent polysomnography study found that 19 % of obese children and adolescents displayed obstructive sleep apnea and 17 % had central sleep apnea with a mean SaO_2 nadir of 82 % [145]. Obese children may also suffer greater consequences of end organ dysfunction related to OSA [146]. Obese children with OSA experience greater daytime sleepiness than lean children even after adjusting for OSA severity [147]. Many overweight and obese children with OSA have tonsillar hypertrophy and do benefit from adenotonsillectomy (AT); however, the most optimal therapy for obese children remains weight loss. The long-term success of AT is reduced in obese children [148] and in those who gain weight following AT [149]. For obese children suffering mild residual OSA following surgery, therapies such as montelukast and nasal steroids have been advocated [150–153]. Nasal continuous positive airway pressure should be implemented for moderate-to-severe residual disease until the patient is able to achieve adequate weight loss [146]. It is important for children and their parents to understand that for many children with obesity and OSA, management approaches such as airway pressure devices and oral appliances may never fully eliminate OSA symptoms and their sequelae.

Obesity Hypoventilation Syndrome (OHS)

Obesity hypoventilation syndrome (OHS) has also become a greater concern among children and adolescents with the increasing prevalence of severe obesity. The syndrome classically is associated with extreme obesity (usually BMI >35) and awake alveolar hypoventilation ($PaCO_2$>45 mmHg). The population prevalence of OHS among children is unknown. However, prospective adult studies suggest that 13–20 % of patients evaluated for OSA [154, 155] (and 31 % with BMI>35 kg/m^2) [156] have OHS. In children, the prevalence is difficult to determine, but extrapolating from these adult data and work in children by Rosen [157], the prevalence of OHS among obese children may be as high as 3–5 %. When suspected, clinicians should establish the presence of wakeful hypoventilation by arterial blood gas analysis and evaluate for possible contributing causes such as muscle weakness, parenchymal lung disease, or hypothyroidism. OHS can lead to acute cardiorespiratory failure and can be life-threatening. The evaluation typically will include polysomnography, arterial blood gas analysis, lung function testing (spirometry, plethysmography, and maximal inspiratory/expiratory pressures), thyroid function, and chest imaging. A high prevalence of children with OHS will have significant sleep-disordered breathing and may benefit from nocturnal positive airway pressure or adenotonsillectomy, or both. Hypoventilation related to obesity may be more common with truncal obesity [158] and may occur with sleep unassociated with upper airway obstruction. These sleep-related central apneas and hypopneas can lead to hypoxemia. Other comorbidities such as metabolic syndrome and pulmonary hypertension with right-sided heart failure may also contribute to the development of OHS and should be considered in the evaluation of patients with OHS.

Conclusions

Obesity in children is a significant public health problem that clearly can affect quality of life and lung health. Obesity does appear to worsen breathing function is many children and appears to increase the risk for new asthma through currently unknown mechanisms. Larger epidemiologic studies involving in-depth disease characterization and more accurate measures of adiposity may be needed to determine how obesity impacts asthma phenotype. In asthmatic children, obesity appears to be associated with greater airflow obstruction and reduced response to controller therapy. Obesity also significantly increases the risk for obstructive sleep apnea and obesity-hypoventilation syndrome. For each of these conditions, weight loss appears to be an effective treatment. Prevention of obesity should continue to be a major public health priority and primary strategy for addressing all obesity-related sequelae including obesity-related lung disease.

References

1. Eaton DK, Kann L, Kinchen S, Shanklin S, Ross J, Hawkins J, et al. Youth risk behavior surveillance–United States, 2007. MMWR Surveill Summ. 2008;57(4):1–131.
2. Ogden CL, Carroll MD, Curtin LR, McDowell MA, Tabak CJ, Flegal KM. Prevalence of overweight and obesity in the United States, 1999–2004. JAMA. 2006;295(13):1549–55.
3. Selassie M, Sinha AC. The epidemiology and aetiology of obesity: a global challenge. Best Pract Res Clin Anaesthesiol. 2010;25(1):1–9.
4. WHO: WHO World Health Statistics 2011. Geneva, Switzerland; 2011.
5. Krebs NF, Himes JH, Jacobson D, Nicklas TA, Guilday P, Styne D. Assessment of child and adolescent overweight and obesity. Pediatrics. 2007;120(Suppl 4):S193–228.
6. Cole TJ, Bellizzi MC, Flegal KM, Dietz WH. Establishing a standard definition for child overweight and obesity worldwide: international survey. BMJ. 2000;320(7244):1240–3.
7. Koplan JP, Liverman CT, Kraak VI. Preventing childhood obesity: health in the balance: executive summary. J Am Diet Assoc. 2005;105(1):131–8.
8. Barlow SE. Expert committee recommendations regarding the prevention, assessment, and treatment of child and adolescent overweight and obesity: summary report. Pediatrics. 2007;120(Suppl 4):S164–92.

9. Bibi H, Shoseyov D, Feigenbaum D, Genis M, Friger M, Peled R, et al. The relationship between asthma and obesity in children: is it real or a case of over diagnosis? J Asthma. 2004;41(4):403–10.
10. Kaplan TA, Montana E. Exercise-induced bronchospasm in nonasthmatic obese children. Clin Pediatr. 1993;32(4):220–5.
11. Perez-Padilla R, Rojas R, Torres V, Borja-Aburto V, Olaiz G. The Empece working group. Obesity among children residing in Mexico City and its impact on lung function: a comparison with Mexican-Americans. Arch Med Res. 2006;37(1):165–71.
12. Spathopoulos D, Paraskakis E, Trypsianis G, Tsalkidis A, Arvanitidou V, Emporiadou M, et al. The effect of obesity on pulmonary lung function of school aged children in Greece. Pediatr Pulmonol. 2009;44(3):273–80.
13. Van Gysel D, Govaere E, Verhamme K, Doli E, De Baets F. Body mass index in Belgian schoolchildren and its relationship with sensitization and allergic symptoms. Pediatr Allergy Immunol. 2009;20(3):246–53.
14. Lazarus R, Colditz G, Berkey CS, Speizer FE. Effects of body fat on ventilatory function in children and adolescents: cross-sectional findings from a random population sample of school children. Pediatr Pulmonol. 1997;24(3):187–94.
15. Ulger Z, Demir E, Tanac R, Goksen D, Gulen F, Darcan S, et al. The effect of childhood obesity on respiratory function tests and airway hyperresponsiveness. Turk J Pediatr. 2006;48(1):43–50.
16. Chu YT, Chen WY, Wang TN, Tseng HI, Wu JR, Ko YC. Extreme BMI predicts higher asthma prevalence and is associated with lung function impairment in school-aged children. Pediatr Pulmonol. 2009;44(5):472–9.
17. Li AM, Chan D, Wong E, Yin J, Nelson EA, Fok TF. The effects of obesity on pulmonary function. Arch Dis Child. 2003;88(4):361–3.
18. Gokbel H, Atas S. Exercise-induced bronchospasm in nonasthmatic obese and nonobese boys. J Sports Med Phys Fitness. 1999;39(4):361–4.
19. Ford ES. Asthma, body mass index, and C-reactive protein among US adults. J Asthma. 2003;40(7):733–9.
20. Nystad W, Meyer HE, Nafstad P, Tverdal A, Engeland A. Body mass index in relation to adult asthma among 135,000 Norwegian men and women. Am J Epidemiol. 2004;160(10): 969–76.
21. Camargo Jr CA, Weiss ST, Zhang S, Willett WC, Speizer FE. Prospective study of body mass index, weight change, and risk of adult-onset asthma in women. Arch Intern Med. 1999;159(21):2582–8.
22. Beckett WS, Jacobs Jr DR, Yu X, Iribarren C, Williams OD. Asthma is associated with weight gain in females but not males, independent of physical activity. Am J Respir Crit Care Med. 2001;164(11):2045–50.
23. Chen Y, Dales R, Tang M, Krewski D. Obesity may increase the incidence of asthma in women but not in men: longitudinal observations from the Canadian National Population Health Surveys. Am J Epidemiol. 2002;155(3):191–7.
24. Stanley AH, Demissie K, Rhoads GG. Asthma development with obesity exposure: observations from the cohort of the National Health and Nutrition Evaluation Survey Epidemiologic Follow-up Study (NHEFS). J Asthma. 2005;42(2):97–9.
25. Huovinen E, Kaprio J, Koskenvuo M. Factors associated to lifestyle and risk of adult onset asthma. Respir Med. 2003;97(3):273–80.
26. Guerra S, Sherrill DL, Bobadilla A, Martinez FD, Barbee RA. The relation of body mass index to asthma, chronic bronchitis, and emphysema. Chest. 2002;122(4):1256–63.
27. Guerra S, Wright AL, Morgan WJ, Sherrill DL, Holberg CJ, Martinez FD. Persistence of asthma symptoms during adolescence: role of obesity and age at the onset of puberty. Am J Respir Crit Care Med. 2004;170(1):78–85.
28. Gilliland FD, Berhane K, Islam T, McConnell R, Gauderman WJ, Gilliland SS, et al. Obesity and the risk of newly diagnosed asthma in school-age children. Am J Epidemiol. 2003;158(5): 406–15.

29. Castro-Rodriguez JA, Holberg CJ, Morgan WJ, Wright AL, Martinez FD. Increased incidence of asthmalike symptoms in girls who become overweight or obese during the school years. Am J Respir Crit Care Med. 2001;163(6):1344–9.
30. Gold DR, Damokosh AI, Dockery DW, Berkey CS. Body-mass index as a predictor of incident asthma in a prospective cohort of children. Pediatr Pulmonol. 2003;36(6):514–21.
31. Mannino DM, Mott J, Ferdinands JM, Camargo CA, Friedman M, Greves HM, et al. Boys with high body masses have an increased risk of developing asthma: findings from the National Longitudinal Survey of Youth (NLSY). Int J Obes (Lond). 2006;30(1):6–13.
32. Taveras EM, Rifas-Shiman SL, Camargo Jr CA, Gold DR, Litonjua AA, Oken E, et al. Higher adiposity in infancy associated with recurrent wheeze in a prospective cohort of children. J Allergy Clin Immunol. 2008;121(5):1161–6. e3.
33. Chinn S, Rona RJ. Can the increase in body mass index explain the rising trend in asthma in children? Thorax. 2001;56(11):845–50.
34. Shore SA, Johnston RA. Obesity and asthma. Pharmacol Ther. 2006;110(1):83–102.
35. Shore SA. Obesity and asthma: possible mechanisms. J Allergy Clin Immunol. 2008;121(5):1087–93. quiz 94–5.
36. Lucas SR, Platts-Mills TA. Paediatric asthma and obesity. Paediatr Respir Rev. 2006;7(4): 233–8.
37. Wilson MM, Irwin RS. The association of asthma and obesity: is it real or a matter of definition, Presbyterian minister's salaries, and earlobe creases? Arch Intern Med. 1999;159(21):2513–4.
38. Schachter LM, Salome CM, Peat JK, Woolcock AJ. Obesity is a risk for asthma and wheeze but not airway hyperresponsiveness. Thorax. 2001;56(1):4–8.
39. Schachter LM, Peat JK, Salome CM. Asthma and atopy in overweight children. Thorax. 2003;58(12):1031–5.
40. Aschengrau A, Seage GR. Essentials of epidemiology in public health. 2nd ed. Sudbury: Jones and Bartlett; 2008.
41. Lang JE, Feng H, Lima JJ. Body mass index-percentile and diagnostic accuracy of childhood asthma. J Asthma. 2009;46(3):291–9.
42. Aaron SD, Vandemheen KL, Boulet LP, McIvor RA, Fitzgerald JM, Hernandez P, et al. Overdiagnosis of asthma in obese and nonobese adults. CMAJ. 2008;179(11):1121–31.
43. Weiss ST, Shore S. Obesity and asthma: directions for research. Am J Respir Crit Care Med. 2004;169(8):963–8.
44. Beuther DA, Weiss ST, Sutherland ER. Obesity and asthma. Am J Respir Crit Care Med. 2006;174(2):112–9.
45. Simopoulos AP. Importance of the ratio of omega-6/omega-3 essential fatty acids: evolutionary aspects. World Rev Nutr Diet. 2003;92:1–22.
46. Simopoulos AP. Evolutionary aspects of diet, the omega-6/omega-3 ratio and genetic variation: nutritional implications for chronic diseases. Biomed Pharmacother. 2006;60(9): 502–7.
47. Simopoulos AP. Overview of evolutionary aspects of omega 3 fatty acids in the diet. World Rev Nutr Diet. 1998;83:1–11.
48. Mantzioris E, Cleland LG, Gibson RA, Neumann MA, Demasi M, James MJ. Biochemical effects of a diet containing foods enriched with n-3 fatty acids. Am J Clin Nutr. 2000;72(1):42–8.
49. Calder PC. Dietary modification of inflammation with lipids. Proc Nutr Soc. 2002;61(3): 345–58.
50. James MJ, Gibson RA, Cleland LG. Dietary polyunsaturated fatty acids and inflammatory mediator production. Am J Clin Nutr. 2000;71(1 Suppl):343S–8S.
51. Caughey GE, Mantzioris E, Gibson RA, Cleland LG, James MJ. The effect on human tumor necrosis factor alpha and interleukin 1 beta production of diets enriched in n-3 fatty acids from vegetable oil or fish oil. Am J Clin Nutr. 1996;63(1):116–22.
52. Toborek M, Barger SW, Mattson MP, Barve S, McClain CJ, Hennig B. Linoleic acid and TNF-alpha cross-amplify oxidative injury and dysfunction of endothelial cells. J Lipid Res. 1996;37(1):123–35.

53. Toborek M, Lee YW, Garrido R, Kaiser S, Hennig B. Unsaturated fatty acids selectively induce an inflammatory environment in human endothelial cells. Am J Clin Nutr. 2002;75(1):119–25.
54. Pepe S. Effect of dietary polyunsaturated fatty acids on age-related changes in cardiac mitochondrial membranes. Exp Gerontol. 2005;40(8–9):751–8.
55. Ghosh S, Kewalramani G, Yuen G, Pulinilkunnil T, An D, Innis SM, et al. Induction of mitochondrial nitrative damage and cardiac dysfunction by chronic provision of dietary omega-6 polyunsaturated fatty acids. Free Radic Biol Med. 2006;41(9):1413–24.
56. Weiland SK, von Mutius E, Husing A, Asher MI. Intake of trans fatty acids and prevalence of childhood asthma and allergies in Europe. ISAAC Steering Committee. Lancet. 1999;353(9169):2040–1.
57. Nagel G, Linseisen J. Dietary intake of fatty acids, antioxidants and selected food groups and asthma in adults. Eur J Clin Nutr. 2005;59(1):8–15.
58. Strom K, Janzon L, Mattisson I, Rosberg HE, Arborelius M. Asthma but not smoking-related airflow limitation is associated with a high fat diet in men: results from the population study "Men born in 1914", Malmo, Sweden. Monaldi Arch Chest Dis. 1996;51(1):16–21.
59. Soutar A, Seaton A, Brown K. Bronchial reactivity and dietary antioxidants. Thorax. 1997;52(2):166–70.
60. Emelyanov A, Fedoseev G, Krasnoschekova O, Abulimity A, Trendeleva T, Barnes PJ. Treatment of asthma with lipid extract of New Zealand green-lipped mussel: a randomised clinical trial. Eur Respir J. 2002;20(3):596–600.
61. Okamoto M, Mitsunobu F, Ashida K, Mifune T, Hosaki Y, Tsugeno H, et al. Effects of perilla seed oil supplementation on leukotriene generation by leucocytes in patients with asthma associated with lipometabolism. Int Arch Allergy Immunol. 2000;122(2):137–42.
62. Nagakura T, Matsuda S, Shichijyo K, Sugimoto H, Hata K. Dietary supplementation with fish oil rich in omega-3 polyunsaturated fatty acids in children with bronchial asthma. Eur Respir J. 2000;16(5):861–5.
63. Villani F, Comazzi R, De Maria P, Galimberti M. Effect of dietary supplementation with polyunsaturated fatty acids on bronchial hyperreactivity in subjects with seasonal asthma. Respiration. 1998;65(4):265–9.
64. Dry J, Vincent D. Effect of a fish oil diet on asthma: results of a 1-year double-blind study. Int Arch Allergy Appl Immunol. 1991;95(2–3):156–7.
65. Castro-Rodriguez JA, Garcia-Marcos L, Alfonseda Rojas JD, Valverde-Molina J, Sanchez-Solis M. Mediterranean diet as a protective factor for wheezing in preschool children. J Pediatr. 2008;152(6):823–8. 8 e1-2.
66. Daniel CR, McCullough ML, Patel RC, Jacobs EJ, Flanders WD, Thun MJ, et al. Dietary intake of omega-6 and omega-3 fatty acids and risk of colorectal cancer in a prospective cohort of U.S. men and women. Cancer Epidemiol Biomarkers Prev. 2009;18(2):516–25.
67. Karlsson M, Marild S, Brandberg J, Lonn L, Friberg P, Strandvik B. Serum phospholipid fatty acids, adipose tissue, and metabolic markers in obese adolescents. Obesity (Silver Spring). 2006;14(11):1931–9.
68. Wood LG, Garg ML, Gibson PG. A high-fat challenge increases airway inflammation and impairs bronchodilator recovery in asthma. J Allergy Clin Immunol. 2010;127(5):1133–40.
69. Belcher BR, Berrigan D, Dodd KW, Emken BA, Chou CP, Spruijt-Metz D. Physical activity in US youth: effect of race/ethnicity, age, gender, and weight status. Med Sci Sports Exerc. 2010;42(12):2211–21.
70. Rasmussen F, Lambrechtsen J, Siersted HC, Hansen HS, Hansen NC. Low physical fitness in childhood is associated with the development of asthma in young adulthood: the Odense schoolchild study. Eur Respir J. 2000;16(5):866–70.
71. Ram FS, Robinson SM, Black PN. Effects of physical training in asthma: a systematic review. Br J Sports Med. 2000;34(3):162–7.
72. van Veldhoven NH, Vermeer A, Bogaard JM, Hessels MG, Wijnroks L, Colland VT, et al. Children with asthma and physical exercise: effects of an exercise programme. Clin Rehabil. 2001;15(4):360–70.

73. Welsh L, Kemp JG, Roberts RG. Effects of physical conditioning on children and adolescents with asthma. Sports Med. 2005;35(2):127–41.
74. Button B, Boucher RC. Role of mechanical stress in regulating airway surface hydration and mucus clearance rates. Respir Physiol Neurobiol. 2008;163(1–3):189–201.
75. Shore SA, Fredberg JJ. Obesity, smooth muscle, and airway hyperresponsiveness. J Allergy Clin Immunol. 2005;115(5):925–7.
76. Fredberg JJ. Frozen objects: small airways, big breaths, and asthma. J Allergy Clin Immunol. 2000;106(4):615–24.
77. Trost SG, Kerr LM, Ward DS, Pate RR. Physical activity and determinants of physical activity in obese and non-obese children. Int J Obes Relat Metab Disord. 2001;25(6):822–9.
78. Marshall SJ, Biddle SJ, Gorely T, Cameron N, Murdey I. Relationships between media use, body fatness and physical activity in children and youth: a meta-analysis. Int J Obes Relat Metab Disord. 2004;28(10):1238–46.
79. Weiss ST. Obesity: insight into the origins of asthma. Nat Immunol. 2005;6(6):537–9.
80. Tantisira KG, Weiss ST. Complex interactions in complex traits: obesity and asthma. Thorax. 2001;56(2):ii 64–73.
81. Howard TD, Meyers DA, Bleecker ER. Mapping susceptibility genes for asthma and allergy. J Allergy Clin Immunol. 2000;105(2 Pt 2):S477–81.
82. Yang W, Kelly T, He J. Genetic epidemiology of obesity. Epidemiol Rev. 2007;29:49–61.
83. Litonjua AA, Gold DR. Asthma and obesity: common early-life influences in the inception of disease. J Allergy Clin Immunol. 2008;12(5):1075–84. quiz 85–6.
84. Murphy A, Tantisira KG, Soto-Quiros ME, Avila L, Klanderman BJ, Lake S, et al. PRKCA: a positional candidate gene for body mass index and asthma. Am J Hum Genet. 2009;85(1): 87–96.
85. Expert panel report 3 (EPR-3): Guidelines for the diagnosis and management of asthma-summary Report 2007. J Allergy Clin Immunol. 2007;120(5 Suppl):S94–138
86. Pianosi PT, Davis HS. Determinants of physical fitness in children with asthma. Pediatrics. 2004;113(3 Pt 1):e225–9.
87. Michelson PH, Williams LW, Benjamin DK, Barnato AE. Obesity, inflammation, and asthma severity in childhood: data from the National Health and Nutrition Examination Survey 2001–2004. Ann Allergy Asthma Immunol. 2009;103(5):381–5.
88. Tai A, Volkmer R, Burton A. Association between asthma symptoms and obesity in preschool (4–5 year old) children. J Asthma. 2009;46(4):362–5.
89. Vargas PA, Perry TT, Robles E, Jo CH, Simpson PM, Magee JM, et al. Relationship of body mass index with asthma indicators in head start children. Ann Allergy Asthma Immunol. 2007;99(1):22–8.
90. Carroll CL, Bhandari A, Zucker AR, Schramm CM. Childhood obesity increases duration of therapy during severe asthma exacerbations. Pediatr Crit Care Med. 2006;7(6):527–31.
91. Carroll CL, Stoltz P, Raykov N, Smith SR, Zucker AR. Childhood overweight increases hospital admission rates for asthma. Pediatrics. 2007;120(4):734–40.
92. Cassol VE, Rizzato TM, Teche SP, Basso DF, Centenaro DF, Maldonado M, et al. Obesity and its relationship with asthma prevalence and severity in adolescents from Southern Brazil. J Asthma. 2006;43(1):57–60.
93. van Gent R, van der Ent CK, Rovers MM, Kimpen JL, van Essen-Zandvliet LE, de Meer G. Excessive body weight is associated with additional loss of quality of life in children with asthma. J Allergy Clin Immunol. 2007;119(3):591–6.
94. Luder E, Melnik TA, DiMaio M. Association of being overweight with greater asthma symptoms in inner city black and Hispanic children. J Pediatr. 1998;132(4):699–703.
95. Ross KR, Hart MA, Storfer-Isser A, Kibler AM, Johnson NL, Rosen CL, et al. Obesity and obesity related co-morbidities in a referral population of children with asthma. Pediatr Pulmonol. 2009;44(9):877–84.
96. Ginde AA, Santillan AA, Clark S, Camargo Jr CA. Body mass index and acute asthma severity among children presenting to the emergency department. Pediatr Allergy Immunol. 2010;21(3): 480–88.

97. Hom J, Morley EJ, Sasso P, Sinert R. Body mass index and pediatric asthma outcomes. Pediatr Emerg Care. 2009;25(9):569–71.
98. Kwong KY, Rhandhawa I, Saxena J, Morphew T, Jones CA. Ability to control persistent asthma in obese versus non-obese children enrolled in an asthma-specific disease management program (breathmobile). J Asthma. 2006;43(9):661–6.
99. Mansell AL, Walders N, Wamboldt MZ, Carter R, Steele DW, Devin JA, et al. Effect of body mass index on response to methacholine bronchial provocation in healthy and asthmatic adolescents. Pediatr Pulmonol. 2006;41(5):434–40.
100. Tantisira KG, Litonjua AA, Weiss ST, Fuhlbrigge AL. Association of body mass with pulmonary function in the Childhood Asthma Management Program (CAMP). Thorax. 2003;58(12):1036–41.
101. van Veen IH, Ten Brinke A, Sterk PJ, Rabe KF, Bel EH. Airway inflammation in obese and nonobese patients with difficult-to-treat asthma. Allergy. 2008;63(5):570–4.
102. Lessard A, Turcotte H, Cormier Y, Boulet LP. Obesity and asthma: a specific phenotype? Chest. 2008;134(2):317–23.
103. Dixon AE, Shade DM, Cohen RI, Skloot GS, Holbrook JT, Smith LJ, et al. Effect of obesity on clinical presentation and response to treatment in asthma. J Asthma. 2006;43(7):553–8.
104. Lang JE, Hossain J, Dixon AE, Shade D, Wise RA, Peters SP, et al. Does age impact the obese asthma phenotype?: Longitudinal asthma control, airway function and airflow perception among mild persistent asthmatics. Chest. 2011;140(6):1524–33.
105. Sutherland ER, Goleva E, Strand M, Beuther DA, Leung DY. Body mass and glucocorticoid response in asthma. Am J Respir Crit Care Med. 2008;178(7):682–7.
106. Boulet LP, Franssen E. Influence of obesity on response to fluticasone with or without salmeterol in moderate asthma. Respir Med. 2007;101(11):2240–7.
107. Camargo Jr CA, Boulet LP, Sutherland ER, Busse WW, Yancey SW, Emmett AH, et al. Body mass index and response to asthma therapy: fluticasone propionate/salmeterol versus montelukast. J Asthma. 2010;47(1):76–82.
108. Lavoie KL, Bacon SL, Labrecque M, Cartier A, Ditto B. Higher BMI is associated with worse asthma control and quality of life but not asthma severity. Respir Med. 2006;100(4): 648–57.
109. Saint-Pierre P, Bourdin A, Chanez P, Daures JP, Godard P. Are overweight asthmatics more difficult to control? Allergy. 2006;61(1):79–84.
110. Forno E, Lescher R, Strunk R, Weiss S, Fuhlbrigge A, Celedon JC. Decreased response to inhaled steroids in overweight and obese asthmatic children. J Allergy Clin Immunol. 2011;127(3):741–9.
111. Boulet LP, Hamid Q, Bacon SL, Bergeron C, Chen Y, Dixon AE, et al. Symposium on obesity and asthma – 2 Nov 2006. Can Respir J. 2007;14(4):201–8.
112. Laprise C, Laviolette M, Boutet M, Boulet LP. Asymptomatic airway hyperresponsiveness: relationships with airway inflammation and remodelling. Eur Respir J. 1999;14(1):63–73.
113. Koskela HO, Hyvarinen L, Brannan JD, Chan HK, Anderson SD. Sensitivity and validity of three bronchial provocation tests to demonstrate the effect of inhaled corticosteroids in asthma. Chest. 2003;124(4):1341–9.
114. Covar RA, Spahn JD, Martin RJ, Silkoff PE, Sundstrom DA, Murphy J, et al. Safety and application of induced sputum analysis in childhood asthma. J Allergy Clin Immunol. 2004;114(3):575–82.
115. Huang SL, Shiao G, Chou P. Association between body mass index and allergy in teenage girls in Taiwan. Clin Exp Allergy. 1999;29(3):323–9.
116. Hancox RJ, Milne BJ, Poulton R, Taylor DR, Greene JM, McLachlan CR, et al. Sex differences in the relation between body mass index and asthma and atopy in a birth cohort. Am J Respir Crit Care Med. 2005;171(5):440–5.
117. von Mutius E, Schwartz J, Neas LM, Dockery D, Weiss ST. Relation of body mass index to asthma and atopy in children: the National Health and Nutrition Examination Study III. Thorax. 2001;56(11):835–8.

118. von Kries R, Hermann M, Grunert VP, von Mutius E. Is obesity a risk factor for childhood asthma? Allergy. 2001;56(4):318–22.
119. Irei AV, Sato Y, Lin TL, Wang MF, Chan YC, Hung NT, et al. Overweight is associated with allergy in school children of Taiwan and Vietnam but not Japan. J Med Invest. 2005;52(1–2):33–40.
120. Vieira VJ, Ronan AM, Windt MR, Tagliaferro AR. Elevated atopy in healthy obese women. Am J Clin Nutr. 2005;82(3):504–9.
121. Leung TF, Li CY, Lam CW, Au CS, Yung E, Chan IH, et al. The relation between obesity and asthmatic airway inflammation. Pediatr Allergy Immunol. 2004;15(4):344–50.
122. Santamaria F, Montella S, De Stefano S, Sperli F, Barbarano F, Spadaro R, et al. Asthma, atopy, and airway inflammation in obese children. J Allergy Clin Immunol. 2007;120(4):965–7.
123. Chow JS, Leung AS, Li WW, Tse TP, Sy HY, Leung TF. Airway inflammatory and spirometric measurements in obese children. Hong Kong Med J. 2009;15(5):346–52.
124. Wong GW, Liu EK, Leung TF, Yung E, Ko FW, Hui DS, et al. High levels and gender difference of exhaled nitric oxide in Chinese schoolchildren. Clin Exp Allergy. 2005;35(7):889–93.
125. Buchvald F, Baraldi E, Carraro S, Gaston B, De Jongste J, Pijnenburg MW, et al. Measurements of exhaled nitric oxide in healthy subjects age 4 to 17 years. J Allergy Clin Immunol. 2005;115(6):1130–6.
126. Scott HA, Gibson PG, Garg ML, Wood LG. Airway inflammation is augmented by obesity and fatty acids in asthma. Eur Respir J. 2011;38(3):594–602.
127. Giouleka P, Papatheodorou G, Lyberopoulos P, Karakatsani A, Alchanatis M, Roussos C, et al. Body mass index is associated with leukotriene inflammation in asthmatics. Eur J Clin Invest. 2011;41(1):30–8.
128. Drazen JM. Asthma therapy with agents preventing leukotriene synthesis or action. Proc Assoc Am Physicians. 1999;111(6):547–59.
129. Drazen JM, Israel E, O'Byrne PM. Treatment of asthma with drugs modifying the leukotriene pathway. N Engl J Med. 1999;340(3):197–206.
130. Kaaman M, Ryden M, Axelsson T, Nordstrom E, Sicard A, Bouloumie A, et al. ALOX5AP expression, but not gene haplotypes, is associated with obesity and insulin resistance. Int J Obes (Lond). 2006;30(3):447–52.
131. Lima JJ, Zhang S, Grant A, Shao L, Tantisira KG, Allayee H, et al. Influence of leukotriene pathway polymorphisms on response to montelukast in asthma. Am J Respir Crit Care Med. 2006;173(4):379–85.
132. American Lung Association Asthma Clinical Research Centers. Clinical trial of low-dose theophylline and montelukast in patients with poorly controlled asthma. Am J Respir Crit Care Med. 2007;175(3):235–42.
133. Dwyer JH, Allayee H, Dwyer KM, Fan J, Wu H, Mar R, et al. Arachidonate 5-lipoxygenase promoter genotype, dietary arachidonic acid, and atherosclerosis. N Engl J Med. 2004;350(1):29–37.
134. Peters-Golden M, Swern A, Bird SS, Hustad CM, Grant E, Edelman JM. Influence of body mass index on the response to asthma controller agents. Eur Respir J. 2006;27(3):495–503.
135. Komakula S, Khatri S, Mermis J, Savill S, Haque S, Rojas M, et al. Body mass index is associated with reduced exhaled nitric oxide and higher exhaled 8-isoprostanes in asthmatics. Respir Res. 2007;8:32.
136. Simard B, Turcotte H, Marceau P, Biron S, Hould FS, Lebel S, et al. Asthma and sleep apnea in patients with morbid obesity: outcome after bariatric surgery. Obes Surg. 2004;14(10): 1381–8.
137. Spivak H, Hewitt MF, Onn A, Half EE. Weight loss and improvement of obesity-related illness in 500 U.S. patients following laparoscopic adjustable gastric banding procedure. Am J Surg. 2005;189(1):27–32.
138. Stenius-Aarniala B, Poussa T, Kvarnstrom J, Gronlund EL, Ylikahri M, Mustajoki P. Immediate and long term effects of weight reduction in obese people with asthma: randomised controlled study. BMJ. 2000;320(7238):827–32.

139. Aaron SD, Fergusson D, Dent R, Chen Y, Vandemheen KL, Dales RE. Effect of weight reduction on respiratory function and airway reactivity in obese women. Chest. 2004;125(6): 2046–52.
140. Mougey EB, Chen C, Tantisira K, Blake KV, Peters SP, Wise RA, Weiss ST, Lima JJ. Response to fluticasone and montelukast therapies are inversely associated with a common variant of the corticotropin releasing hormone receptor 1 (CRHR1) gene [publication page: A4080]. Proc Am Thoracic Soc – ATS. 2011:A4080.
141. Price D, Musgrave SD, Shepstone L, Hillyer EV, Sims EJ, Gilbert RF, et al. Leukotriene antagonists as first-line or add-on asthma-controller therapy. N Engl J Med. 2011;364(18): 1695–707.
142. Mastronarde JG, Anthonisen NR, Castro M, Holbrook JT, Leone FT, Teague WG, et al. Efficacy of esomeprazole for treatment of poorly controlled asthma. N Engl J Med. 2009;360(15):1487–99.
143. Lemanske Jr RF, Mauger DT, Sorkness CA, Jackson DJ, Boehmer SJ, Martinez FD, et al. Step-up therapy for children with uncontrolled asthma receiving inhaled corticosteroids. N Engl J Med. 2010;362(11):975–85.
144. Redline S, Tishler PV, Schluchter M, Aylor J, Clark K, Graham G. Risk factors for sleep-disordered breathing in children. Associations with obesity, race, and respiratory problems. Am J Respir Crit Care Med. 1999;159(5 Pt 1):1527–32.
145. Verhulst SL, Schrauwen N, Haentjens D, Suys B, Rooman RP, Van Gaal L, et al. Sleep-disordered breathing in overweight and obese children and adolescents: prevalence, characteristics and the role of fat distribution. Arch Dis Child. 2007;92(3):205–8.
146. Gozal D, Kheirandish-Gozal L. The multiple challenges of obstructive sleep apnea in children: morbidity and treatment. Curr Opin Pediatr. 2008;20(6):654–8.
147. Gozal D, Kheirandish-Gozal L. Obesity and excessive daytime sleepiness in prepubertal children with obstructive sleep apnea. Pediatrics. 2009;123(1):13–8.
148. Mitchell RB, Kelly J. Outcome of adenotonsillectomy for obstructive sleep apnea in obese and normal-weight children. Otolaryngol Head Neck Surg. 2007;137(1):43–8.
149. Amin R, Anthony L, Somers V, Fenchel M, McConnell K, Jefferies J, et al. Growth velocity predicts recurrence of sleep-disordered breathing 1 year after adenotonsillectomy. Am J Respir Crit Care Med. 2008;177(6):654–9.
150. Kheirandish-Gozal L, Gozal D. Intranasal budesonide treatment for children with mild obstructive sleep apnea syndrome. Pediatrics. 2008;122(1):e149–55.
151. Berlucchi M, Salsi D, Valetti L, Parrinello G, Nicolai P. The role of mometasone furoate aqueous nasal spray in the treatment of adenoidal hypertrophy in the pediatric age group: preliminary results of a prospective, randomized study. Pediatrics. 2007;119(6):e1392–7.
152. Goldbart AD, Goldman JL, Veling MC, Gozal D. Leukotriene modifier therapy for mild sleep-disordered breathing in children. Am J Respir Crit Care Med. 2005;172(3):364–70.
153. Kheirandish L, Goldbart AD, Gozal D. Intranasal steroids and oral leukotriene modifier therapy in residual sleep-disordered breathing after tonsillectomy and adenoidectomy in children. Pediatrics. 2006;117(1):e61–6.
154. Kessler R, Chaouat A, Schinkewitch P, Faller M, Casel S, Krieger J, et al. The obesity-hypoventilation syndrome revisited: a prospective study of 34 consecutive cases. Chest. 2001;120(2):369–76.
155. Mokhlesi B, Tulaimat A, Faibussowitsch I, Wang Y, Evans AT. Obesity hypoventilation syndrome: prevalence and predictors in patients with obstructive sleep apnea. Sleep Breath. 2007;11(2):117–24.
156. Nowbar S, Burkart KM, Gonzales R, Fedorowicz A, Gozansky WS, Gaudio JC, et al. Obesity-associated hypoventilation in hospitalized patients: prevalence, effects, and outcome. Am J Med. 2004;116(1):1–7.
157. Rosen CL. Clinical features of obstructive sleep apnea hypoventilation syndrome in otherwise healthy children. Pediatr Pulmonol. 1999;27(6):403–9.
158. Malhotra A, Hillman D. Obesity and the lung: 3. Obesity, respiration and intensive care. Thorax. 2008;63(10):925–31.

159. Centers for Disease Control and Prevention (CDC). CDC grand rounds: childhood obesity in the United States. MMWR Morb Mortal Wkly Rep. 2011;60(2):42–6.
160. Barbiero SM, Pellanda LC, Cesa CC, Campagnolo P, Beltrami F, Abrantes CC. Overweight, obesity and other risk factors for IHD in Brazilian schoolchildren. Public Health Nutr. 2009;12(5):710–5.
161. Lazzeri G, Rossi S, Pammolli A, Pilato V, Pozzi T, Giacchi MV. Underweight and overweight among children and adolescents in Tuscany (Italy). Prevalence and short-term trends. J Prev Med Hyg. 2008;49(1):13–21.
162. Nakano T, Sei M, Ewis AA, Munakata H, Onishi C, Nakahori Y. Tracking overweight and obesity in Japanese children; a six years longitudinal study. J Med Invest. 2010;57(1–2):114–23.
163. Al-Isa AN. Body mass index, overweight and obesity among Kuwaiti intermediate school adolescents aged 10–14 years. Eur J Clin Nutr. 2004;58(9):1273–7.
164. Utter J, Scragg R, Schaaf D, Fitzgerald E, Wilson N. Correlates of body mass index among a nationally representative sample of New Zealand children. Int J Pediatr Obes. 2007;2(2):104–13.
165. El Mouzan MI, Foster PJ, Al Herbish AS, Al Salloum AA, Al Omer AA, Qurachi MM, et al. Prevalence of overweight and obesity in Saudi children and adolescents. Ann Saudi Med. 2010;30(3):203–8.
166. Malik M, Bakir A. Prevalence of overweight and obesity among children in the United Arab Emirates. Obes Rev. 2007;8(1):15–20.

Index

A.E. Dixon and E.M. Clerisme-Beaty (eds.), *Obesity and Lung Disease: A Guide to Management*, Respiratory Medicine, DOI 10.1007/978-1-62703-053-3,

FSC
www.fsc.org
MIX
Papier | Fördert gute Waldnutzung
FSC® C083411

Kolibri 360 GmbH
Ferdinand-Jühlke-Straße 7
99095 Erfurt, Deutschland
produktsicherheit@kolibri360.de